GENDER PERSPECTIVES ON REPRODUCTION AND SEXUALITY

ADVANCES IN GENDER RESEARCH

Series Editors: Vasilikie Demos
and Marcia Texler Segal

Recent Volumes:

Volume 1: Theory, Methods and Praxis – Edited by Vasilikie Demos and Marcia Texler Segal, 1996

Volume 2: Cross-Cultural and International Perspectives – Edited by Vasilikie Demos and Marcia Texler Segal, 1997

Volume 3: Advancing Gender Research Across, Beyond and Through Disciplines and Paradigms – Edited by Vasilikie Demos and Marcia Texler Segal, 1998

Volume 4: Social Change for Women and Children – Edited by Vasilikie Demos and Marcia Texler Segal, 2000

Volume 5: An International Feminist Challenge to Theory – Edited by Vasilikie Demos and Marcia Texler Segal, 2001

Volume 6: Gendered Sexualities – Edited by Patricia Gagné and Richard Tewksbury, 2002

Volume 7: Gender Perspectives on Health and Medicine: Key Themes – Edited by Marcia Texler Segal, Vasilikie Demos with Jennie Jacobs Kronenfeld, 2003

ADVANCES IN GENDER RESEARCH VOLUME 8

GENDER PERSPECTIVES ON REPRODUCTION AND SEXUALITY

EDITED BY

MARCIA TEXLER SEGAL

Indiana University Southeast, Indiana, USA

VASILIKIE DEMOS

University of Minnesota-Morris, Minnesota, USA

with

JENNIE JACOBS KRONENFELD

Department of Sociology, Arizona State University, AZ, USA

2004

ELSEVIER

JAI

Amsterdam – Boston – Heidelberg – London – New York – Oxford – Paris
San Diego – San Francisco – Singapore – Sydney – Tokyo

ELSEVIER B.V.	ELSEVIER Inc.	**ELSEVIER Ltd**	ELSEVIER Ltd
Sara Burgerhartstraat 25	525 B Street, Suite 1900	**The Boulevard, Langford**	84 Theobalds Road
P.O. Box 211	San Diego	**Lane, Kidlington**	London
1000 AE Amsterdam	CA 92101-4495	**Oxford OX5 1GB**	WC1X 8RR
The Netherlands	USA	**UK**	UK

First edition 2004

British Library Cataloguing in Publication Data
A catalogue record is available from the British Library.

ISBN: 0-7623-1088-X
ISSN: 1529-2126 (Series)

♾ The paper used in this publication meets the requirements of ANSI/NISO Z39.48-1992 (Permanence of Paper). Printed in The Netherlands.

CONTENTS

GENDER PERSPECTIVES ON REPRODUCTION AND SEXUALITY: INTRODUCTION

Marcia Texler Segal and Vasilikie Demos with Jennie Jacobs Kronenfeld

HORMONE THERAPY

In 2002 when we began reviewing papers for possible inclusion in *Advances in Gender Research* volume 7: *Gender Perspectives on Health and Medicine: Key Themes*, and Volume 8: *Gender Perspectives on Health and Medicine: Reproduction and Sexuality*, the popular press was full of headlines about Hormone Replacement Therapy (HRT) (for references and extended and detailed discussion by researchers and physicians see the editorial by Ronald C. Hamdy, MD, FRCP, FACP (2002) and the letters to the editor (Mikhail, 2003) in the *Southern Journal of Medicine*).

The controversy over HRT, or as referred to by the National Drug Administration, hormone therapy (HT), began on July 9, 2003 when the Women's Health Initiative (WHI) announced it was ending the largest study ever of the use of hormone therapy for menopausal women. The WHI had found that the risks of continuing the study outweighed the benefits.

As reported in the *New York Times* on July 10, 2002, "A rigorous study found that the drugs, a combination of estrogen and progestin, caused small increases in breast cancer, heart attacks, strokes and blood clots. Those risks outweighed

Gender Perspectives on Reproduction and Sexuality
Advances in Gender Research, Volume 8, 1–9

ISSN: 1529-2126/doi:10.1016/S1529-2126(04)08001-4

the drugs' benefits – a small decrease in hip fractures and a decrease in colorectal cancer."

The WHI announcement was widely circulated and sent shock waves throughout the nation. Hormone therapy for relieving symptoms of menopause such as hot flashes had been in existence since the 1940s. In 1966, a physician, Robert A. Wilson, teamed up with the Wyeth-Ayerst pharmaceutical company to market the estrogen therapy, Premarin. In his book, *Feminine Forever*, Wilson described menopausal women and changes associated with menopause as undesirable. Hormone therapy he argued would reverse the undesirable effects of menopause and make women young and therefore, sexually attractive. When in 1975, two respected studies found that women taking estrogen therapy faced a risk of cancer to the uterine lining, doctors and drug companies began recommending taking estrogen along with progestin, a hormone which would counteract the effect of estrogen on the lining. The marketing strategy was enormously effective. Sales climbed again in the 1980s when the pharmaceutical industry advertised hormone therapy for the prevention of osteoporosis. Despite questions raised by feminist health activists, by the time of the announcement millions of women were taking hormone therapy, and most were taking Prempro, Wyeth-Ayerst's estrogen progestin therapy.

The discussion about H(R)T continues. As Gina Kolata reported in the *New York Times* on March 18, 2003, the latest findings suggest that taking hormones is counter-indicated not only to reduce risks of breast cancer and heart attack but even to feel better and be more sexually responsive. Further, Peggy Peck (2003: http://www.medscape.com/viewarticle/453299) reports that Heart Estrogen/Progestin Replacement Study (HERS) researchers found a significantly higher rate of urinary incontinence among women taking a combination of estrogen and progestin than among women who did not take the therapy.

In Volume 7 of *Advances in Gender Research*, Erica S. Breslau (2003), a researcher at the National Cancer Institute, wrote about her research on somatic distress in women to the medicalization of breast cancer. Shortly after the announcement of the WHI study, Breslau (2003) and her colleagues conducted a national telephone survey of households that included women 40–79 years old. Of the 819 women interviewed, 64% had learned of the announcement from either the media or in talking with others. A larger number, 74%, were confused about the use of hormone therapy. Fifty-seven percent expressed worry about how the findings applied to them, and 79% were interested in obtaining additional information about hormone therapy. Of those who had heard of the study, only 24% had actually sought additional information. More educated women were more likely to be aware of the study, less likely to be confused by hormone therapy, and more likely to seek additional information. Breslau et al. concluded,

"The Women's Health Initiative" study provided a clear message about health risks and benefits of HT use. An important next step is to continue to convey accurate information to women, health providers, and the media so that women can make informed decisions about HT (Breslau et al., 2003, p. 33).

Also in Volume 7 of our series, Heather Hartley (2003) demonstrated the questionable links pharmaceutical companies make with physicians and researchers. She argued that the pursuit of profit on the part of pharmaceutical companies is often more pressing than the assurance of the products being marketed. Clearly, the history of hormone therapy provides a good example of this issue.

Because this volume focuses on sexuality and reproductive health, we thought it appropriate to ask the contributors to state their reactions to the hormone therapy announcement. We offer some of their comments here. The announcement is no longer headline news, but as the comments reveal, brought to the public's attention were issues of long-standing concern among feminist researchers of health and medicine. The comments clearly tie the announcement and the resulting media coverage to points raised in this volume.

An examination of the reactions reveals four major issues. First, none of the contributors was surprised by the announcement. Chikako Takeshita, noted "It is disturbing that HRT was widely circulated before its risk was established. Yet it does not surprise me considering the history of medicine. The same thing has happened with, for example, the contraceptive pill and breast implants." Carol Warren stated, "... I am not surprised that messing with the body can result in all kinds of problems; I would not be surprised if the current epidemic of auto-immune deficiency diseases among middle aged women was not related to the birth control pill." Lara Foley simply said, "It did not surprise me at all."

While Tracy B. Cieroni and Alejandro Cervantes-Carson were not surprised by the findings of the Women's Health Initiative, they were shocked by the announcement. They said, "... despite our extensive knowledge about the history and politics of HRT, we were shocked when NIH suspended the clinical trail. We were not surprised by the findings themselves, but rather by the presence of critical discussions of HRT and the menopause industry in mainstream popular media."

Second, the contributors tend to agree that the recommendation of hormone therapy for women is a typical part of the history of women's health in the United States. Terri Winnick related her paper to the announcement. She stated, "My paper explores the long tradition of meddling with women's bodies so characteristic of the modern medical profession. I argue that because the profession is male dominated, its orientation is often interventionist. Their goal is to 'manage' and control the body, rather than follow its rhythms and respect its innate power." Denise Copelton, observes, "The redefinition of menopause, a normal bodily process, into a 'hormone deficiency disease' represents yet another example of the medicalization of women's lives." She argues that just as menstrual extraction is a political issue so is menopause. Cervantes and Citeroni observe, "The history of HRT in the United States has been one of exaggerated and unsubstantiated claims that menopause is an illness that women desperately need to treat/cure. The name alone implies that hormones are something 'missing' in (peri-and post-) menopausal women, something crucial that needs to be 'replaced.' The entire hormone industry is predicated on sexist and ageist assumptions concerning the post-reproductive phase of women's lives."

The third point pertains to the application of study results to the lives of individual women. Making this point, Takeshita cautions that studies of large populations necessitate careful interpretation. She notes, "If read carefully, the July 9th announcement considers individualized prescription of HRT for short-term relief of climacteric symptoms acceptable though the overall risk of breast cancer would be deemed too high if the method were applied long term and indiscriminately to women. HRT may still be an option for treating difficult menopause, while balancing the risks individually." Kathryn Yount and Deborah Balk argue, "In an information age, researchers have a responsibility to make new information about the costs and benefits of HRT treatment widely available. At the same time, such information should be relayed in a way that enables women to weigh potentially alarming population-level risks with their individual circumstances."

Fourth, Citeroni and Cervantes-Carson point to the lack of attention to women's rights in the discourse surrounding the study. They observe, "It is very troubling to witness a public discussion on hormone replacement therapy in which a discourse of rights is completely absent. The manufacturing of needs and markets not only undermines the required separateness of biomedical research from corporate interests, but it constitutes an institutionalized platform where the rights of women are systematically violated."

PAPERS IN THIS VOLUME

In his paper, "Reproductive Rights: An Analytical Proposal," Alejandro Cervantes-Carson examines the issue of reproductive rights on an international level. His focus is on United Nations policies. Cervantes-Carson begins with an explanation of changes in the United Nations' position on reproductive rights. Initially the United Nations identified the family unit as the appropriate focus of such rights. Then it shifted to the identification of the parental unit, followed by the unit of the "couple." Its current focus is on the individual. In the first part, too, Cervantes-Carson makes the critical point that while reproduction actually consists of three realms: sexuality, procreation and rearing, reproduction law focuses on procreation. This he argues is highly problematic for procreation is dependent on sexuality and rearing.

In the second part of the paper, Cervantes-Carson identifies entitlement, responsibility, and inequality as three concrete issues surrounding reproduction rights. Of the three, two – entitlement and responsibility – are particularly problematic: According to the United Nations, individuals are entitled to reproductive freedom; but because they are enjoined to reproduce "responsibly," the nation-state may make policies that circumscribe the exercise of reproductive freedom when it perceives that such freedom is detrimental to the goals of the state. Further, structured social inequality means that all individuals are not equally free to exercise reproductive rights.

In the third part of the paper, Cervantes-Carson proposes a solution to the dilemma posed in the second part. He suggests responsibility be eliminated from the definition of reproductive rights, and that nation-states ensure equal reproductive rights for their citizens.

Terri Winnick's paper, "Delivery: Gender and the Language of Birth," is also on reproduction. Her focus, however, is on the *language* of reproduction. Winnick argues that contemporary child-bearing women have been defined in terms of the "biologically impossible," as passive in the birthing process. Taking up the use of the medical term, "delivery," Winnick points out that because doctors are said to *deliver* babies, language relegates women to a passive role in childbirth. She argues that this contemporary linguistic practice represents a departure from past practices, and that in the bible, for example, language referring to women's role in childbirth is active.

Winnick specifically identifies the emergence of the male medical model of birth and the decline of midwifery and non-scientific birth as responsible for the language shift. She observes that an ideological shift occurred as the obstetrician replaced the midwife and the scientific birth replaced the non-scientific one. Winnick attributes the shift to fear of pain in childbirth. With their ability to use medicine to reduce pain, physicians were able to use women's fear to attract them to a medicalized birth.

Winnick addresses the tenacity of the male medical model of birthing. She explains that even as hospitals allow for the decoration of rooms and the presence of midwives, it is the attendant male physician who is the *deliverer* (savior) freeing the woman from children. She argues that the male medical language of birth is an embedded part of culture, and that this holds true more for the United States than other nation-states.

In "How I Became a Midwife: Identity, Biographical Work, and Legitimation in Midwives' Work Narratives," Lara Foley examines the narratives of twenty-five direct entry and nurse-midwives in Florida. She adds to Winnick's history of the identification of the American south as a critical site of midwifery. As does Winnick, Foley underscores the importance of language in the construction of reproduction.

In her examination of the narratives, Foley uses the women's voices to present a re-definition of the concept of "work." In addition, she finds that the major factor differentiating the narratives is the women's passage to midwifery. Nurse midwives provided succinct stories of how they entered midwifery and referenced nursing as their base. By contrast, direct-entry midwives provided longer and more complicated narratives. They used mothering as a relevant context to their midwifery and were more likely than nurse-midwives to have been involved in counterculture movements.

In her article, on "Menstrual Extraction, Abortion and the Political Context of Feminist Self-Help," Denise Copelton provides an historical account of such a counterculture movement, a radical feminist health group, or more specifically, a women's self-help abortion group that learned and used the method of menstrual extraction. For her study, Copelton relied on the extensive media coverage of such groups as well as scholarly articles. In addition, she interviewed two women involved in a menstrual extraction self-help group. Given the borderline legality of menstrual extraction self-help groups and the associated problems in obtaining human subjects consent, the interviews provide a privileged inside view of the groups.

Copelton found that menstrual extraction groups first emerged within the feminist health care movement of the 1960s in 1971 when the safety and legality of abortions was threatened. The groups re-emerged in the 1980s and early 1990s in reaction to the conservative anti-abortion political climate of that time.

Maintaining that menstrual extraction groups are feminist and pro-woman, Copelton notes that the media is generally critical of the groups by juxtaposing menstrual extraction to scientific medical abortion while linking it to back-alley abortions. Further, she observes that pro-choice feminists claiming a concern for safety and legality were also critical of the groups. Thus, she argues that menstrual extraction self-help feminists challenged the large institutional model of medicine – described by Winnick as patriarchal – while many other feminists accepted it.

Copelton explains the difference between the two types of feminists by considering the political climate and the strategies feminists used to deal with birth control. In the conservative anti-abortion context of the time, menstrual extraction feminists took a pro-woman stance. Pro-choice feminists did not want to take a pro-woman stance at a time when anti-abortionists were arguing for fetal rights. Rather, their concern for the right to abortion was based on a safety and legality position. The menstrual extraction self-help groups faded out because the political climate changed, and the right to abortion became relatively secured.

Copelton's analysis points to the potential for social change that radical self-help groups embody. Further, her work is easily tied into that of Foley. Both Copelton and Foley examine approaches to reproductive health from a perspective critical of the medical model. They each, also, discuss women as empowered active practitioners of life processes. In addition, they each identify nursing as a site from which women begin to challenge the scientific practice of medicine.

In "Genital Surgeries and Stimulation In Nineteenth Century Psychiatry," Carol Warren provides further support of medicine as a patriarchal practice. She describes physicians' use of genital stimulation as a treatment for mental illness in women. While men were subject to such treatment, it was women who were the major subjects. Noting that the "medical suppression of female sexuality in Victorian society" is well documented, Warren examines the history of medical treatments to *enhance* sexuality.

Warren begins by tracing the identification of hysteria as a condition affecting women to Ancient Greece and Rome. She notes that Galen, the ancient Greek physician, provided an account of a widow whose hysteria was successfully treated by rubbing an ointment on her genitals. Observing that documentation of this treatment disappeared from reference during the Middle Ages, but re-surfaced in the Renaissance, Warren establishes a history of genital stimulation in the western world. By the 19th century and the emergence of scientific medicine and gynecology, the treatment for women whose mental illness or hysteria was defined as deficient in sexuality included rubbing of the clitoris, female genital mutilation (FMG), and genital electrical treatment. Moreover, FMG, continued to be used as a treatment in the West into the twentieth century, ending between the 1920s and 1940s, and female circumcision and Galen's Widow's Treatment continued to be used into the middle of the century. Thus, Warren clearly shows that genital treatments including FMG and female circumcision have been a part of Western cultural practices dating back to the Ancient Greeks and Romans and continued to be a part of those practices through the European Enlightenment and the rise of scientific medicine.

In their paper "A Demographic Paradox: Causes and Consequences of Female Genital Cutting in Northeastern Africa," Kathryn M. Yount and Deborah L. Balk delve into the demographic and theoretical literature on contemporary practices of genital cutting. They observe that such practices are found throughout Africa, and that though they predate the birth of Christianity and Islam, in Northeastern Africa they spread with Islamification.

Yount and Balk identify five different types of genital cutting and observe there is considerable cross-cultural difference in this practice. Acknowledging that the topic of genital cutting is value-laden, they refrain from using the term, "female genital mutilation (FGM)." Yount and Balk discuss the various psychological and physical consequences of genital cutting for women. With respect to physical pain, the least severe of the practices is symbolic circumcision. Infibulation is the most invasive of the practices and can result in urinary conditions, infections, painful intercourse and sterility.

Yount and Balk argue that genital cutting involves paradox. Its practice is held in place by cultural traditions surrounding marriage. At the same time, the practice can lead to marital difficulties. In places such as the Sudan, men do not derive pleasure from having intercourse with women who have been infibulated, and consequently the practice can result in divorce or polygyny.

Yount and Balk note that women play a critical role in the institution of genital cutting. It's maintenance is associated with mothers wishing to secure the marriageability of their daughters, while its discontinuance is associated with mother's educational attainment.

In her article, "Contraceptive Technology and Reproductive Rights: The IUD at Historical and Geographical Junctures," Chikako Takeshita takes us full circle to the beginning of the introduction and Cervantes-Carson's concern with reproductive rights on an international level. Takeshita juxtaposes the birth control movement to population control policies. The two, she argues, are at cross-purposes. While the birth control movement puts women and their personal control over reproduction at the center of its program, population control policies seek to minimize women's freedom to reproduce. She identifies the use of the inter-uterine device (IUD) in developing nations as critical to state population control policies. Because the IUD is fitted and removed most safely by a medical practitioner, the state is able to insure that the "unmotivated woman" (to control birth) factor is removed.

Takeshita provides a western history of the IUD, and explains that women in the west have rejected its use because it can negatively affect reproductive health. She, also, considers ethnographic documentation, and argues that women in non-western societies exercise their own will with respect to the IUD by negotiating the terms of its use or non-use or by secretly resisting attempts to control their fertility.

CONCLUSION

We conclude this introduction with a reminder that until 1990 when the Office of Research on Women's Health at the National Institutes of Health was established to include women and minorities in medical research, such research focused on white, primarily middle-class men. Dr. Nancy S. Hardt, obstetrician/gynecologist, pathologist and the first director of the Institute for Women's Health in Memphis,

Tennessee in an interview (see, "Hardt Leads Institute," 2003) noted the critical part women's health plays in society. She said, "A wide realm of social issues have an impact on health.... Women's health is related to women's ability to sustain a health home environment, including affordable housing, child care, mentoring in job-related skills, negotiation skills and leadership training," ("Hardt Leads Institute," 2003, p. 6). Noting the importance of interdisciplinary research in defining domestic violence as a medical issue, not simply a criminal one, Hardt points to the critical role of interdisciplinary, and particularly social scientific work, in the future of health and health care delivery for women.

Volume 7 of *Advances in Gender Research* focused on the relevance of gender to general health issues. It revealed many ways in which women and people of color have been overlooked in medical research and health care delivery. The theme of this volume, reproduction and sexuality, is one traditionally associated with women's health. The medical specialization, gynecology, literally the study of women, but, practically,the study of women's reproduction and sexuality, has been the one area of medicine along with the related area of obstetrics in which women have been the focus. Yet, even in this area there are many medical and social justice issues that remain (see Wortmann, S., "Fact Sheet on Women's Reproduction," 2003). As the articles in this volume reveal, there is yet much work to be done.

REFERENCES

Breslau, E. (2003). The continuum: Somatic distress to medicalization in women with breast cancer: Theoretical and empirical assessment. In: V. Demos & M. Texler Segal (Eds), *Advances in Gender Research* (Vol. 7). Oxford, England: JAI Press.

Breslau, E., Davis, W. W., Doner, L., Eisner, E. J., Goodman, N. R., Meissner, H. I., Rimer, B. K., & Rossouw, J. E. (2003). The hormone therapy dilemma: Women respond. *Journal of the American Women's Association*, *58*, 33–43.

Hamdy, R. C. (2002). Lessons learned from the women's health initiative study. *Southern Medical Journal*, *95*, 951.

Hardt Leads Institute for Women's Health (2003). The University of Memphis center for research on women. *Standpoint*, *21*(Spring), 1 & 6.

Hartley, H. (2003). "Big pharma" in our bedrooms: An analysis of the medicalization of women's sexual problems. In: V. Demos & M. Texler Segal (Eds), *Advances in Gender Research* (Vol. 7). Oxford, England: JAI Press.

Kolata, G. (2003). Hormone therapy is now said to lack benefits. *New York Times*, March 18.

Mikhail, N. (2003). Lessons learned from the women's health initiative study. *Southern Medical Journal*, *96*, 940–941.

Peck, P. (2003). *Medscape Today*. April 30. http://www.medscape.com/viewarticle/453299.

Wortmann, S. (2003). SWS fact sheet on women's reproduction: Issues and inequalities in the 21st Century. *SWS Network News*, *XX*(Spring), 19–22.

REPRODUCTIVE RIGHTS: AN ANALYTICAL PROPOSAL☆

Alejandro Cervantes-Carson

1. INTRODUCTION: STRUCTURE OF THE PROPOSAL

The central objective of this chapter is to develop a theoretical reading of the international and contemporary discourse of reproductive rights. My hope is that the perspective and analytical proposal set forth represent a contribution to the expansion and consolidation of the field of study, and renders useful for the analysis and evaluation of the situation of reproductive rights within national contexts.

The chapter is divided into three sections. In the first section, I explore the basic structures of what defines the concept of reproductive rights. From the perspective of the foundation of a field of study, and using a genealogical approach I attempt to reconstruct the central meanings and basic questions of reproduction as rights. This effort has the purpose of establishing some very elementary cognitive boundaries for the field, and identifying some issues that have political and sociological relevance for the analysis of the international discourse of reproductive rights.

In the second section I identify three contentious and problematic areas: entitlement, responsibility, and inequality. From this vantage point I engage the international definition of reproductive rights and assess its virtues and limitations. Both the definition of entitlement and the concept of responsibility have been the most contentious issues of the evolution of reproductive rights. While the definition of who constitutes the subject of these rights has been altered and changed

☆For Tracy Citeroni.

Gender Perspectives on Reproduction and Sexuality
Advances in Gender Research, Volume 8, 11–49

ISSN: 1529-2126/doi:10.1016/S1529-2126(04)08002-6

numerous times, the concept of responsibility has generated a constant debate that, up to this day, remains unresolved. Countries that have chosen not to endorse international covenants on reproductive rights have precluded their citizens, through a normative marginalization, from their protection and enjoyment. Within endorsing nations, however, social inequality is the single most important factor in determining the exercise of reproductive rights. I end the section by arguing that how and even who gets to enjoy and exercise these rights is contingent on the systems of social inequality and the structure of opportunities in these societies.

Finally, in the third section, I develop a normative reading and a sociological interpretation of the process of making reproductive decisions. I start by exploring the assumptions embedded in the international definition and its concurrent discourse. There are a series of assumptions that can be derived and made explicit from the definition and its historical development. However, there are others that are not easily derived and thus have remained basically implicit and unthematized. Yet these are not secondary. I contend that these sets of assumptions are fundamental for the exercise of reproductive rights, both in the private and public realms, and decisive for reproductive decision-making processes. But, what would be the ideal situation and process for making a reproductive decision? Taking Habermas' lead (1984, 1987, 1990, 1993), I use the analytical intention of his "ideal speech situation" to produce an "ideal reproductive decision-making process."[1] Informed by the standards of justice and equality suggested by contemporary human rights[2] and feminist theory,[3] I thematize the required elements, the key social relations, and the necessary conditions for an "ideal process." Once established the ideal normative, I turn my attention to the sociological dimension. Social structures and social relations represent a permanent jeopardy for the actualization of the ideal normative. I conclude the section (and the chapter) by assessing the disturbances that the ideal reproductive decision-making process suffers when placed in contemporary societies; that is, within social contexts that are structured unequally, and where the prevailing form of social relations is domination. For both the private and the public realms, I identify two main sources of disturbances: power relations and systems of social inequality. I examine the distortions these create to the ideal process, the constraints they impose over individuals and couples, as well as the effects they have on the process of formulating and carrying out reproductive decisions.

2. REPRODUCTION AS RIGHTS

This first section can be thought of as an effort to lay the basic building blocks of the analytical proposal. I begin by engaging in an abstract examination of the fundamental components of the discourse of reproductive rights, and will suggest some routes of interpretation of its sociological and political meaning.

2.1. Charting a Relation

An utterance with two related conceptual components, like "reproductive rights" (in which one can read the pretense or foundation effort of being placed at the center of a cognitive field), contains conceptual proposals that go beyond a mere intellectual exploration. At first, this means that the projected images, the implied connections, and the conceptual interactions suggested in the one utterance are neither general nor uncertain. It is not that the connection between two conceptually autonomous universes is being hypothesized (as an utterance in the style of "rights and reproduction" would reflect), but rather that the utterance already implies a selective process of reasoning where false hypotheses and spurious relations have been discarded. That is to say, in the non-theorized utterance of "reproductive rights" previous conceptual work of differentiation and association is already summed up.

In "reproductive rights" we find the presence of two big components and of a relationship of bilateral qualification. On the one hand, "reproduction" as an event or central action is qualified and delimited by the concept of "rights." On the other, "rights" as a social and legal condition confer a specific entitlement, and protect the same event that grants them their reference: the process of "reproduction."

The component of "reproduction" finds its basis in biology. It does not allude to processes of reproduction in the social, economic, cultural or symbolic dimensions but to one that occurs in the sphere of the biological, even when this process might be provoked by forces, movements, and events from other spheres of life. In addition, the qualification of "rights" points to the fact that elements of this process are recognized by the legal or political word. Indeed, from the great process of biological reproduction certain aspects and dimensions are identified and given life within the sphere of the legal discourse, and others are deemed as worthy political projects of civil mobilization and social movements.

On this last point it is worthwhile to insist that what creates the qualification of "rights" does not have an engulfing effect over the entire process. That is, the qualification of "rights" does not transform the whole process of reproduction into legal or political discourse. Only some parts and some particular instances are targeted by legal thought and chosen by civil organizations and social movements. In addition to being a qualification that sets boundaries, "rights" is for "reproduction" a mechanism that filters and modifies certain elements of the process from the domain of biology to the domain of law, and to the domain of social and political struggles.

From this first look we can already derive at least two distinct alternatives for the development of research:

(a) What dimensions, elements, or aspects of the process of reproduction have been legally recognized and transformed into rights? What are the reasons behind the selection of these dimensions, elements, or aspects of reproduction? What were the social, political, and cultural conditions that allowed and explain the legal recognition of selected dimensions, elements, or aspects, and their transformation into rights?
(b) What dimensions, elements, or aspects of the process of reproduction become part of political agendas and struggles? Who are the social agents, groups, and organizations that acknowledge the need to include and expand or to restrict and eliminate reproductive rights? What kind of tactics and strategies are used to promote and push for specific agendas? How do rights become institutionalized (and de-institutionalized)?

In addition to delimiting and qualifying the concept of "reproduction," the component of "rights" implies itself a relationship, a relationship that actually defines it. The concept of "rights" represents the crystallization of a historically grounded process of continuous or discontinuous interactions, exchanges, and clashes between state and civil society. That is, "rights" are the juridical product of social processes that attempt to negotiate the tension between the needs and perspectives of national states and their civil societies.

The implied relationship in the component of "rights" directly introduces the notion of tension. It is a notion that is permanent, because as a source it never disappears. Yet, at the same time it is transitive, to the extent that an agreement is always possible. It is a social tension with history and a result of different needs that, at certain points in time, may or may not be recognized, may or may not be open to negotiation.

In that sense, the qualification that "rights" grants to reproduction should be understood, also, as the conceptual inclusion of the two fundamental social actors, state and civil society, and the complex social relations that they hold in the generation of laws and regulations within a national society, and at a given historical period. What the inclusion of state and civil society does, in effect, is to raise and acknowledge the social (and if I may, sociological) nature of "rights."

From this second look, it is possible to propose two additional routes of research, that seem to be intimately related to the previous ones:

(c) A first one that has to do with the historical and social reconstruction of the formation, formulation, and recognition of reproductive rights within the boundaries of national societies. What were the specific conditions that gave birth to them? What were the specific processes that generated the possibilities of their recognition and formulation? What were the social needs and political forces behind their recognition and formulation?

(d) A second that is driven by the study of the social agents that participated in their formation, formulation, and the possibilities of their social and legal recognition. What were the social forces, groups of power, groups of representation, and the particular actors that were instrumental to the process? What explicit and implicit agendas were put in motion? Which were the open and hidden needs that were argued and negotiated? What relationship did the particular actors and social groups establish and maintain throughout the process?

2.2. The "Reproduction" Component

As a process, human reproduction is a multidimensional and multifaceted phenomenon where vital forces of different orders intervene and whose complex dynamics is constituted by the interweaving of multiple domains: biological, social, cultural, psychological, linguistic, symbolic, and mythical.

From a formal point of view, in the process of human reproduction we can distinguish three large realms: sexuality, procreation, and rearing (Fig. 1). While the realm of procreation is constituted by three events that happen in a sequential way and with a successive order (conception, pregnancy, and childbirth), in the initial realm (sexuality), and in the terminal one (rearing) the constituent events do not present occurrences in a certain order. This is such, that the realm of sexuality like that of rearing can be described, formally speaking, as a sequential mesh of simultaneous events, and that of procreation as a trajectory of sequential and successive events.

The first realm, that of sexuality, can be understood as a universe of libidinal impulses, symbolic structures, and signifying processes where masses of energy, forces, and movement permanently interact to produce the internal logic of its dynamics. In this universe we would find an incredibly diverse collection of attributes from symbolic and sociolinguistic images like sexual fantasies and libidinal repressions; the development of ideas, judgments, and individual forms of introjecting and interacting with norms and social controls; ways to symbolize, to separate, to administer, and to regulate bodies, activities, and expressions according to socially significant differentiation (gender, age, class, and race); behavioral expressions like sexual practices and their particular forms of corporal manifestation (skin, oral, anal, genital, etc.); elusive terrains like eroticism, courtship, and seduction, and even socio-corporal notions like carnal love along with its social forms of permissiveness, toleration, and subjection.

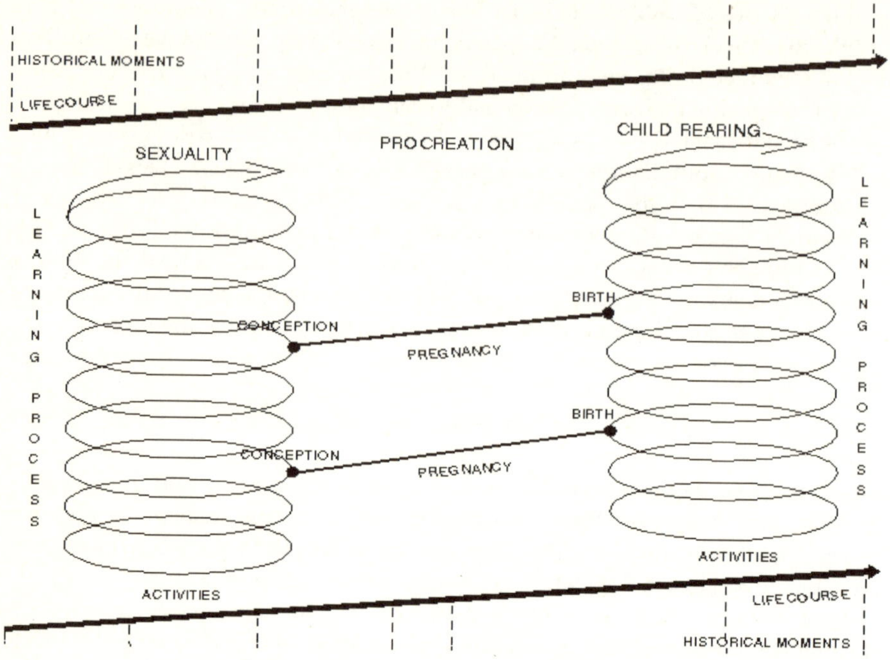

Fig. 1. Process of Human Reproduction.

If we turn our attention to the last realm, that of rearing, I would also propose to describe it in the same sense: as an universe of emotional bonds, also with their symbolic dimensions and signifying processes, where (as is the case with sexuality) masses of energy, forces, and movements permanently interact to produce the internal logic of its dynamics. In this universe we would also find a tremendously diverse group of qualities from the very basic and emotionally significant dyadic relationship between children and their parents, and that carry such a heavy representational weight through images, for example, like maternal love and paternal responsibility; spaces of communicative and affective interactions, of tensions and emotional conflicts, of negotiation of space and presence, of identity construction, and of consolidation of self and ego; ongoing processes that assure the transmission of perceptual, value, and behavioral frameworks like socialization, education, and communicative competence; even activities that are both practical and emotional linked to physical care (feeding, cleaning, body and health protection, organizing the immediate environment, etc.), and also linked to emotional care (affective protection, sentimental stimulation, loving, respecting, comforting, etc.).

An interesting similarity between the realm of sexuality and that of rearing (both of which I have assigned a spiral image in Fig. 1) has to do with their internal dynamics and their processes of development. They both appear as vital spaces where a finite series of activities are organized, executed and repeated; they are exposed to permanent and changing signifying processes; are constantly affected by the historical moments of society, and by the life course events of individuals.

As vital spaces of finite activities, both sexuality and rearing have the possibility of being experienced as renovated life processes, and at the same time as learning processes. On the one hand, while the activities are well known and are experienced repeatedly, either in specific series or articulated in groups, they can be experienced as renovated life processes if they are left open or exposed to new symbols and new ways of attributing meaning. The activities themselves might not change, but new sets of symbols and forms of interpretation transform the ways in which they are lived. On the other, the execution and repetition of activities, adjusted to the demands and needs of the life of individuals, and developed under certain contextual conditions, can benefit from past experiences and, in this sense, can produce the basic conditions to generate a continuous learning process. Thus, both the symbolic renovation and the possibility of learning from the past are presented to individuals as options in their everyday life experiences, and as ways to guide and interpret those experiences in their lives.

While sexuality and rearing can be relatively self-contained realms with relations, events, forces, and dynamics that maintain certain level of autonomy from each other, procreation substantially depends on the existence of each one of these realms. Sexuality generates the possibilities of its beginning, through conception, and rearing can only be a reality when the experience of procreation is complete through a successful birth. From this vantage point, procreation lacks relative autonomy, but instead becomes an experiential bridge that connects the realms of sexuality and rearing.

Procreation is constituted by a chain of events with a predetermined sequence and within specific ranges of time: childbirth does not happen before conception, and pregnancy, that it is taken to term, only happens after conception, and it leads to childbirth. In contrast with sexuality and rearing, procreation is a relatively simple process of understanding and of predicting, because it is constituted by less variables, its elements have well-known forms of appearing, and because in the constitution of its dynamics there are also less forces that intervene.

The temporal classification of its events and the linearity of their trajectory become a natural foundation for the possibility of programming and intervening in the process of procreation by different instances of society: family, community, and institutions. It is in this sense that procreation can be thought of as a territory, within the process of human reproduction, that is open and susceptible to the efficiency of normalization and to the diverse systems of social control. To be clear, I am not suggesting that sexuality and rearing are realms that escape the forces of social normalization – in one way or another, the patterns of behavior, the prevalence of traditions, and the existence of legal codes are signs contrary to this. Rather, what I am arguing and advancing as a hypothesis is that from a theoretical and formal point of view procreation is, because of the linearity and orderly nature of its events, a territory more prone to intervention and normalization than the realms of sexuality and rearing.

Another characteristic that sets procreation apart from the other two realms has to do with the cultural signs and social markers of this process. In a complete sequence the events of conception, pregnancy, and childbirth produce cultural signs that tie the personal experience with social forms of interpretation, classifying, and labeling. At the same time, these events produce social markers that are visually confirmed by the extended social environment, and that are shared by more immediate groups of social membership. These vital experiences that have privileged record in the biographies of individuals, become social spaces of public opinion, of moral judgment, of recognition, and of condemnation; their visibility transforms the sequence of events into social spaces of intervention. In this route of reflection, I do not find fortuitous that, in comparison with the realms of sexuality and rearing, it is in the realm of procreation where we find a more constant and diverse presence of social rituals, and their associated traditions and histories. That is to say, the social visibility of the events in the process of procreation has made them good cultural material for the establishment of "rites of passage."

The description and formal analysis of the characteristics of the three realms of reproduction and their differences has allowed us to understand their qualities and specificities, dynamics and movements, relationships and dimensions, and to identify their specific contributions to the process of human reproduction.

To engage and develop this theoretical exercise it has been necessary to make abstraction of the social conditions and determinants that affect reproduction, in general, and of each one of its realms, in particular. However it should be stated with all clarity that the abstraction of this sociological dimension has only been a methodological recourse, and in no way is meant as an analytic argument.

To be clear, the process of human reproduction is embedded and deeply marked by the systems of social differentiation and inequality of a society (age/generation, sex/gender, race/ethnicity, and class). These systems do not only work as mechanisms of inclusion and exclusion, as forms of prestige and disadvantage, or as ways of assigning activities and distributing responsibilities, but in addition as the fundamental conditions that structure the experience itself. In this way, the systems of social differentiation and inequality of a society serve as normative criteria for the construction of moral judgments about, for example, who can "rightfully" exercise their sexuality and when, who can decide to get pregnant and under what circumstances, or who should be in charge of rearing children. But it also means that belonging to certain social groups (by a combination of age, sex, ethnicity/race, and class), at different stages of the life course, will generate specific forms of perceiving and of interpreting the events of reproduction, and will define the social spaces from where individuals are to live (in an advantageous or disadvantageous way) their reproductive experiences. The systems of social differentiation and inequality will also define the social territory where individuals establish their meaningful relationships, and are able to negotiate the circumstances and certain conditions under which they make their reproductive decisions. Thus, power relations not only submit, exclude, and dominate but also structure social experience.

2.3. The "Rights" Component

It was in 1968 when reproductive decisions were, for the first time, declared as human rights. Article 16 of the Proclamation of Teheran established that all decisions concerning the number of children and their spacing should occur under conditions of freedom, and be taken responsibly. Subsequently it was ratified in 1969 by the Declaration of Social Progress and Development (Articles 4 and 22), as well as by other decrees thereafter. It became part of the Convention on the Elimination of All Forms of Discrimination Against Women (article 16, section 1e), which was passed in 1979 by the United Nations General Assembly, and forced as an international standard of procedure in 1981 (Cook, 1992, 1993; Dixon-Mueller & Germain, 1994; United Nations, 1990).

The core elements of the international definition of reproductive rights were established during that eleven-year period and were materialized in the Convention's document. Article 16(1e) resolves that "State Parties . . . shall ensure, on a basis of equality of men and women . . . the same rights to decide freely and responsibly on the number and spacing of their children and to have access to the information, education and means to enable them to exercise these rights" (Boland, 1997; Boland, Rao & Zeidenstein, 1994; Cook, 1994; CRLP, 2000; United Nations, 1990).

From its emergence in the late sixties the formulation has undergone four types of changes that are worth noting. The first was in regard to the category of persons possessing the rights. It was transformed multiple times from the decade of the sixties to that of the eighties. The figure of entitlement shifted from "family" and "parents" at the beginning of the period, and settled on "couples and individuals" in 1984, as a consequence of the International Conference on Population, that took place in Mexico City. The second change occurs during the eighties and throughout the nineties, when the concept of "responsibility" is qualified to mean "consideration of the needs of living and future children as well as a recognition of community responsibilities." The third and fourth changes take place in the nineties and through various international conferences. On the one hand, while being ratified in its core elements, the definition is largely enhanced to include the "right to attain the highest standard of sexual and reproductive health." On the other, a human rights maxim is asserted as the right "to make decisions concerning reproduction free of discrimination, coercion and violence" (Boland, 1997; Boland, Rao & Zeidenstein, 1994; Cook, 1994; CRLP, 2000; Dixon-Mueller, 1993; Petchesky, 1998; United Nations, 1990, 1994, 1995).

I will analyze the meaning and the effects of those changes over the international discourse and the interpretation of reproductive rights in the next section. For the time being, however, I would like to turn to the analysis of the central definition (and its core elements) that was established in 1979 and has been ratified since then numerous times through international conferences and forums.

Reproductive rights are by nature multidimensional because they involve more than one moment and more than one decision. Three dimensions define them centrally: the decision to have a child, the decision of when to have a child, and the decision of regulating ones fertility. That is, they are rights that enable decisions about the possibility of progeny, and decisions in regard to ones own body.

Furthermore, reproductive rights are social rights (as we will see later on) because they imply and require the presence of a national state. The full and free exercise of the reproductive rights of individual citizens imply and require the presence of their national state in functions of supervision, protection, regulation, administration, service, and provision.

If we subject the fundamental postulates that define reproductive rights to the analysis of reproduction thus far advanced, it is possible to reveal some interesting characteristics. First, what has been enacted as reproductive rights in the world of international declarations is circumscribed to the realm of procreation. Second, it is the possibility to decide about procreation, that is, to decide about conception, pregnancy, and childbirth what is essentially enabled and protected by these rights. Third, being that the decisions on the events of procreation are the moral and legal center of reproductive rights, what ultimately matters is the enabling and protection of the capacity to make those decisions. Finally, it is not enough to enable and protect the capacity to make the decisions. The decisions made need to be enacted in an environment of material quality, required services, and under an absolute respect of the social diversity and identity of the individuals involved.

To the extent that "reproductive rights" are concentrated in the events of conception, pregnancy, and childbirth to that extent is that there is a legal exclusion of the realms of sexuality and rearing. Both in the international norms and in their national translations, reproduction is not only defined as the conceptual equivalent of procreation, but it consequently implies the absence of sexuality and rearing in the legal discourse of "reproductive rights."

Indeed, the possible links that we can trace between "reproductive rights" and the realms of sexuality and rearing are, in any event, secondary. With the realm of sexuality the link is established through the institutional functions of formal instruction such as: (a) access to information about sexual and reproductive physiology; (b) the right to receive relevant information from qualified personnel and institutional services, when required and needed; (c) access to medical information and services in sexual health; and (d) access to preventive and curative technologies. In the case of rearing, the possible links are even scarcer and weaker, whereas they depend on the existence of other rights, such as labor rights. The access to childcare services and maternity leaves, for example, are granted only to women that work in those sectors protected by specific legislation.

From this analysis I would like to make a two-fold argument. On the one hand, it is important to acknowledge the discursive disparity between "reproductive rights" and their current effect of enabling only rights connected to the events of procreation. Not because I am suggesting we should reduce the legal terrain of their influence or confine them to be only procreative rights. But, I believe it is important to point out their current limitations and the need to expand their protection beyond the limits of procreation, to areas and elements in the realms of sexuality and rearing. On the other hand, however, I believe it would be a mistake to subsume the entire realms of sexuality and rearing to the legal protection of "reproductive rights." The fact that "reproductive rights" have international recognition and protection does not mean that they are capable of responding to the needs of rights connected with sexuality and rearing or that they should be a protective legal umbrella of these two realms. Reproduction while obviously linked with sexuality and rearing should continue to be kept separate from these two realms. Sexual rights and the rights involved in the rearing of children require their own analyses and deserve separate processes of recognition and entitlement.

3. ENTITLEMENT, RESPONSIBILITY, AND INEQUALITY

Entitlement is a crucial aspect of the discursive and legal constitution of a right. The determination and assignment of entitlements for human rights has normally been a straightforward and relatively uncomplicated process. This, however, has not been the case for reproductive rights. In this section I will explore the reasons of this unique discursive and legal history. Additionally, I will explore the "social character" of reproductive rights, the concept of responsibility in their definition, and the meaning that social inequality has for the possibilities of their exercise.

3.1. Entitlement and Its Transformations

From their inception the transformations that reproductive rights have undergone have been fundamentally tied to the definition of their entitlement. Who is the subject of these rights? Do reproductive rights protect and entitle individuals, couples, parents or families? Who should be the beneficiary of these rights, women, men, couples, parents, or families? These were the kind of questions that lead the discussions and the efforts to define the persons that possessed these rights.

While in the mid-60s the family was perceived to be the social unit who should be the recipient of these rights, by 1968 this figure had been replaced by parents, however. During the 70s the entitlement was changed to that of the couple, and remained this way until the mid-80s. Currently, however, entitlement has moved away from the idea of the family or parents as the central recipient, has established the couple as a basic unit, and has fundamentally enhanced the definition to include, protect, and empower individuals as well (Boland, 1997; CRLP, 2000; Dixon-Mueller, 1993; Fincancioglu, 1990; Freedman & Isaacs, 1993; United Nations, 1997, 2000).

The need for the first major transformation in the entitlement can be readily understood because the family was a very imprecise and diffuse legal reference, and because it allowed the inclusion of people not directly involved in the process of reproduction. The imprecision had to do with the definition of family itself and its variations across societies and cultures. But the central concern was that entitling the family jeopardized the autonomy and self-determination of those individuals directly involved in the decisions regarding reproduction. These problems made the abandonment of the figure of the family a logical move, but replacing it with parents opened up another series of problems.

The choice of entitling parents over families was by comparison a better choice, to the extent that it granted rights to persons directly involved in the process of reproduction, but it was an ambiguous alternative because it introduced a troubling exclusion. This form of entitlement made parenthood a prerequisite to these rights, disabling their enjoyment and exercise as a way to delay or avoid parenthood all together. While formally this change moved away from the intervention of a diffuse yet powerful set of kin-related people in the decisions about reproduction, it still made basic assumptions about the constitution of families through reproduction. In this way, parenthood was not presented as a choice but as a normative assumption.

The multiple steps from entitling the family, and then parents, to entitling couples represented an evolution toward a more precise reference. People not directly involved in the process of reproduction were left outside the domain of decisions, and parenthood was no longer assumed as a condition for granting these rights. However, the entitlement of couples was still problematic to the extent that the autonomy of individuals, in particular of women, was relativized and not protected. Granting the entitlement to couples assumed equal standing, participation, and responsibility in reproduction. This assumption is highly problematic given the social dynamics of gender power relations. The changes in entitlement and the demands for further specification required a much more complex discussion, however.

The fundamental concern can be summarized in the following way. Under patriarchal structures of social organization gender relations disable women in the exercise of their rights. Gender relations create a constant and systematic disadvantage for women that prevent them from making decisions about reproduction, and from exercising their rights in an autonomous way across different social spheres and throughout their life courses.

In light of this problem of a sociological order, the response, however, was not sociological but from the domain of legal discourse. Since gender relations put women at a disadvantage, the solution rested – it was thought – in originating rights and entitlements capable of counteracting or reversing that situation. The question was how best to design rights and curtail their entitlements so as to grant women differential legal power, as a way of equalizing with men their capacity to make decisions and of protecting them from male domination. Women required legal protection and a discourse capable of empowering them during the decision-making process, and in the exercise of their reproductive rights.

A route that was chosen proposed modifications in the definition of entitlement. Rights should be granted first and foremost to individual women, and only then should they be extended to their partner or significant other. The intention was to privilege women over men, to create the legal structures to empower them as decision makers and to fortify the possibility for them to exercise their rights. The problem was how to justify this unequal entitlement of two individuals participating in the same process. The argument found suggested that this was justifiable to the extent that the participation of women and men in the process of reproduction was not at all equal. While genetically men participate as much as women during conception, from a biological point of view women have the central role and carry a larger responsibility during pregnancy and birth. Thus, women are fundamental for the most part of the process of reproduction, an experience that has no parallel in the life of men. Because of this fact and the right to self-determination over one's own body, women – it was argued – should have a primordial place in the definition of reproductive rights and their entitlements (Azzolini, 1993; De Barbieri, 1985, 1990; Fincancioglu, 1990; Macklin, 1990).

This type of argumentation has the grave problem of supporting, unintentionally all be it, social practices and reinforcing reasoning of a patriarchal character. On the one hand, by centering the decision only on one person (childbearing women) it minimizes the participation, responsibility, and accountability of the other member of the reproductive couple, precluding all potential contributions to the decision-making process and to the enrichment of the experience. This exclusion is also unfortunate because it diminishes the importance that decisions can (and should) be a product of communicative processes between both members of the reproductive couple, where individual rights are exercised freely and responsibilities are shared equally. Communicative processes, that are intersubjective, not only allow for mutual understanding of desires and needs, but in addition they are a very effective tool for solving conflicting ideas, positions, plans, and needs. On the other, the attribution of rights represents, at the same time, attribution of obligations. In this sense, to privilege childbearing women in the entitlement has, also, the subtext of making procreation, from beginning to end, their exclusive responsibility. A normative route that was conceived as a counterbalance to gender inequality and as a way to empower women in the decision-making process turned out to work against women. By excluding men (or the other member of the reproductive couple), it impoverishes our conceptions of reproductive decision-making processes. And while the design of the entitlement might grant women a certain "legal edge," the overall consequence is, in effect, disempowering because it places the whole burden of procreation (yet again) solely on women, pretty much in the fashion that patriarchal reasoning has done for such a long time.

The fact that men and women have a biologically different participation in reproduction, and that there are social practices that systematically discriminate against women does not mean that the remedy, from a normative point of view, is to construct discriminatory rights or exclusionary entitlements. If the objective is to create social conditions of gender equality and to grant equal rights within couples and for individuals, this does not seem to be the route. I believe that the problem stems from confusing the normative dimension with the sociological. It is problematic, at best, to give a normative solution to a sociological problem without recognizing the complex relationship these dimensions hold, and the limits that each one has to produce changes in the other.

The international definition of reproductive rights mitigated the problem and deferred the debate by extending the entitlement to include both the couple and individuals involved in the process of reproduction. The more substantive debate, however, about how to face and deal with the issue of gender inequality, when defining entitlements and rights, remained open until the mid-1990s.

Three consecutive international conferences (World Conference on Human Rights in Vienna, 1993; International Conference on Population and Development in Cairo, 1994; and Fourth World Conference on Women in Beijing, 1995) had a definitive effect over the orientation and content of the debate by moving it away from the domain of entitlement. The problem of gender inequality for the exercise of reproductive rights was no longer seen as resolvable through a normative transformation of entitlement. It was no longer a battle about formally empowering women in an effort to equalize the conditions under which reproductive decisions were made. Now the goal was about embedding the notion of gender equality as a necessary condition for reproductive decisions and the exercise of reproductive rights. This resulted in a substantive and profound change that, in my estimation, transformed the entire landscape of the debate by shifting the framework of reference and interpretation, and positively responding to the need of facing the problem of gender inequality.

Paragraph 96 of the Beijing Declaration and Platform for Action, can be read as a crystallization of that process:

> The human rights of women include their right to have control over and decide freely and responsibly on matters related to their sexuality, including sexual and reproductive health, free of coercion, discrimination and violence. Equal relationships between women and men in matters of sexual relations and reproduction, including full respect for the integrity of the person, require mutual respect, consent and shared responsibility for sexual behavior and its consequences (United Nations, 1995).

I agree with Rosalind Petchesky when she refers to this as an historic international recognition (1998). It represents a conceptual and political landmark because it established the social need for gender equality beyond the previously recognized public realms. Equal relations between men and women need to be assured, protected, and fostered in the private sphere, and in the specific realms of family, reproduction, and intimacy for women's human rights to self-determination and equality to flourish. This international recognition makes gender equality a social issue that cuts across all spheres of life.

3.2. Social Character of Entitlement and the Concept of Responsibility

From an historical and formal point of view, reproductive rights should be included simultaneously under two different categories of human rights: as individual rights and social rights (Cook, 1993, 1994). On the one hand, the right to decide how many, when, or whether to have children is the expression of an individual right to reproductive freedom. It is predicated on the notion of individual liberty, and it implies the right to control one's own body. On the other, the right to have the information and means to regulate (or not) one's own fertility is the expression of a right to social goods. Regardless of the choices people make in regard to their fertility, all individuals have the right to the most current and accurate information, and to the most effective and safe means for the regulation of their fertility.

This connection to both the domains of individual and social rights creates an interesting duality. It introduces a tension between the individual freedom to choose and the conditions that need to be met for that choice to be significant and meaningful. In other words, it establishes the need to assure access to certain social goods as a condition for reproductive freedom.

Ruth Dixon-Mueller describes that dual characteristic in the following way:

> The individual liberty elements consist of the freedom to choose among alternative sexual and reproductive behaviors without coercion from governments or from individuals or social institutions . . . The social entitlement elements consist of the obligation of the state, or of "society," to ensure that everyone can exercise the full range of economic, social, political, and civil rights that infuse reproductive choice with real meaning (1993, pp. 14–15).

The inclusion of reproductive decisions as rights of citizens in the World Plan of Action in Population of 1974 established two types of obligations for national governments. First, governments cannot interfere nor inhibit the decision-making processes of their citizens with regard to reproduction, either through mechanisms of coercion or the concealment of the necessary information for making reproductive decisions. Reproductive decisions are the exclusive and sovereign domain of citizens, and it is the obligation of the state, or the governments in turn, to assure that they are protected and kept this way. Second, governments have the obligation to provide the necessary information so citizens can make knowledgeable decisions, as well as to provide the means for those decisions to materialize in the best way possible (Correa & Petchesky, 1994; Fincancioglu, 1990; Hartmann, 1987; Warwick, 1982).

As Dixon Mueller points out,

> the role of governments, ideally, is to balance in practice the sometimes contradictory demands of individual freedom and social entitlement as abstractly defined . . . Too little state intervention can make it impossible for people to decide freely on the number and spacing of their children, for example, because they lack the economic resources, information, and services to do so or because their rights are violated by other individuals or groups. Too much intervention can infringe on individual choice in the name of collective security or the common good (1993, p. 15).

All rights require a social environment of freedom and respect, or to put it in a negative sense, require the absence of all forms of coercion. However and unlike individual rights, social rights are by definition rights that are also dependent on specific conditions for their exercise to be possible. The lack of these conditions constitutes direct impediments to their expression and exercise: without hospitals, schools, and a productive plant it becomes impossible to exercise the right to health, to education, and to work. Social rights establish a binding contract of the state towards civil society. They imply duties and responsibilities for governments of providing the means and conditions so their populations can fully exercise their rights as citizens of their societies. In this sense, the social rights of a population are dependent on their state's provision and enabling intervention.

What is unique about reproductive rights is that without being exclusively social rights their individual dimension requires access to social goods (information and means), and a social agreement to protect their autonomy from individuals, groups, social institutions, and particularly from government itself.

Why would an internationally supported plan of action (like the one elaborated in 1974) obligate national governments not to interfere in the reproductive decisions of their citizens, by way of coercive measures? Why would governments feel the need to intervene in the reproductive decisions of their citizens? The normative effort could have been a response to governments that were violating the reproductive freedom of their citizens or an anticipation of that possibility. Whether the intention was corrective or preventive, the most interesting issue, it seems to me, is that it was perceived to be a problem that required addressing.

While a liberal framework for international law would require that all governments respect the reproductive freedom of their citizens, the World Plan of 1974 set out to obligate national governments not to be coercive, even if they felt it was justifiable in the name of the common good. In the 1970s population growth had already been articulated as a major obstacle, if not the central reason, for the lack of social and economic development in the so-called "Third World" countries (Duden, 1992). Governments that were concerned about their population growth could only see certain type of reproductive decisions as good for the nation (Finkle & McIntosh, 1994). Reproductive decisions could not be made disregarding the "needs of the nation"; otherwise citizenship freedom would be used irresponsibly. In this sense, reproductive freedom was at odds with national development projects, and ultimately with the common good. Reproductive decisions needed to be not only free – it was thought – but also responsible.

Since their inception, reproductive rights have been accompanied by the idea of responsibility. But the concept was not fully defined until 1974 through the World Plan of Action in Population. According to that formulation, and in the absence of later modifications to this date, responsibility is introduced as a qualifier to the exercise of reproductive freedom. Couples and individuals need to take into consideration their situation, as well as the implications of their decisions for the development of their children, their community, and their society. A revision of the concept in 1984 added that a responsible decision would also require taking into account the well being of future children (Boland, 1997; United Nations, 1990, 1997, 2000).

Defined in that way, the inclusion of the concept of responsibility within reproductive rights seems to create an intrinsic contradiction.

> Does the recognition of the needs of the community, and of society justify the intervention of the state where fertility decision-making processes take place? If the answer is affirmative, to what degree and in what way? This fundamental topic continues being debated in the different instances of the United Nations (United Nations, 1990, p. 59).

While the Cairo Conference in 1994 resulted in important modifications to the interpretation of reproductive rights and meaningful enhancements of its domain, it is somewhat noteworthy that in its core elements the international definition has remained (the entitlement figure being the exception) as it was formulated in 1968 and reformulated in 1979. This includes the concept of responsibility, and its subsequent qualifiers. In effect, the Cairo Program of Action "moved reproductive rights away from only family planning and access to these services towards a broader focus on sexual and reproductive health . . . It also emphasized the principle that the right to reproductive self-determination is a right that is to be exercised freely, without discrimination, violence, or coercion" (Boland, 1997, p. 16). Both of these modifications were not only ratified but also further developed and specified in 1995 at the Beijing Conference and in its Program of Action.

In light of all these modifications that have enhanced reproductive rights, it is quite remarkable and somewhat unsettling that the concept of responsibility has not been challenged or changed in any way.

The inclusion and permanence of the idea of responsibility in the definition of reproductive rights can be interpreted – I am suggesting – as a product of a political compromise between state interventionists and reproductive rights defenders. From the state's perspective it can work as a corrective to "deviant behavior" and as an avenue to protect the discretionary power to intervene when the project of the nation is threatened. From the rights' perspective it situates the whole decision-making process in the sphere of individual freedom, and therefore under the control of individuals and couples, including the interpretation of what is best for their communities and societies. But neither the tension nor the contradictions disappear.

The rights' perspective has always manifested a concern with state intervention in the decision-making processes of individuals and couples. And while there has been a certain level of consensus around the idea of restricting this type of state intervention, the concept of responsibility has produced debate and divisions. The discussion has been divided on two fronts: those that support an initiative where the boundaries of freedom and responsibility are clearly delineated and, those that believe in the omission of the concept of responsibility from the international definition. The first position understands the problem as transitory: the source of conflict is a direct result of the lack of conceptual clarity. All that is required is a clear definition of where freedom ends and responsibility begins. A clearly established definition of responsibility – they would argue – not only would restrict state intervention, but also would obligate individuals to think in terms of the common good. In contrast, the second position defends the idea that individuals having the means and the necessary knowledge will achieve reproductive decisions in accordance not only to their needs, but to their social reality as well. Thus, there is no need to establish responsibility beforehand because the decisions would be contextually situated responding differentially to different sectors of the population. Of course, this assumes that the project of the nation would be receptive and inclusive of a wide array of reproductive decisions, and would respect the content of those decisions.

To what extent, then, is it a wise idea that an international definition of reproductive rights includes the concept of responsibility? Is it possible to reconcile the freedom of individuals and couples with the needs of their communities, their societies, and their nation states? Should there even be an effort to reconcile differences between these spheres? And if so, is the concept of responsibility capable of achieving this?

The debates surrounding the concept of responsibility have suggested that there are different plausible interpretations of the concept, and that these can lead to dramatically different expressions of reproductive rights. Furthermore, I believe that the opposing interpretations of the concept of responsibility are symptoms of conceptual contradictions that are not only worth exploring but that need to be faced and solved.

The fact that the concept of responsibility is still part of the international definition of reproductive rights, and that it still remains without clarification has, in my opinion, serious implications. In its current form, the concept of responsibility allows states to intervene "legitimately" in the reproductive decisions of their citizens, on the grounds that their decisions or actions are irresponsible. The scenario is not a difficult one to imagine. A governmental plan evaluates the possible implications of a certain rate of population growth as negative for the economic development and future viability of the nation. Fertility is identified as the variable that has the most weight in producing that population growth, and contraception as the most effective tool to bring down the fertility rate. Caring about the future of the nation the government would organize efforts and structure plans with the objective of reversing the trend and avoiding its negative consequences. In this way fertility is linked to economic development and high fertility is perceived to be an obstacle to a better future. Contraception and reproductive choices become the social space where government meets citizens, the administrative and political "battle ground" where decisions will be sanctioned as responsible or not. How much a government is willing to push for what they have determined to be a "responsible" decision, and to encroach on the autonomy of individuals and couples will ultimately depend on how authoritarian or democratic a country is. But an active government that "cares" about the future of the nation will aggressively pursue administrative goals, becoming a permanent threat to free and autonomous reproductive decisions.

Without a clear international definition, the interpretation that governments make of the concept of responsibility will be dependent on the prevailing political culture and the political relations of that society. At the center of this question we have the problem of the potential or real contradiction between state needs and the needs of social groups and individuals; of how tolerant of difference and even of dissent governments are; of how important the autonomy and freedom of citizens is to governments, and how representative the administration of state is of the will of the people (Fig. 2). Also at the center is the crucial problem of how

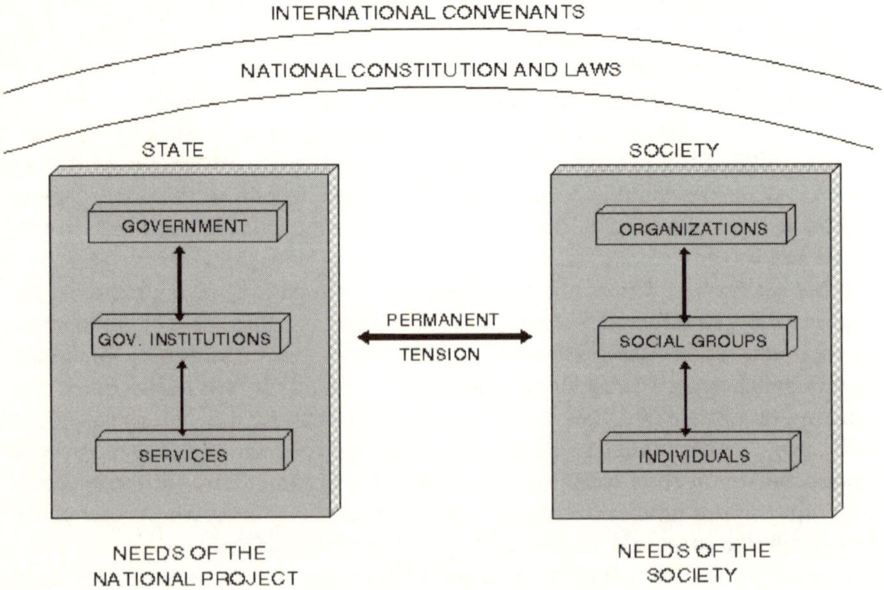

Fig. 2. Rights within Nations.

and who defines, at certain historical junctions, what is a national need, what is in the best interest of a nation, and what constitutes a social and political priority. Ultimately, it is about how democratic a society is, and how participatory and representative the political system really is (Habermas, 1996; Hirschmann, 1992; Seligman, 1992; Taylor, 1995).

Population policies are specific and historical expressions of how states and governments interpret the relation between development and demographic phenomena. In turn, the establishment of demographic goals represent quantitative ways in which the interpretation of that relation is translated into plans and programs. It is the state and its concrete governments who determine what is the best population scenario for the development of the nation, and who design it into programmatic practice. It is within this interpretative frame that reproductive responsibility is contextually defined (Duden, 1992; Foucault, 1990; Sen, Germain & Chen, 1994).

Given the centrality of fertility for population growth, demographic goals find their translations into fertility level goals, regardless if the intention is to reduce or increase growth. The national goal for population growth becomes a national goal for fertility, and then an ideal number of children to have. The establishment of demographic goals and their translation into number of children sets the normative boundaries for reproduction, and determines in a numerical form the criteria for responsible reproductive behavior (Shapiro, 1985; Warwick, 1982, 1990, 1994).

The free exercise of reproductive rights is defined and determined within these programmatically fixed limits. Anything outside these limits might be considered from an individual or couple's perspective a free decision, an unconstrained reproductive act, but from the perspective of the state it is deemed as irresponsible, or at best as a reproductive freedom used irresponsibly. In this way, responsibility appears as the process by which individuals and couples incorporate in their reproductive decisions the historical "needs of the nation" (Ginsburg & Rapp, 1995; Hartmann, 1987). It is not enough, for individuals and couples, to take into consideration their situation, as well as the implications of their decisions for the development and well-being of their (current and future) children, a responsible decision will require considering and incorporating the "demographic demands" and the "developmental needs" of their community and their society, such that the decision itself reflects the "needs of the nation." Because no other sphere provides such a precise measure to judge a reproductive decision as do population policies and their demographic goals, ultimately it is the "needs of the nation," expressed in a programmatic ideal number of children to have, that provides the criteria for responsibility. The concept of responsibility becomes the metamorphosis of the will of the state into individual will; it creates the precise limits within which women and men, couples can be sanctioned as "free and responsible" when exercising their rights and making their reproductive decisions.

Whether or not the inclusion of the concept of responsibility was a product of a political compromise, its presence results in a lopsided definition that favors state intervention and disempowers citizens in the exercise of their reproductive rights. The lack of a definitive and forceful challenge to rid the definition of the concept of responsibility may suggest a tacit agreement with the need for state intervention and a patronizing politics: "People can't be trusted to do the right thing, to make adequate reproductive decisions; that is why we have to appeal to their sense of obligation and force them to be responsible for their own reproductive actions. And if people can't be trusted, who is going to assure the nation's future?"

Even in the absence of this last perverse political possibility, I believe there are enough reasons to completely eliminate the concept of responsibility from the international definition of reproductive rights. The concept of responsibility allows, invites, and justifies state intervention; it reflects a politics of disdain and not of trust, and it advocates normalization and intolerance rather than respect and acceptance of reproductive diversity.

3.3. Entitlement, Inequality, and the Exercise of Rights

Due to the universal criteria that define the concept of justice in a society, all individuals are equal. They are equal because the only condition that an individual requires to be entitled to laws and regulations, and to the protection of a system of justice is to be a member of that society (Ferry & Renaut, 1994; Hirschmann, 1992; Lummis, 1992).

From a strictly formal perspective, "if the same norms and rules are applied to each and every one of the members of a society (independently of the social group to which they belong), these norms and rules make all equal from the point of view of the norms and rules in question" (Heller, 1987, p. 16). It is the social existence of a system of laws and their pervasive application that allows all citizens in a formal democracy to be members of that society. A system of laws provides equal rights and equality of all citizens under them. In turn, citizenship appears as the legal form of social membership (Hirschmann, 1992; Lummis, 1992; Turner, 1990).

In the particular case of reproductive rights, all individuals are entitled to the inalienable rights over their own bodies, and to be able to decide freely about their fertility and when or whether to have children. The only condition that they require is having been born in this world, for they are international rights granted to all human beings. Furthermore, if individuals were born in a country where these rights are protected legally, that is to say, where the condition of being a citizen allows for the translation of a human right into a constitutional right, then their national state will have the obligation of assuring that the circumstances are suitable for the free and full exercise of reproductive decisions. From this vantage point, the citizens of the world that are also citizens of these nations turn out to hold a rights' privilege because they have a double legal and moral protection, one from an international legal frame and from a national one as well. These citizens would have "doubly" insured the entitlement to rights that seek to safeguard their reproductive life.

However, the fact that belonging to a society will grant individuals with a series of rights and obligations, and that these will work as equalizers between all individuals of that society, does not mean that all will have the same possibilities or be in equality of circumstances to exercise those rights that (formally) define them all as equal. Having rights does not mean that one can exercise them. Between the entitlement to a formal right that all individuals have due to their membership to a society and the possibility of their exercise stand social constraints specific to that society (structural, systemic, ideological, symbolic).

In contemporary societies, social inequality is foundational to social relations and central to the organization of social life and opportunities. The system of inequality in a given society changes from one historical period to another, and is a product of a complex articulation of different (sub)systems of social inequality based on class, gender, race and ethnicity, and age. The weight that each one of these (sub)systems has on the profile of the overall stratification and inequality depends on the specific history and internal dynamics of a society. These complex articulations are unique to the social formation of each society, yet they are permanently undergoing transformations and re-articulations (Andersen & Collins, 1992; Marger, 1999; Ore, 2000).

Social inequality, as a result of these complex articulations, determines the manner in which individuals participate in the production and benefit from the distribution of social wealth, as well as the structure of options within which individuals construct their lives and exercise their personal will. And, conversely, in the exercise of their personal will and the construction of their lives individuals create and re-create the structure of options and the related social determinations, as well as their own insertion into the production and distribution of social wealth (Bourdieu, 1977, 1990; Giddens, 1984; Habermas, 1984, 1987; Luhmann & De Georgi, 1993).

Trying to explain the relationship of multiple determinations between agency and structure, Giddens uses the concept of duality to assess that unique characteristic and quality of all social structures: "Structure (is) the medium and outcome of the conduct it recursively organises; the structural properties of social systems do not exist outside of action but are chronically implicated in its production and reproduction" (1984, p. 374).

It is not only that people's actions are constantly confronted by social structures or that social structures permanently impose constraints over people's actions, but also that the different (sub)systems of inequality (class, gender, race and ethnicity, and age) have a foundational effect over the relationship that people and social groups establish with each other. The action of individuals and groups, as well as the multiple constraints of social structure operate through the mesh of social inequality and its different (sub)systems.

Consequently, the exercise of rights happens in accordance with the options and conditions arranged by the relative position individuals and groups occupy within the mesh of (sub)systems of social inequality. The specificity of the exercise of those rights, then, is generated by the exercise of personal will within the context of the options that social inequality offers to individuals and groups.

All individuals are equal under the law because as citizens of a nation they are entitled to the same rights. This equality is only but formal; as members of a society their equal entitlement does not assure equal enjoyment. The formal equality is completely shattered when equal rights are realized as unequal exercise, and equal entitlement becomes unequal enjoyment. For some individuals the exercise of rights will happen in a social environment full of possibilities, and saturated with diverse alternatives. For others, the choices will be given in a context of restricted possibilities, and a small array of alternatives. For yet others, the choice might not even be a possibility.

Although formally all citizens of a nation, that recognizes reproductive rights, are entitled to the same set of rights not all will be able to exercise them in a context of multiple options and diverse alternatives; some will not even have a chance to exercise them at all. For example, if we take the issue of access to medical services, we find that some citizens will be able to choose a specialized, highly qualified, and private medical practice according to their resources, and the amount of money they are willing to pay for them. Others will be immediately precluded from these options because resources cannot be made readily available for these purposes; they will be obligated to make use of services partial or totally subsidized and provided by state institutions. Yet others, in stark contrast, will be excluded from access to reproductive medical services all together.

In the previous example, the effect of social inequality over access to medical services is presented as a problem linked to economic resources. But the issue is larger than economic resources and has crucial effects over other important dimensions of the possibility of exercising reproductive rights and the social experience involved in that exercise. Taking into account variations across social contexts, having access to a private medical service or only to a public one is gaining access to two very different medical environments. Aside from the issues of quality and specialization that are affected by economic resources, each one of the environments will produce very distinct experiences due to differences in the type of physician-patient relationship, normative practices, institutional orientations, social expectations, sense of entitlement, and capacity for negotiation.

Also the dynamics of the interaction might be altered in ways that affect the quality of the experience, and the decision-making process. Allowing for social and cultural variations, physicians in a private practice, for example, will tend to view their patients as clients that need to be catered to, and perhaps make efforts to preserve the clientelistic relationship to the extent that they are personally profiting from it. This might translate into a more receptive physician to the specific needs and demands of the patient. In turn, a patient that has purchased a service might feel more empowered to expect and demand a certain level of quality, that would range anywhere from the amount and type of information demanded to feeling comfortable when accepting or declining a medical suggestion or procedure. This sense of empowerment could work as a potentiating force of the level and quality of the information the person brings into the medical service, and would allow for arriving at a reproductive decision more suited to the life and the needs of the patient.

Access to medical services is only but one area of the whole set of reproductive rights. Although in different ways, all areas are affected by social inequality once we place entitlement within a specific social context and we explore the differential possibilities that citizens would have of actualizing these rights.

The vital social experience of individuals permanently questions the level of feasibility of formal equality granted by the law, and it challenges the notion that formal equality translates in anyway into the social conditions of their every day life existence. Legal discourse asserts not only that all citizens are equal under the law, but also that all citizens have equal possibilities of enjoying and exercising all rights, as well as being equally protected by the law. Formal equality encounters stark forms of inequality; the all-inclusive promise of rights clashes with the pervasive forms of exclusion and marginalization creating a schizophrenic split between the discursive promises of the law and the social experiences of individuals.

4. REPRODUCTIVE DECISIONS: A NORMATIVE AND SOCIOLOGICAL INTERPRETATION

Using a Habermasian methodology (1984, 1987, 1990, 1993),[4] this section explores the concept of reproductive rights in two analytical dimensions: as a normative phenomenon and as a social reality. The analysis is developed from the perspective of the decision-making process involved. The international definition of reproductive rights is based on a series of complex assumptions about decisions pertaining to reproduction. I start by briefly presenting the basic assumptions of this definition, and reconstruct the meaning these assumptions have for decisions. Then, I propose an ideal process of reproductive decision making as a normative frame for reproductive rights. Once I have established the ideal normative process, in the final part of this section I turn my attention to the identification and analysis of possible disturbances. By disturbances I mean the social, political, and economic conditions that interfere with the development of an ideal process of decision making. Two main sources of disturbances are assessed for both the private and the public realms: power relations and systems of social inequality.

4.1. On the Assumptions

According to the components that define the legal parameters of reproductive rights in a national context or a specific country, certain conditions are required so that these rights can be fully exercised by their citizens. On the one hand, the state is under the obligation of providing to its population of current, truthful, general and specific information, as well as the appropriate means for the regulation of fertility. On the other, in order for citizens to carry out their reproductive decisions freely, the state should not only abstain from intervening in the process of decision making but in addition make sure that the social conditions that surround this process allows for the generation of autonomous decisions (Boland, 1997; CRLP, 2000; Dixon-Mueller, 1993; Petchesky, 1998; United Nations, 1990, 1995).

In that sense, the state plays the double role of general supplier and of guardian of the freedom and autonomy of its citizens. That is why the full exercise of reproductive rights, in particular, but of all the social rights, in general, depends on concrete provisions and actions from the state to assure autonomy and freedom. While the role of supplier is directly tied to the availability and distribution of resources, the role of guardian is more closely linked to political will and the relationship it has with civil society. For the provision of information and means the state requires material and human resources, but their availability does not assure that the state has the political will of distributing them or that society has access to them; resources are a necessary condition but they are not enough to satisfy the obligation of providing or the need for the provision. In contrast, for the protection of autonomy and freedom in the exercise of citizens' rights, the state is required to have an unrestricted respect for their private processes and to trust that their decisions will ultimately be good for the nation, regardless if they approve or not of them. In any one of the two cases, the key resides in that the state is able to recognize the political virtue of one of the maxims of democracy: ultimately, the power of the state is located in civil society, and in the decisions that citizens make. These, of course, can be expressed as preferences while voting, while determining what is the common good or through intersubjective public deliberations.

The full exercise of the reproductive rights of the citizens of a nation can only be developed in relation with the state: on the basis of its provisions and under the help of its guardianship.

The legal definition of reproductive rights and their explanatory (international) discourse has been constructed on the basis of a series of normative assumptions that are not, necessarily, made explicit or submitted to analytical and public scrutiny. Nevertheless, these assumptions have greatly informed and guided their interpretation. In this way, for example, the right to make free and informed decisions about when or whether to have children presupposes two simultaneous conditions. On the one hand, the process of making decisions needs to develop in the absence of all forms of coercion. In other words, the decisions made by citizens should be carried out in a fully autonomous way and in correspondence to the reasons and needs determined by them. On the other, the state is responsible for assuring that all citizens have access to accurate and relevant information on reproduction, such that their decisions are made with full knowledge of the current alternatives to regulate fertility and to protect pregnancies. Reproductive rights are envisioned on the basis of a network of assumptions that precede them, and at the same time explain their legal discourse.

In an effort to clarify the assumptions that exist behind the international definition of reproductive rights, and to advance in their discussion I would like to propose a reading from a normative perspective. The objective is two-fold. First, it allows opening the discussion about the content of reproductive rights by making their justification and explanation explicit, and enables an evaluation of their discursive legitimacy. That is to say, it allows for an analytical scrutiny of some of their underpinnings, the uncovering of veiled elements, and an opportunity to thematize the taken-for-granted reasoning behind them. Second, once we have defined the normative parameters it is not only possible to establish goals to pursue, but in addition to use normative agreements as an organized way to evaluate current practices, and to discover the impediments for the realization of the desired norm.

4.2. Ideal Process for Making Reproductive Decisions

Following a Habermasian approach,[5] I propose the reconstruction of a normative framework for reproductive rights as an ideal decision-making process, where the end product is a decision about reproduction able to fulfill all the conceptual

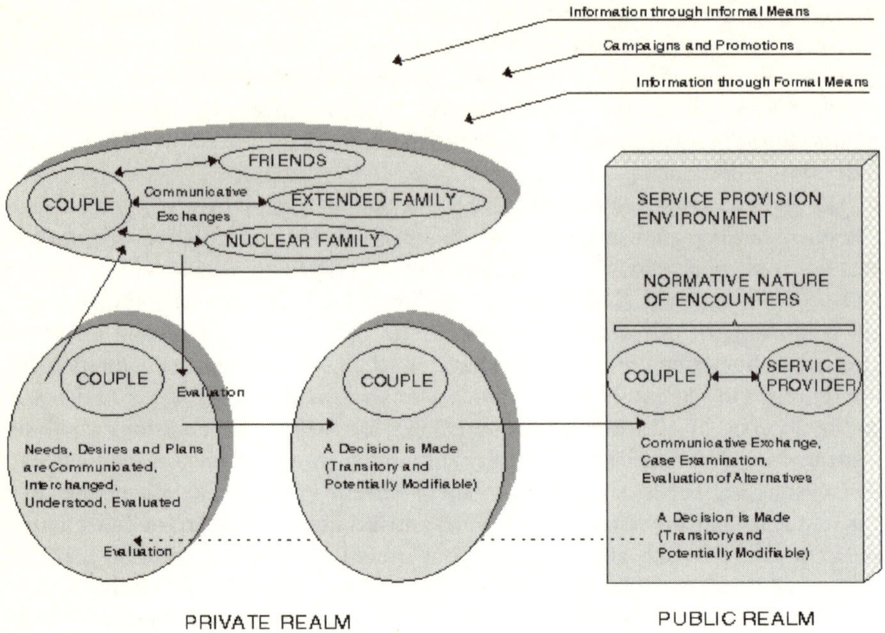

Fig. 3. Ideal Reproductive Decision-Making Process.

and procedural requirements that would be demanded by the current international definition of reproductive rights.

The ideal decision-making process takes place in the private dimension of social life as much as it does in the public dimension (Fig. 3). In each one of these dimensions differentiated dynamics are generated that contribute in different moments of the process to produce general, as well as particular resolutions. The process begins in the private sphere, it moves toward the public domain and returns back to the private where resolutions are taken (although always transitory and potentially modifiable) in specific moments of the life course.

It is in the dimension of the private that couples face their need of regulating or not their fertility, of becoming or not pregnant, of interrupting or not a pregnancy, of having or not a child. Couples develop their decision-making processes in their private worlds, through communicative interactions between them and with other people that are significant for their social and affective life and that are able to become emotional, moral, and cultural interlocutors. Through these interactions, couples discover, develop, and make explicit their desires, expectations, interests, and plans. This group of representations will constitute a constant source of meaning and the symbolic material from which couples can elaborate their reproductive decisions, and compare them against other social representations and decisions made by others: family members, friends, acquaintances or other people with whom they interact.

The elements and criteria used for the elaboration of the decisions should be chosen and determined autonomously by each couple. If these elements and criteria come from history, tradition, science, or magic and if they are affective, moral, rational, religious, or economic depends ultimately on the needs and preferences of the couple.

To the extent that all decisions are potentially exposed to reconsideration and evaluations, these should always be appreciated as transitory and modifiable. For example, through communicative interactions the couple can discover new elements, standards, or ideas that modify their position or perspective in relation to certain reproductive decisions. Likewise, the discovery of new information and alternatives can constitute important ground that can lead to evaluations of past positions and perhaps partial or total reconsideration.

In this dimension and in regard to the dynamics of the private, the freedom to make a reproductive decision is fundamentally determined by the exercise of individual and couple autonomy. Within the couple, free and equal individuals engage in explorations and conversations that are fair and respectful of each other's needs. These conditions are extended to other private contexts to sustain the autonomy of the couple so that we can assure that the communicative interactions, with other significant interlocutors, are developed in the absence of impositions or coercion.

Once a reproductive decision is elaborated in the private domain, the couple meets with the logic and nature of social relations, in the public sphere, when they require and look for the provision of professional and specialized services. The type of service that is required depends on the type of decision that the couple has taken.

Public institutions (governmental or not) should provide three different types of services: (1) information that is both general, and specific, as well as professional and specialized; (2) advice that is comprehensive and particular, and recommendations that are supported by professional and specialized knowledge; and (3) the most appropriate, current, and safe means that allow the couple to carry out their decisions. The provision of these services should not only be of the best possible quality, but they should be offered with an unrestrained recognition and respect for the couple's autonomy and their decisions.

The participation of institutions in the process of reproductive decisions should be, fundamentally, to facilitate the realization of the desires, needs, and determinations of the couple. It is neither the function nor the charge of institutions to intervene in the determination of the judgments, criteria or elements of a decision and, much less, to determine the type or content of the decision for the couple. Institutions should assure that the couple has elaborated their decision aware of all relevant information and in light of professional recommendations that are impartial, of quality, and current. Additionally, they should offer the necessary means so that, once the decision is taken, couples can carry it out under the best and most healthy conditions.

The meeting between couples with demands and providers of services take place within the realm of specific institutions that are regulated by national legislation, as well as by administrative norms and internal regulations. Even when institutions work according to the law and with arrangement to regulations, they hold a certain degree of autonomy that allows them to define the characteristics of the services they want to offer. Furthermore, this relative autonomy allows them to determine the basic profile of their internal organization, dynamics, and the structure within which social relations are established. It is in this sense that the freedom to make decisions requires not only of the protection from legal discourse, apparent in laws, but also from institutional norms that guide the action of the providers of services, and that regulate the relationship with citizens that require of their services.

On the basis of the previous arguments we can conclude that the full exercise of reproductive rights is assured through two basic conditions: freedom and access.

Decisions can be elaborated freely if the process of decision making is developed with absolute autonomy and in the absence of all forms of coercion. This has a different significance for the private dimension than for the public realm. In the private sphere freedom begins with self-determination and the control of one's own body. This principle is extended to the relationship of the couple (regardless of its daily, sexual, affective, legal or social arrangement), but it requires to be paired with the equality of rights and responsibilities in the decision-making process, in its realization, and in its consequences. Also, the presence of significant others in making decisions need to be carried out through free and respectful exchanges, and never as the imposition of approaches, perspectives, and interpretations that disregard the needs and desires of the couple. In the public realm, freedom is carried out from the private when the couple obtains an institutional service that is complete, of quality, and respectful of the autonomy of their decision.

The condition of access also has different meanings depending on the dimension in which the decision-making process is occurring. In the private, it begins with a positive perception of the right to have access to the provision of services, and it extends to the possibility of obtaining relevant and necessary information throughout the process, and in the different moments of the life course of individuals and couples. In the public, access also refers to information, that is professional and specialized, and that can aid the couple in the evaluation of alternatives and in the elaboration of their decisions. Additionally, institutions represent the access to the most appropriate, current, and safe means for the realization of the decisions made with regard to fertility and reproduction. Both in the private as in the public sphere it is crucial that access be universal, unrestricted, and equal for all citizens.

4.3. Disturbances in the Ideal Process for Making Reproductive Decisions

Once we have established the general structure of the normative ideal of the process of making reproductive decisions, now we can identify and analyze, in a very general way, the type of disturbances that the process suffers or to which it can be exposed or subjected (Fig. 4).

By disturbances I am referring to all those social, political, and economic conditions that interfere or can potentially interfere in the development of an ideal process of decision making. Therefore, these disturbances represent serious obstacles for the full exercise of the reproductive rights of citizens in specific national contexts.

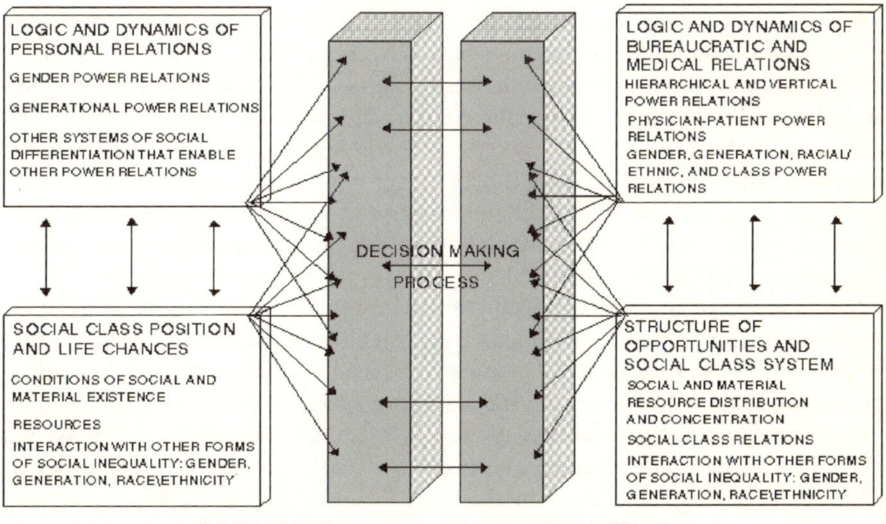

Fig. 4. Disturbances in the Ideal Decision-Making Process.

The sources of these interferences are basically two: power relations and systems of social differentiation that produce social inequality. The concept of power is understood here in its negative sense, that is to say, as domination. That is, power relations are conceptualized as relations of domination, where the will of some is imposed on others. In turn, I use systems of social differentiation when referring to a network of perceptions and interpretations that make differences significant, and that generate and legitimate multiple social actions based on those forms of explaining and interpreting differences. These are forms that are prevalent and pervasive in societies, and that have a certain historical stability. However, not all forms of social differentiation become forms of social inequality. Together social inequality and relations of domination, produce the fundamental disturbances in the ideal process of making decisions, and constitute the central obstacles for the full exercise of reproductive rights.

These disturbances occur both in the private and public sphere, although the specific ways in which they interfere and affect decisions will vary according to the dimension and to the social interactions through which they manifest their destructive force.

For the part of the process that occurs in the private sphere, the interferences have two origins. One can be located in the logic and the dynamics of personal relationships, and the other linked to the class position and the place occupied within the structure of opportunities.

For personal and intimate relationships, gender and generational domination (and perhaps other forms as well) are constant threats for developing decisions based on communicative interactions between equals. The imposition of perspectives, needs, and desires of one individual over the other transform decisions into unilateral outcomes that fracture the right to decide about one's own body, and relativize the free determination about one's own fertility and reproduction. In the world of intimacy, the self-determination over one's own body and the freedom to decide over one's own reproduction can only be fully exercised when there is absolute respect for the other, intersubjective understanding, and communicative interactions that are free and equal.

We have basically the same problem when the couple or their individuals share their desires, needs, and plans with friends and members of their nuclear and extended families. If the communicative exchanges become instruments of domination and vehicles for the imposition of other's will by means of gender, generation, or kinship relationships the self-determination over the body and the freedom to make reproductive decisions disappears in a complex net of manipulation and subjection. In this way communities ratify and reproduce their membership through bonds of domination and subordination, instead of becoming enriching resources for the affective and symbolic world, and for the construction of individual identity, at the time that they consolidate a sense of belonging.

Class position and the structure of opportunities have a disturbance effect in the private sphere because it interferes with access to information and the capacity to manage it. The most obvious and direct relationship is linked to schooling and formal education: the higher the education, the more exposure the individual will have to complete, truthful, current, and relevant information. But other associations might be underlying, perhaps connected with the formation of analytic and critical judgment, with the capacity to discern and discriminate, as well as with the possibilities of constructing autonomous and independent positions.

As for the part of the process that is developed in the public realm, the interferences have two origins. One can be found in the logic and dynamics of medical and bureaucratic relations and, the other in the system of classes and structure of opportunities. To the extent that the provision of services happens, generally, in medical institutions, the relations that are established between citizens and providers are constantly exposed to different kinds of systems of power. The doctor-patient relation transforms reproductive knowledge into a specialized and professional knowledge that is concentrated in the social figure of physicians and medical personnel. It also transforms individuals that require a service into ignorant patients that depend on medical knowledge and their will to provide. This distribution of knowledge structures the relation in a hierarchical and vertical fashion, granting physicians and medical personnel a great deal of discretional power and influence over the reproductive decisions of individuals and couples.

In turn, the structure and organization of institutions, the internal logic of their administrative systems and their specific forms of exercising power, the vertical flow of information and control, as well as their authoritarian practices and forms of distributing privileges are all brought to the forefront when citizens are forced to deal with the bureaucrats that represent those institutions. The content of the relation that the institutional employee offers to the citizen depends on how the institution defines its functions of service provision, perceive their responsibility towards citizens, and interpret their obligations in the provision of that service. To the extent that bureaucratic and medical institutions are intertwined in an administrative complex the supply of services, the doctor-patient and bureaucrat-citizen relation appear linked and interwoven in their practices.

The disturbances produced by the exercise of medical and bureaucratic power take place in combination and through other forms of social domination. In this way, systems of inequality and of social discrimination based on social class, race/ethnicity, sex, and age become vehicles of the exercise of medical and bureaucratic power or additional systemic forms to distribute attention, respect, services, and resources in a systematic, differential, and unequal way.

The social class system and the structure of opportunities of a given society, in a specific period of its history, have profound effects over access to services. It not only determines the chances of having access, but also the characteristics and the quality of the services offered by the non-governmental (private sector), of course, but also over those offered by governmental institutions.

The patterns of concentration and distribution of material and social wealth generate favorable conditions of access for certain sectors of the population, while restricting or precluding access for others. It is in this sense that the amount and quality of alternatives, on the basis of which reproductive decisions are made, depend on the amount of social and material resources that individuals and couples are capable of mobilizing during decision-making processes throughout their life course.

This complex of power relations and systems of social inequality constantly threaten the two central conditions for the exercise of reproductive rights in the public domain: freedom and access. On the one hand, the universal entitlement of obtaining services is seriously disabled. Nation states fall short from their obligation to provide basic services to its entire population, and not all citizens have the possibility of obtaining them or of benefiting from the same service quality. On the other, the singular characteristic of the right to self-determination and freedom is deeply questioned. Institutions abandon their charge to protect and encourage individuals and couples to develop free and autonomous reproductive decisions, and instead allow for the imposition of criteria that is guided by the logic of the exercise of specific powers and the intrusion of institutional programs and policies, that may or not coincide with the needs and desires of citizens.

5. CONCLUSION

Throughout this chapter, I developed a series of arguments and put forward some theoretical elaborations with the intention of offering a sociological framework for the analysis of reproductive rights in their different social, political and legal dimensions, both at an international level and within specific national contexts.

I started by examining the two main components that define reproductive rights. First, I introduced an interpretation of the process of human reproduction and signaled the segments that have become the basis for the construction of the normative discourse. Second, I explored the sociological and political significance, as well as the implications that these rights have been defined as "social rights," that is rights that imply a certain type of relationship between nation states and their citizens. Third, I identify two contentious issues in the history of their definition: entitlement and responsibility. While the debate around entitlement has allowed for the emergence of a thoughtful and more refined definition, the problem with the concept of responsibility that qualifies these rights remains, in my estimation, largely unresolved and politically problematic, because it formally allows states to intervene, with discretionary power, in the reproductive lives and decisions of citizens.

Next, I moved to the analysis of the assumptions that are embedded in the current international definition of reproductive rights. There are a series of assumptions that can be derived and made explicit from the definition and its historical development. However, there are others that are not easily derived and thus have remained basically implicit and unthematized. Yet these are not secondary. I argued that these sets of assumptions are fundamental for the exercise of reproductive rights, both in the private and public realms, and decisive for reproductive decision-making processes.

Using Habermas' "ideal speech situation," I reconstructed the "ideal reproductive decision-making process," informed both by human rights standards of social justice, and feminist theory. This ideal normative reconstruction identifies the process of making autonomous, unrestricted, and informed decisions, both in the private and the public sphere, as the center of the exercise of reproductive rights.

Once I established the ideal normative, my analysis turned to the factors that might impede the full realization of these rights. Within the contexts of nation states, I find two sources of disturbances: power relations and social inequality. Both power and inequality create profound distortions to the decision-making process in the private, as well as in the public domain.

From a cognitive point of view, the objective is to contribute to the expansion and development of this field of study, as well as to participate in the consolidation of an emergent academic community interested in studying population policies from a critique of power relations.

From a political point of view, in turn, the proposal seeks to offer some analytical guidelines to civil organizations that work in favor of the protection and defense of reproductive rights and on the generation of processes that can empower individual citizens and groups.

NOTES

1. Jürgen Habermas uses the "idealization" of conditions and forms of communication both as an argumentative and a methodological recourse. On the one hand, he reconstructs

processes that already take place in everyday communication and in situations of argumentation. On the other, he uses these insights to argue for normative standards of ethical and democratic communicative interactions. Thus, his "ideal speech situation" as a genealogical reconstruction and a normative procedure is fundamental for his theory of communicative action, his discourse ethics, as well as for his interventions in the contemporary debate about the limits and virtues of deliberative democracy (Habermas 1984, 1987, 1990, 1993).

2. The human rights literature that informs my perspective and analysis is included in the references. Special mention, however, should be given to Bobbio (1990), Dews (1999), Donnelly (1989), Freeman (1994), Macfarlane (1985), Palumbo (1982), Robertson (1999), Savic (1999), Shute and Hurley (1993), Sjoberg (1996), Sjoberg and Vaughan (1993), Taylor (1996, 1999), and Turner (1993).

3. In addition to my piece (Cervantes-Carson, 1997) published in Vol. 2 of this series, which critically organizes the feminist theory that informs my work, I would like to mention in particular Benhabib (1992, 1996), Bourdieu (2001), Cornell (1998), Correa (1994), Fraser (1989), McAfee (2000), Nicholson (1995), Oliver (1993), and Petchesky (1995, 1998).

4. By this I mean the process by which Habermas reconstructs the ideal normative of speech situations, and uses this framework to evaluate the socially restricted conditions under which communication is realized. What I am doing here is extending this methodology to the terrain of reproductive decisions (Habermas 1984, 1987, 1990, 1993).

5. See Notes 1 and 4.

ACKNOWLEDGMENTS

I want to wholeheartedly thank my editors Vasilikie Demos and Marcia Texler Segal for their support, understanding, and empathy, in this what has turned out to be a very difficult year for me. In the middle of my battles against bureaucracies and the bureaucratic mind, their unmitigated support was an island of hope (where I was able to survive) in a bleak horizon. I am indebted to both of them.

REFERENCES

Andersen, M. L., & Collins, P. H. (Eds) (1992). *Race, class, and gender: An anthology*. Belmont, CA: Wadsworth Publishing Co.

Azzolini, A. (1993). Legalidad y legitimidad en torno al derecho de la mujer a la reproducción. In: *Foro: Políticas Públicas, Mujeres y Maternidad: Un Debate Urgente*. México, DF: Grupo Educacion Popular con Mujeres, A. C.

Benhabib, S. (1992). *Situating the self: Gender, community, and postmodernism in contemporary ethics*. New York, NY: Routledge.

Benhabib, S. (Ed.) (1996). *Democracy and difference: Contesting the boundaries of the political*. Princeton, NJ: Princeton University Press.

Bobbio, N. (1990). *El tiempo de los derechos*. Madrid, España: Editorial Sistema.

Boland, R. (1997). *Promoting reproductive rights: A global mandate*. New York: Center for Reproductive Law and Policy.

Boland, R., Rao, S., & Zeidenstein, G. (1994). Honoring human rights in population policies: From declaration to action. In: G. Sen, A. Germain & L. Chen (Eds), *Population Policies*

Reconsidered. Health, Empowerment, and Rights (pp. 89–106). Cambridge, MA: Harvard University Press.
Bourdieu, P. (1977). *Outline of a theory of practice*. Cambridge: University Press.
Bourdieu, P. (1990). *The logic of practice*. Stanford, CA: Stanford University Press.
Bourdieu, P. (2001). *Masculine domination*. Stanford, CA: Stanford University Press.
The Center for Reproductive Law and Policy (2000). *Reproductive rights 2000: Moving forward*. New York: CRLP.
Cervantes-Carson, A. (1997). Disentangling consensus: The social dimension of women's gender identity. In: V. Demos & M. Texler Segal (Eds), *Advances in Gender Research* (Vol. 2, pp. 9–36). London, England: JAI Press.
Cook, R. J. (1992). International protection of women's reproductive rights. *Journal of International Law and Politics*, *24*(2), 645–728.
Cook, R. J. (1993). Women's international human rights law: The way forward. *Human Rights Quarterly*, *15*, 230–261.
Cook, R. (Ed.) (1994). *Human rights of women: National and international perspectives*. Philadelphia: University of Pennsylvania Press.
Cornell, D. (1998). *At the heart of freedom: Feminism, sex, and equality*. Princeton, NJ: Princeton University Press.
Correa, S. (1994). *Population and reproductive rights: Feminists perspectives from the South*. London and New Jersey: Zed Books Ltd.
Correa, S., & Petchesky, R. (1994). Reproductive and sexual rights: A feminist perspective. In: G. Sen, A. Germain & L. Chen (Eds), *Population Policies Reconsidered. Health, Empowerment, and Rights* (pp. 107–123). Cambridge, MA: Harvard University Press.
De Barbieri, T. (1985). Las mujeres, menos madres. Control de la natalidad, control de la mujer? *Nueva Sociedad*. (enero-febrero).
De Barbieri, T. (1990). Derechos humanos y políticas de población: La decisión sobre el cuerpo propio. In: *Cuarta Reunión Nacional sobre la Investigación Demográfica en México* (Abril). México, DF: El Colegio de México.
Dews, P. (1999). Law, solidarity and the tasks of philosophy. In: O. Savic (Ed.), *The Politics of Human Rights* (pp. 84–100). London, England: Verso.
Dixon-Mueller, R. (1993). *Population policy and women's rights. Transforming reproductive choice*. Westport, CT and London, England: Praeger.
Dixon-Mueller, R., & Germain, A. (1994). Population policy and feminist political action in three developing countries. In: J. L. Finkle & A. C. McIntosh (Eds), *The New Politics of Population: Conflict and Consensus in Family Planning* (pp. 197–219). New York, NY: Population Council. (Population and Development Review: A Supplement to Vol. 20.)
Donnelly, J. (1989). *Universal human rights in theory and practice*. Ithaca, NY and London, England: Cornell University Press.
Duden, B. (1992) Population. In: W. Sachs (Ed.), *The Development Dictionary: A Guide to Knowledge as Power* (pp. 146–157). London and New Jersey: Zed Books Ltd.
Ferry, L., & Renaut, A. (1994). How to think about rights. In: M. Lilla (Ed.), *New French Thought: Political Philosophy* (pp. 148–154). Princeton, NJ: Princeton University Press.
Fincancioglu, N. (1990). Contraception, family planning and human rights. In: *Population and Human Rights: Proceedings of the Expert Group Meeting on Population and Human Rights (Geneva, 3–6 April, 1989)* (pp. 87–103). New York, NY: United Nations.
Finkle, J. L., & McIntosh, A. C. (1994). Introduction: The new politics of population. In: J. L. Finkle & A. C. McIntosh (Eds), *The New Politics of Population: Conflict and Consensus in Family Planning* (pp. 3–34). New York, NY: Population Council. (Population and Development Review: A Supplement to Vol. 20.)

Foucault, M. (1990). *The history of sexuality: An introduction* (Vol. 1). New York: Vintage Books.

Fraser, N. (1989). *Unruly practices. Power, discourse and gender in contemporary social theory*. Minneapolis, MN: University of Minnesota Press.

Freedman, L. P., & Isaacs, S. L. (1993). Human rights and reproductive choice. *Studies in Family Planning, 24*(1), 18–30.

Freeman, M. (1994). The philosophical foundations of human rights. *Human Rights Quarterly, 16*(3), 491–514.

Giddens, A. (1984). *The constitution of society: Outline of the theory of structuration*. Cambridge: Polity Press.

Ginsburg, F. D., & Rapp, R. (Eds) (1995). *Conceiving the new world order: The global politics of reproduction*. Berkeley, CA: University of California Press.

Habermas, J. (1984). *The theory of communicative action. Vol. 1: Reason and the rationalization of society*. Boston, MA: Beacon.

Habermas, J. (1987). *The theory of communicative action. Vol. 2: Lifeworld and system: A critique of functionalist reason*. Boston, MA: Beacon.

Habermas, J. (1990). *Moral consciousness and communicative action*. Cambridge, MA: MIT Press.

Habermas, J. (1993). *Justification and application. Remarks on discourse ethics*. Cambridge, MA: MIT Press.

Habermas, J. (1996). *Between facts and norms: Contributions to a discourse theory of law and democracy*. Boston, MA: MIT Press.

Hartmann, B. (1987). *Reproductive rights and wrongs: The global politics of population control and contraceptive choice*. New York, NY: Harper & Row.

Heller, A. (1987). *Beyond justice*. Oxford, UK and New York, NY: Blackwell.

Hirschmann, N. J. (1992). *Rethinking obligation. A feminist method for political theory*. Ithaca, NY: Cornell University Press.

Luhmann, N., & De Georgi, R. (1993). *Teoría de la sociedad*. Guadalajara, México: Universidad de Guadalajara.

Lummis, C. D. (1992). Equality. In: W. Sachs (Ed.), *The Development Dictionary: A Guide to Knowledge as Power* (pp. 38–52). London and New Jersey: Zed Books Ltd.

Macfarlane, L. J. (1985). *The theory and practice of human rights*. London, England: Maurice Temple Smith.

Macklin, R. (1990). Ethics and human reproduction: International perspectives. *Social Problems, 37*(1), 38–51.

Marger, M. N. (1999). *Social inequality: Patterns and processes*. Mountain View, CA: Mayfield Publishing Co.

McAfee, N. (2000). *Habermas, Kristeva, and Citizenship*. Ithaca, NY and London, England: Cornell University Press.

Nicholson, L. J. (1995). Interpreting gender. In: L. J. Nicholson & S. Seidman (Eds), *Social Postmodernism. Beyond Identity Politics* (pp. 39–67). Cambridge, Great Britain: Cambridge University Press.

Oliver, K. (1993). *Reading Kristeva. Unraveling the double-bind*. Bloomington and Indianapolis, IN: Indiana University Press.

Ore, T. E. (2000). *The social construction of difference and inequality: Race, class, gender, and sexuality*. Mountain View, CA: Mayfield Publishing Co.

Palumbo, M. (1982). *Human rights: Meaning and history*. Malabar, FL: Robert E. Krieger Publishing Co.

Petchesky, R. P. (1995). The body as property: A feminist re-vision. In: F. D. Ginsburg & R. Rapp (Eds), *Conceiving the New World Order: The Global Politics of Reproduction* (pp. 387–406). Berkeley, CA: University of California Press.

Petchesky, R. P. (1998). Introduction. In: R. P. Petchesky & K. Judd (Eds), *Negotiating Reproductive Rights: Women's Perspectives Across Countries and Cultures* (pp. 1–30). International Reproductive Rights Research Action Group, London and New York: Zed Books Ltd.

Robertson, G. (1999). *Crimes against humanity: The struggle for global justice*. New York, NY: New Press.

Savic, O. (Ed.) (1999). *The politics of human rights*. London, England: Verso.

Seligman, A. B. (1992). *The idea of civil society*. New York, NY and Toronto, Canada: Free Press.

Sen, G., Germain, A., & Chen, L. (Eds) (1994). *Population policies reconsidered. Health, empowerment, and rights*. Cambridge, MA: Harvard University Press.

Shapiro, T. M. (1985). *Population control politics. Women, sterilization, and reproductive choice*. Philadelphia: Temple University Press.

Shute, S., & Hurley, S. (Eds) (1993). *On human rights*. New York, NY: Basic Books (The Oxford Amnesty Lectures, 1993).

Sjoberg, G. (1996). The human rights challenge to communitarianism: Formal organizations and race and ethnicity. In: D. Sciulli, N. Y. Armonk & M. E. Sharpe (Eds), *Macro Socio-Economics: From Theory to Activism* (pp. 273–298).

Sjoberg, G., & Vaughan, T. R. (1993). The ethical foundations of sociology and the necessity for a human rights perspective. In: T. R. Vaughan, G. Sjoberg & L. T. Reynolds (Eds), *A Critique of Contemporary American Sociology* (pp. 114–159). Dix Hills, NY: General Hall.

Taylor, C. (1995). *Philosophical arguments*. Cambridge, MA: Harvard University Press.

Taylor, C. (1996, Summer). A world consensus on human rights? *Dissent, 17*.

Taylor, C. (1999). Conditions of an uninforced consensus on human rights. In: O. Savic (Ed.), *The Politics of Human Rights* (pp. 101–119). London, England: Verso.

Turner, B. S. (1990). Outline of a theory of citizenship. *Sociology, 24*(2), 189–217.

Turner, B. S. (1993). Outline of a theory of human rights. *Sociology, 27*(3), 489–524.

United Nations (1990). *Population and human rights: Proceedings of the expert group meeting on population and human rights (Geneva, 3–6 April, 1989)*. New York, NY: United Nations Publications.

United Nations (1994). *Programme of Action of the International Conference on Population and Development. Report of the International Conference on Population and Development, Cairo*. New York, NY: United Nations Publications.

United Nations (1995). *Beijing Declaration and Platform for Action. Adopted by the Fourth World Conference on Women, Beijing*. New York, NY: United Nations Publications.

United Nations (1997). *The state of world population, 1997. The right to choose: Reproductive rights and reproductive health*. New York, NY: UNFPA, United Nations Publications.

United Nations (2000). *The state of world population, 2000. Lives together worlds apart: Men and women in a time of change*. New York, NY: UNFPA, United Nations Publications.

Warwick, D. P. (1982). *Bitter pills: Population policies and their implementation in eight developing countries*. Cambridge, MA and New York, NY: Cambridge University Press.

Warwick, D. P. (1990). The ethics of population control. In: G. Roberts (Ed.), *Population Policy: Contemporary Issues* (pp. 21–37). New York, NY: Praeger.

Warwick, D. P. (1994). The politics of research on fertility control. In: J. L. Finkle & A. C. McIntosh (Eds), *The New Politics of Population: Conflict and Consensus in Family Planning* (pp. 179–195). New York, NY: Population Council. (Population and Development Review: A Supplement to Vol. 20.)

DELIVERY: GENDER AND THE LANGUAGE OF BIRTH

Terri A. Winnick

> The man had relations with his wife Eve, and she conceived and bore Cain, saying, "I have produced a man with the help of the Lord."
>
> Genesis 4: 1,2.

> Without assistance from doctors or mid-wives, Rosenberger delivered his son Caleb into the world at 9 pounds, 2 ounces . . . "I like doing it at home," Rosenberger said. "To watch and be the one that does it."
>
> Anderson Independent-Mail: December 31, 1986

Since Eve, language granting women ownership of childbirth has slowly eroded. In our American culture, as in other industrialized societies, words such as "bear" or "give birth to" are falling out of usage, and we now speak of birth as "delivery." In this paper, I argue that this new language accomplishes linguistically the biologically impossible: birth becomes an increasingly *masculinized* activity. It positions the childbearing woman in the passive role and assigns agency to the attendant, who, as often as not in the United States, is likely to be male. In the language used in the second snippet shown above, taken from a newspaper article bearing the title, "Son's Birth Marks Third Time Man Has Delivered His Own Child," the woman is more than passive – she is referentially absent from the entire activity. Her input seems not important enough to even be noted by the journalist. The text of the article in its entirety primarily focuses on John Rosenberger, what he does for a living, his philosophy toward home birth, and his skill in bringing life into the world. Is this way of thinking about John Rosenberger, this captivation with his essentially peripheral participation in his wife's birth experience, an

Gender Perspectives on Reproduction and Sexuality
Advances in Gender Research, Volume 8, 51–85

ISSN: 1529-2126/doi:10.1016/S1529-2126(04)08003-8

anomaly? I think not, for a closer examination shows that even Mrs. Rosenberger, who couches all references to herself in terms of "we," also defers to her husband as the active participant in the undertaking (Giddens, 1986).

In this paper, I develop a theoretical model that argues that the medical model of childbirth now has a masculine orientation which is the logical result of the appropriation and transformation of childbirth by men. Further, as birth became male-dominated and male-controlled, it also became a male-*centered* undertaking. As a result, even now as women increasingly join the ranks of obstetricians, they enter what has been for several generations an essentially male preserve, one in which the attendant to the event, be it doctor, husband, or taxi-driver, whether attending in fact or just happening to be there, is assumed to be the active participant – the "deliverer." The forces which allowed men to claim, through the portal of obstetrics, what is perceived as the important, conspicuous, *necessary* role in birth include hegemonic control of the systems of politics and power in our society, and through that mechanism, control of systems of cultural influence, most specifically, language.

THE NEW LANGUAGE OF BIRTH

Language is a fundamental and yet extraordinarily powerful medium. Language is more than the primary feature distinguishing humans from other species. As our principle means of communication, language links us to culture, and in so doing, shapes our perceptions and determines the way in which we think (Clark, Eschholz & Rosa, 1981; Thorne, Kramarae & Henley, 1983). Language is inseparable from social life. Through language, individuals learn cultural patterns and political and social values (Mueller, 1973). Language also reflects the prejudices of society, with assumptions about relative status, power or appropriate behavior often built into the words we use to talk about different groups of people. As Frank and Anshen (1983) note, ageism, racism, and most importantly for this discussion, sexism, are all perpetuated by our language, even among those who consciously reject those prejudices.

If the "dividedness of our minds is etched into our language" (Griffen, 1989, p. 7), it may be because the language that we use causes us to be divided in our minds. For example, a careful examination of the words used in the two excerpts shown above demonstrates how we have over time increasingly become divided in our minds in the way in which we view woman's participation in the childbearing process. Early writings, such as the passage from *Genesis* in which Eve boasts, "I have produced a man with the help of the Lord," is typical of biblical passages using language that depicts the birthing woman as playing an autonomous, active role in the process of birth. Eve "bore" Cain; she was not "delivered of" Cain.

Woman's role in maternity as recorded in scripture and other early literature was inherently active. Women are described as *bearing, giving birth*, and *bringing forth children*, ironically despite strongly patriarchal cultures where childbirth was viewed as a service performed for men.[1] In both the Old and New Testaments, other women, called midwives (a word which literally means "with" women), stood by to offer comfort and support to the laboring woman, but their service was not described as "delivering" children, nor was it common for the process of birth to be intruded upon. It is noteworthy that even the dragon in the *Book of Revelation* did not interfere with childbirth, despite its otherwise pernicious intent. With unseemly patience, "the dragon stood before the woman about to give birth, ready to devour her child when it should be born."[2] Words like "deliver," which had no place in scriptural references to reproduction, have only recently developed meanings in regard to childbirth. These new meanings derive from a context of intrusion. Only late in the second millennium, when men became the primary managers of childbirth and technological advances made possible active intervention in the birth process, did new language develop to describe that activity. This new language has become the common language of birth.

"To give birth," to be sure, can still being used interchangeably with the term "to deliver," for subject-active verbs such as "bear" and "give birth" have not fallen completely out of use. However, terms such as "deliver" and "delivery," which position the childbearing woman in the passive or objective role, have become more familiar. Perhaps the new language is replacing the old because the new language more accurately reflects the activity described. As the childbearing role becomes more passive in act or deed, the passive form of the words gain greater currency until *the passive deed now is understood as an active experience*, for passivity has become the way in which, for many subjects, the activity is now enacted. Agency in this convoluted manner then is essentially passive. If, in time, the incongruous subject-object inversion should right itself, the notion of agency may fall out of the understanding of the process altogether.

The word "deliver" likewise is caught up in the process of redefinition vis-à-vis birth. We still say that a woman delivers the child, but it is also acceptable to say that her attendant at the same time and in the same situation *also* delivers the child. The term "deliver" has become so corrupt that it carries little or no reference to the woman's active role in the birth process. In cursory searches of the word "deliver" in a variety of books and articles on childbirth, I was able to locate only one example in which the woman referentially plays an active role – a derogatory reference to the alleged brutishness of a certain ethnic group about whom the "opinion is not uncommon that a mother should be able to practically deliver herself" (quoted in

Shorter, 1982, p. 143). Is it possible that our culture has grown so comfortable with the image of the woman in a passive role that the notion of a woman "performing her own delivery" now seems absurd? Or *unfeminine*? Ann Oakley (1993, p. 24) observes, "Women's imputed need for medical care and control is demanded by the very premise of obstetrical science – women can only be 'delivered of' their babies: childbirth cannot be allowed to be an autonomous act."

Similarly, in the new language of birth, "delivery" has two distinct meanings. The first refers to the attendant's active role. Delivery in this instance is the act on the part of the attendant of relieving the woman of her child. Thus, we say, "The legal requirement that a doctor [be] present to *'do' a delivery* implies that bad and dangerous things can happen without him and with him (emphasis added)" (Shaw, 1974, p. 81). The other use refers to the process of birth in an object sense: "She was nonetheless satisfied with her forceps delivery because she believed that her baby would have died without this intervention" (Klee, 1986, p. 13).

If other language for birth were to fall away and only *deliver* and *delivery* remain – which may be the way our language is evolving – we would have no other way of describing, or even thinking about, the experience of birth other than as something that exists outside of a woman – an act, done not *by* a woman, but *to* her or *for* her instead.

The word "deliver" masculinizes birth in and of itself by definition and through its connotations. "To deliver" is a verb literally meaning "to free," according to the *Oxford English Dictionary*. The image of one who "delivers" or frees, without too much of a stretch of the imagination, is the image of savior, a term that can continue on a steady trajectory of meaning from a messiah to a superhero who flies in just in time to save the day. All are distinctly male representations in our culture, coincidentally quite compatible with the image that has developed around the role of the obstetrician, the "hero who rescued mothers and infants from almost certain death" (Donegan, 1978, p. 166; see also Shorter, 1982). So comfortable is society with this depiction that it is common to routinely ask following a birth occurring outside of a hospital setting (where a physician's attendance is taken for granted), "Who delivered the baby?" overlooking completely what should be fairly obvious, that the woman herself did.

THE LANGUAGE OF MIDWIFERY

Those not part of or else strongly opposed to the medical model of childbirth have developed yet another way of speaking about birth. Notable among them are midwives, especially those who serve home birth enthusiasts. In their practice, they shun "delivery" in favor of expressions such as "be there for her birth," "attend a birth," or even "catch the baby." In this paper, I will detail how their social history and ongoing constraints have helped shape their philosophy, choice of words, and the way they practice. Since many midwives politically endorse women's right to an active, assertive role in birth (Howell-White, 1999; O'Connor, 1993; Sacks & Donnenfeld, 1984), they intuitively understand that in order for the childbearing woman to be the active participant, the attendant must be yielding. They have a keener awareness of the connotations in the word "deliver," and as a result tend to carefully monitor their language so as to stress the autonomy of the childbearing woman and the merely supportive role of the attendant. The typical midwifery philosophy is deferential: "The midwife is a servant, not a goddess. She's there to serve . . . and to bring her skills and knowledge, but beyond that, it's not her business. The birth belongs to the parents" (Oakley & Houd, 1990, p. 4).

Midwives, whether certified nurse-midwives who tend to practice in hospitals, or direct entry (or "lay" midwives) who often assist women in planned home births, currently serve only a minuscule fraction of the American population (McClain, 1987; Sullivan & Weitz, 1984). Yet prior to the nineteenth century, midwives were the typical birth attendants both in this country and abroad. In other countries as industrialized as the United States, such as Russia and all of Europe, sufficient social, economic and political support for midwives exists, and they continue to manage most routine births, both in and out of hospitals (Rooks, 1997). Only in the U.S. does the hospital-based, physician-controlled medical model prevail, and this has led to a dramatic decline in midwife-managed births in this country. The decline began with the ascendancy of male-dominated obstetrics which began early in the nineteenth century and continued throughout, so that by 1900 midwives were only attending about half the nation's births, and by the early part of the twentieth century, only a small fraction (Dye, 1980; Litoff, 1978). Midwifery's nadir occurred in the 1970s when midwives served fewer than 1% of all childbearing women, and, despite a recent move toward professionalization and increased public exposure, today only assist in fewer than 10% of all births in the U.S. (Rooks, 1997). From a feminist point of view, this is a misfortune since the midwife greatly contributes to woman's autonomy in reproduction. Rothman (1989, p. 70), referring to midwifery as form of feminist "praxis," a Marxist term for activism, asserts:

> Midwifery works with the labor of women to transform, to create, the birth experience to meet the needs of women. It is a social, political activity, dialectically linking biology and society, the physical and social experiences of motherhood . . . it is an ideological and political stance.

Midwives "respect the natural birth-giving abilities of women's bodies" (Rooks, 1997, p. 128), and in so doing, empower women. But more than that, they keep in circulation a unique language used to describe birth, a language which I will argue shapes both practice *and* praxis and reinforces the feminist ideological and political stance.

By deliberately choosing terms that self-consciously position childbearing women in the subject-active role, the midwife may inadvertently be the last protector of the concept that birth is a feminine activity *accomplished* by women. By her deferential use of the term "assists," or "helps," or the more colloquial "catches the baby" in reference to her own role, the midwife using this language grants to the laboring woman *active* participation in the birth process (Oakley & Houd, 1990; Peterson, 1983; Rooks, 1997). An apt illustration is provided by Beth Rushing (1993, p. 58) who interviewed a lay midwife who claimed she tells her clients: "I'm not going to deliver your baby, *you're* the one who delivers. I'll be there to help you, but you are going to do the work."

This deliberate avoidance of the word "deliver" in reference to their own actions reflects the midwives' philosophy which combines the feminist principles of shared empowerment and solidarity with other women (Rooks, 1997; Rothman, 1989). Often an aspiring midwives' interest in and pursuit of this occupation begins with their own feeling of enlightenment after experiencing a midwife-assisted home birth (Rooks, 1997; Rushing, 1993). They grow conscious of the need to deprogram other pregnant women away from passive acquiescence in matters surrounding maternity that have been built up in the last century or so by generations of women who have followed daughter after mother in the male-dominated, medicalized model of childbirth that is so typical of American style birth (Davis-Floyd, 1992; Mitford, 1992). As one of the midwives interviewed remarked: "With home birth, it's not 'Here's my body, take care of it for me.' They have to do it" (Peterson, 1983, p. 275).

The legal system which grants hegemony in matters of maternity to obstetricians, general practitioners, and other licensed members of the medical profession may also play a role in the development of the midwives' more deferential language. Legal injunctions have restricted the practices of licensed midwives solely to non-interventionist techniques, and have caused lay midwives, because they are at risk for being charged with practicing medicine without a license, to work underground in most states (Kitzinger, 2000; Mitford, 1992; Weitz & Sullivan, 1984). While midwives often ask parents to share the risks (Peterson, 1983), emergencies can expose them to public scrutiny and sanctions. For example, stillbirth and neonatal deaths in a hospital setting are often dismissed with the assumption that everything that can be done had been done. Civil malpractice cases may be filed, but rarely are criminal charges brought in these cases (Corea, 1985; Oakley, 1993). But woe to the non-licensed midwife who assists a woman who loses a child. In 1988, Bloomington, Indiana lay midwife Vickie Smith was charged with manslaughter following her involvement in a home birth that resulted in a neonatal death (Whyde,

1988). Even taking emergency life saving measures may be criminal. Millersburg, Ohio midwife Frieda Miller who gave a drug to stop hemorrhaging was charged with practicing medicine without a license, an offense punishable by imprisonment (AP, 2002). Thus, deliberate avoidance of the active term "deliver," in favor of more non-commital expressions such as "be there for" or "help" may be a self-protective device on the part of these women. Indeed, fear of legal culpability may pose a powerful constraint on speech.

The contrast in language reference and use is striking between those who practice autonomously and those who do not. As the previous discussion has pointed out, a midwife's tone is generally deferential, but in the following sections I will outline how the language of obstetrics has become strikingly operative (i.e. "I'll deliver her now" (in Shaw, 1974, p. 136)) as it became dominated and controlled by male attendants. Indeed, in her intensive investigation of a maternity center in the late 1960s, Shaw describes the customary demeanor of the obstetrician, a role then almost exclusively occupied by males. Empowered by legitimacy, social status and privilege, the attitude of the obstetrician toward the birth process during that period of medical hegemony appears just short of pomposity. From her field notes she writes: "The doctor is the star delivering a baby from a woman. Instead of the doctor assisting the woman with the birth, she *may*, if he allows, assist him" (p. 82).

Arrogance can easily arise in an arena in which power is reinforced by structural arrangements which give physicians not only a legal monopoly on all medical care (Friedson, 1970, 1994), but that also allow them to work in an hierarchical institution where they make all decisions because "the doctor *does the delivery* (emphasis added) and therefore has the right to decide *how* it will be done" (Shaw, 1974, p. 85). Indeed, some scholars (Dye, 1980; Leavitt, 1986) point out that whatever measure of autonomy women managed to retain in childbearing before hospitalization became the preferred birthplace was sacrificed with the wholesale transfer of parturition to the hospital. This loss of autonomy is expressed in the language of birth:

> The active role taken by the doctor and the passive role imposed on the woman made it appear that it was men, not women, who delivered babies; that women could not deliver babies without men; that it was terribly irresponsible, even a form of child abuse, to attempt to do so. The propaganda on these points has been so thorough in recent decades that most people believe it and would be afraid to have a baby outside the male-controlled hospital" (Corea, 1985, p. 306).

In short, structural arrangements and language mutually reinforce the acceptance of the attendant as the active and *necessary* participant in the undertaking.

In the historical analysis which follows, I will show how language, ironically, played as much a part in the early rejection of the male in the role of childbirth attendant as it does today in his acceptance. "Man-midwife," the first term to describe males in the occupation, displays the dissonance with the gendered connotations that surround the word midwife which, in reference to a female, still requires no modifier. As the new term "obstetrician" replaced the term "man-midwife" in industrialized societies, it too has, for the most part, picked up gendered connotations, and often carries a modifier (i.e. female or woman obstetrician) to differentiate a woman in the role (Donegan, 1978).

Gender role reversals have occurred in a number of occupational roles. Secretaries, school teachers, bank tellers and tailors were once male-dominated occupations, and as women appropriated them, there was a corresponding decrease in status. Conversely, when males enter a female-dominated field, such as nursing, they usually enhance the status of the occupation. The rise of man-midwifery, and its transformation into the science of modern obstetrics, represents what may be arguably the most important, socially defined gender role reversal ever to occur. The appropriation of midwifery by men reversed more than the gender of the occupation and its status – *it also inverted the balance of power between service providers and clients*. What is especially intriguing is that it occurred in the context of the sole biological difference that exists between males and females – a once inviolate, sacred realm, worshiped as a source of women's strength and power.

How did it come to happen that this unique sphere of femininity was usurped, and whom did this usurpation benefit most? Before answering these questions, we must first digress and examine the social contexts, both historical and contemporary, surrounding childbirth. In the sections that follow, I will show how this extreme role reversal developed and offer two explanations for why it occurred. First, the political and structural circumstances were favorable to, and supportive of, the appropriation of midwifery by men. Of no small import was the identification of medicine with science and rationality, nor could the control of institutions of power and influence be ignored. Second, the appropriation was successful because the activity, when performed by males, incorporated a *method* of action and a context of *meaning* that completely identified and defined the activity in male terms. By this I mean, in general, that male participation in *any* otherwise feminine activity not only changes the way the activity is performed, it also changes cultural views of how that activity *should* be performed. As Key (1975, p. 15) succinctly points out, the idea that "man does, woman is" is built into our language through our cultural beliefs regarding gender role expectations which "correlate with language structures and control the syntax of language as they control the behavior of a people" (Key, 1975, p. 19). Language "aids construction of the male supremacist society," including male dominion in birth, because it shapes our perceptions and behaviors in subtle but extremely pervasive ways

(Thorne, Kramarae & Henley, 1983, p. 8). Thus, shifting structural arrangements surrounding birth led to changes in language describing birth. Structure and language mutually reinforced orientation toward the medical model and acceptance of that orientation in culture.

FROM MIDWIFERY TO OBSTETRICS

The marked differences in orientation between obstetricians and midwives, the philosophies that "midwives care for women, and obstetricians control and master childbirth" (Oakley, 1993, p. 72) developed as a result of how each group came to view and practice their roles. Midwifery, now somewhat of a quaint term to the American ear, is perhaps one of the world's oldest occupations, whereas obstetrics as a profession developed only within the last two centuries. Obstetricians developed a view of birth as a medical *problem*, a potentially high risk event, while midwives clung to the belief that birth was a natural phenomenon best managed through "watchful waiting" (Rooks, 1997). It is difficult to sufficiently grasp the marked discrepancies in orientation, ideology and language use typical of each group and its relation to the gender of the participants without first examining at some length the historical circumstances and opportunity structures in which these similar, yet discrepant, roles developed.

As the biblical references to birth attest, from earliest known history, childbirth once was woman's exclusive sphere. Especially in the period before the male contribution to reproduction was completely understood, males, as outsiders, for the most part were barred from participation in this activity (Arms, 1975; Donegan, 1978; Dye, 1980; Leavitt, 1986; Wertz & Wertz, 1989). Midwives, but also female family members and friends, assisted other women in childbirth (Arms, 1975; Kitzinger, 2000; Wertz & Wertz, 1989). Goddesses representing female fertility were the first known deities, and a certain sacredness and mystery surrounded birth (Kitzinger, 2000). Not surprisingly, womb envy and male concern over paternity emerged during this ancient period, sometimes becoming a major obsession, spawning at different periods of history curious practices, phallocentric theories, and repressive laws designed to control women's sexual behavior.

In some less technologically advanced cultures, anthropologists have identified a widespread male-simulated labor and delivery charade known as *couvade*. Kitzinger (2000, p. 44) reports that typically the expectant father enacts the birth himself, dramatizing the sufferings "with a great deal of noise and fuss." It is he who receives the special attention and consideration, while the mother of his child gives birth alone and unattended. Kitzinger points out some functional aspects of the practice, such as acknowledgment of paternity and the diversion of evil spirits from the mother and child. However, a form of couvade persists even in more technologically advanced societies. Wilson (1977), a Seattle psychiatrist writing in the *American Family Physician*, describes a "couvade syndrome" in which modern expectant fathers undergo sympathetic morning sickness and labor pains. He attributes these symptoms to deep empathy, envy and/or resentment of their partner. Regardless of its source or function, couvade's untoward effect, nonetheless, is to diminish the importance of the woman's role in birth (Corea, 1985).

The earliest quasi-scientific thinking (Aristotle's humunculus theories, for instance, in which it was thought that the child was deposited, in miniature, into the womb where it grew as if a seed in fertile soil) at first dismissed women's part in reproduction outright and later admitted it only grudgingly. Similarly, the Judeo-Christian culture viewed women's bodies as mere vessels for the male's child. Laws enforcing paternity rights are still common across the globe, and even today in U.S. culture, children more often than not carry their father's last name (Frank & Anshen, 1983). Access to birth control and abortion, a recent achievement in the U.S., is still unavailable in some other countries, and everywhere reproductive rights remain challenged by fundamentalist factions. Less striking but nonetheless suggestive is the observation by Rothman (1989) that some infertile couples will forego potentially successful artificial insemination and opt instead for a surrogate mother to propagate the male partner's seed. But to some observers, the *coup de grace* in the battle to control women by controlling their reproduction at its most basic level, was the appropriation of midwifery and its transformation into obstetrics and gynecology by men. Corea (1985, p. 303) suggests, "In the obstetrician, this male desire to take control of childbearing is expressed."

The emergence of scientific thought provided the catalyst for the positioning and acceptance of males in this role. Science was an overarching endeavor dominated and controlled by men. At first, women were excluded from scientific study and other intellectual pursuits because it was assumed that only males had the capability to engage in rational thought (Todd, 1989). As early as the twelfth century, European universities began offering courses in the science of medicine for aspiring physicians, training primarily upper class male students in philosophy, theology and Latin, the language of medicine. Acquiring a medical education at that time was a far more cerebral than empirical achievement, the experience being devoid of patients, experiments, and dissection. Nor was common healing, including midwifery, part of the curriculum (Ehrenreich & English, 1979; Rooks, 1997). Common healing and midwifery, then as in the past, were usually left to women who employed folk remedies such as herbal and other household concoctions, hence the term "old wives' tales." Following these diverse streams, by the thirteenth century, European medicine consisted of university-educated physicians in the early stages of professional organization whose purpose was to serve the upper class, and uneducated, unorganized peasant women serving the health needs of the lower classes (Ehrenreich & English, 1973b).

During the fifteenth and sixteenth centuries, the Catholic church took on the supervision of midwives. Their interest in spiritual health at that time was far greater than their interest in physical health. Emphasis was placed on ensuring that midwives knew how to baptize frail infants and to hear the final confession of women dying in childbirth. Midwives were also expected to report to the authorities contraceptive use, abortion and any illegitimate births (Rooks, 1997; Shorter, 1982). Midwives failing to comply with these codes were often suspected of engaging in witchcraft. Between the fifteenth and seventeenth centuries, witch-hunting took on a feverish pace. Associated with the social upheaval accompanying the break-up of feudal society during that period, persons accused of being witches were executed by the thousands. The majority of those executed were women, and at least half of them were thought to be healers and midwives. Their crimes included offering herbs and potions to relieve pain in labor as well as helping women gain some control of their reproductive processes through mysterious, if primitive, methods of birth control and abortion (Ehrenreich & English, 1973a, 1979; Rooks, 1997). In a social world which judged male virility by means of their partner's fecundity, these acts were viewed as demeaning, even castrating, to men (Todd, 1989).

Fear of being accused of witchcraft drove many women healers and midwives underground. Combined with reduced educational opportunities and lack of organization, professional development among women healers and midwives was severely curtailed (Oakley & Houd, 1990; Rooks, 1997). As the early modern period drew to a close, it was clear that no longer would birth and healing be confined to woman's sphere. By the late eighteenth century, the practice of medicine had become a thriving male specialty closely linked with the pursuit of scientific progress. Physicians were especially eager to manage lying-in cases, primarily because they viewed this service as a springboard to family practice. Having gained control of science, men could now become "saviors of women and their health" (Donegan, 1978, p. 39).

THE LANGUAGE OF INTERVENTION

The *Oxford English Dictionary* marks the year 1325 as the first recorded usage of the term "deliver" in reference to childbearing with the words, "be delvuer of hir chylde." This date is somewhat contiguous with the nascent development of the guild of "barber-surgeons." Barber-surgeons, while possessing only rudimentary anatomical training and tools, were usually called as the last resort in emergency lying-in cases, "where [it was understood] . . . one or both must necessarily die" (Donegan, 1978, p. 42). These practitioners used grim tools such as hooks and desperate measures such as embryotomies (or infant dismemberment) to extract an impacted child in order to save the mother's life. The term "deliver" offers an apt, if crude, description in these cases. If the woman survived, she would indeed be "delivered," or freed, of her child. In an age where aseptic techniques and anesthetic were unheard of, Caesarian sections were usually only performed in cases in which the mother was already dead in order to try and save the child. More often, the child was sacrificed to save the mother, but the methods used were unsanitary, if not barbaric, and often both were lost (Shorter, 1982). The barber-surgeon, who, with later specialization in maternity cases came to be called the "man-midwife," "acquired and continued to carry with him the aura of death," a decided impediment to the growth of the profession (Donegan, 1978, p. 49). Not surprisingly, several hundred more years were to pass before the man-midwife was to able to gain much acceptance at all.[3]

Unlike the barber-surgeons' grisly tools of annihilation, the forceps, invented in the late sixteenth century by Peter Chamberlin the Elder, and kept as a "family secret" for another one-hundred years, was the earliest successful interventionist device, the "gentler method of bringing along the head" (Donnison, 1977, p. 21). It is noteworthy that during this period normal births remained the sole concern of the childbearing woman and the midwife; only when extraordinary measures of intervention were needed were males summoned (Ehrenreich & English, 1979; Leavitt, 1986; Wertz & Wertz, 1989). The man-midwives of the Chamberlin family were highly skilled attendants who during this time acquired a reputation for whom the image of savior, or "deliverer," would not be hyperbole. For the select group of women served by these individuals, the arrival of the man-midwife did not necessarily mean certain death, and "delivery" could be associated with a live birth. Once their secret became known, the forceps was eagerly adopted as a routine obstetrical tool by the Chamberlins' male contemporaries and successors, many of whom, unfortunately, exhibited far less sophistication in their application, as we will discuss later. The use of technology, notably operative interventions, the first of which was the forceps, became the first of two features that sharply divided physicians and midwives in terms of philosophy, practice orientation and language used to describe their work. Forceps' use was characteristically absent among midwives for a number of reasons: they could not afford them, they lacked the strength to use them, and/or they disapproved of their use (Donnison, 1977; Litoff, 1978; Shorter, 1982). Hence while physicians employed active measures to "deliver" children, midwives merely "caught" them as they entered the world. The other chasm between the two groups was that midwives faced the typical constraints that women have traditionally faced throughout history in terms of freedom and opportunities for advancement. Male physicians did not and hence encountered few impediments to their professionalization (Donegan, 1978; Leavitt, 1986; Rooks, 1997; Wertz & Wertz, 1989), which aligned them squarely with the emergent structural supports and cultural acceptance that the medical profession would soon come to enjoy.

PROFESSIONALIZATION

Prior to the early part of the twentieth century, medicine was an entrepreneurial field. Anyone who wanted to practice medicine could take up the healing craft. In addition to allopathic (or "regular") medicine, a variety of treatment approaches which today we recognize as "alternative medicine" (e.g. homeopathy, hydrotherapy, herbal therapies) were commonly practiced. Patient preference tended to be largely based upon the class of the practitioner. Upper class patients preferred university-trained regular physicians, mostly because of a desire to be treated by a practitioner of the same social standing as themselves, while lower-class patients sought whatever type of treatment they could afford (Rooks, 1997; Shorter, 1982). Regular medicine, which until the middle of the nineteenth century employed leaches, bleeding and purgatives as standard remedies (even for obstetrical cases), was no more efficacious than any other approach (Caton, 1999; Rooks, 1997).

While universities in the U.S. and abroad provided state-of-the-art medical training, certification, and the title of "physician" following the instruction, the acquisition of a formal university education by healers was the exception rather than the rule (Litoff, 1978). Prior to the early twentieth century, most doctors received either no education at all, or attended proprietary (or profit-making) schools. Between the middle of the eighteenth century and the beginning of the twentieth, more than 800 medical schools were founded, most of them little more than short-lived diploma mills (Rothstein, 1972; Wertz & Wertz, 1989).

Not all medical schools required training in obstetrics, and those that did were diminished considerably in practical value by the prudery of the Victorian era. Concessions to standards of modesty and propriety included the use of leather mannequins and artistic renderings of anatomical parts to teach obstetrical techniques (Donegan, 1978). Even prestigious Harvard Medical School in 1815 taught its first course on obstetrics using dolls as instructional aids! Most physicians, certified and otherwise, began their practice without ever observing a live birth. Often the first maternity case new physicians would see is the first maternity case to which they were called (Caton, 1999; Leavitt, 1986).

By the early part of the twentieth century, however, medicine had become streamlined, and allopathic or regular physicians dominated medical practice, aided by structural arrangements that favored and supported their method of healing over other approaches. Structural factors contributing to the demise of most competing sects were educational reform, licensing, and control of the medical marketplace. The 1911 Flexnor report, which exposed the grave deficiencies of medical education, led to the closing of all but a few (mostly allopathic) medical schools (Larson, 1977). Medical regulation, in terms of licensing and laws governing medical practice, was enacted following educational reform (Friedson, 1970). With allopathy legally established as the standard medical profession and granted a monopoly on practice, control of the medical marketplace was assured (Rothstein, 1977; Starr, 1982).

The "professionalization project" of the nineteenth and early twentieth centuries thinned the ranks and radically altered the status and prestige of men calling themselves physicians (Larson, 1977). Women, as midwives or aspiring physicians, were not part of this project, but continued to face the same obstacles women have always faced based on gender expectations. Women were frequently denied admittance to certified medical training programs,[4] and early efforts to train midwives consisted only of short courses in which they were taught only to recognize what they could not do as attendants and under what circumstances physicians should be summoned (Donegan, 1978). Only a very small number of women took part in these programs for a number of reasons. Few were literate, even fewer could afford the tuition, and most felt it ludicrous to be trained for this work by men (Rooks, 1997). Most midwives received no formal training but merely learned and sharpened their skills through empirical practice. As a result, midwives' skills ranged from abysmal to "highly proficient" (Shorter, 1982, p. 47), which was also the case for physicians of the period, as I will show directly. However, it was clear that a hierarchical order was beginning to emerge (Donegan, 1978).

The appropriation of midwifery and its transformation into obstetrics, a speciality of allopathic medicine, was pivotal to the emergence of the medical profession as a high status, male-dominated occupation (Donegan, 1978). Moving beyond emergency high risk cases to a more routine attendance at uneventful births, where successful outcomes are commonplace and competent performance is likely, became a particularly attractive proposition to the swelling ranks of physicians (Wertz & Wertz, 1989). While midwives seem to be drawn to the profession for numerous reasons, among them a sense of inherent empathy with childbearing women (Peterson, 1983; Rooks, 1997), fledgling male physicians were often attracted to obstetrics because it had the potential to develop into a lucrative family practice. Therefore, physicians took up the profession despite what was viewed as its most formidable obstacle, the cultural prohibitions against male interest in these intimate matters, a trend that was particularly pronounced during the Victorian era (Litoff, 1978; Wertz & Wertz, 1989). As male encroachment in this sphere became more widespread, a veritable social reform movement arose during the middle of the 19th century, fueled by Victorian prudishness and anxiety that men involved with these intimate matters may be tempted to take sexual advantage of the women that he served. The reform movement, intent on driving men out of the midwifery, claimed that man-midwives were amoral, indecent and depraved, licentious practitioners of an altogether "bawdy profession" (Donegan, 1978, p. 167).

SAFETY

In response to charges of impropriety, physicians employed language that lingers today as the most powerful counter-argument to their cause, language that easily overcome the defenses of the most strident objectors, words made more authoritative by the makers' association with science (Todd, 1989). "Deliver" and "delivery," the language of intervention, speaks directly to issues of safety. Using these words, physicians were able to convince the women and their families that childbirth was *dangerous*, that it would be in their best interests to employ a skilled attendant whose ministrations were inherently safer than the uneducated midwives, and, who could, at the same time, offer a less painful birth (Dye, 1980). Certainly, spokespersons for the profession argued, the woman's "well being and safety were more important than preserving decency in the lying-in chamber" (Litoff, 1978, p. 135). Wertz and Wertz (1989, p. 93) assert:

> The doctor's strategy . . . was to tell women that safe delivery was such a deeply imperiled event that they needed doctors constant advice in order to make it a planned and conscious success. At the same time, the doctors endlessly reiterated that each woman's individual and social fulfillment turned basically on being a mother. By calling women to a necessary but threatened destiny, which doctors were best able to aid, doctors make themselves indispensable comforters of women.

These claims of course were somewhat grandiose considering that early obstetrical treatment was typically only one pair of forceps removed from ordinary midwifery. Yet by shrewdly couching childbirth in terms of risk, over which science will eventually prevail, and placing themselves in the role of expert, or "deliverer," male physicians were finally able to take control of obstetrics, and in short order, the medical profession. The first to support the obstetrical specialist, or *accoucheur* (as he was called by the elite), "who campaigned against the profession of midwifery on the grounds that pregnancy was a disease and demanded the care of a doctor," were upper class women, regarded during the Victorian age as "weak invalids" by nature, who found this argument especially convincing (Ehrenreich & English, 1973b, p. 15; Oakley, 1984; Rooks, 1997). Thus, it became fashionable among the elite to have a physician, as a man of science, present and taking control of birth.

Women to be sure were complicit participants in male empowerment in this sphere. The primary reason was self-interest. Recall that childbirth was women's domain throughout most of history – women in consort with other women had the power to control the location and circumstances of the event and all but exclude men from the experience. Seen in this light, women seeking relief of pain in childbirth (indeed, they clamored for this relief!) exhibited how far reaching was the scope of their autonomy (Leavitt, 1986). The rationality of science with its technological advances promised, and eventually delivered, pain-free childbirth (Caton, 1999) and women were not about to be denied this comfort. Moreover, women realistically feared death in childbirth, for it would have been exceedingly uncommon for a woman at that time to not have at least one person in their social network who had not succumbed, so it was only natural for them to seek ways to reduce that risk (Dye, 1980; Leavitt, 1986).

Thus, even the celebrated "social childbirth" in which the support and assistance of other women in labor was part of a shared cultural experience was happily exchanged for less prolonged and painful labors (Wertz & Wertz, 1989). "Women ceded control over physiological processes of birth to the medical profession in order to gain control over their birth experience" asserts Howell-White (1999, p. 9). Of course this desire would undergo revision yet again as later generations began to seek a "peak experience" in birth, one that is enhanced by being awake and aware (Dick Read, 1954). But for childbearing women prior to the twentieth century, "controlling their birth experience" meant demanding an entirely *different*, less painful experience than the one to which they were accustomed. This demand for change, ironically, attests to the autonomy in decisions surrounding childbirth that women previously enjoyed. The ceding of power was essentially an autonomous act – power was theirs to give.

In a patriarchal world, however, childbirth was the only arena in which women had power to spare. In all other spheres, women have far less power than men. The words we use with their connotations and shades of meaning reflect the social organization that exists: *Man does, woman is* (Key, 1975). Men control the language, the culture, the prevailing point of view. Women respond to, but do not always create, the social contexts in which their lives are played out (Davis-Floyd, 1992). Control of a woman in childbirth, once a means of control has been established, becomes yet another appendage of male dominance in other spheres, a reinforcement of her helplessness (Rothman, 1989; Todd, 1989). Once power is relinquished, it is exceedingly difficult to restore.

THE EMERGENCE OF THE MEDICAL MODEL

To say that childbearing women were better off in the care of a physician during the period of obstetrical professionalization, however, would be grossly inaccurate. Ehrenreich and English (1979, p. 97) argue that physicians of that era were less competent, less patient, and far more likely to interfere with birth in order to save themselves time. Indeed, the male entry into the profession coincided with sharp increases in maternal and infant mortality, and rates continued to climb even in the early decades of the twentieth century as physicians managed an ever increasing proportion of the births. Maternal mortality rates rose more than 14% between 1915 and 1929, and neonatal deaths by an astonishing 41% during the same period. The U.S. rates were higher in the 1920s than in all other industrialized countries (Louden, 1992). An escalation in the number of obstetrical operations (including needless use of forceps), the lack of understanding or failure to practice antiseptic techniques, and hospitalization account for many of these deaths (Dye, 1980; Tew, 1990).

Leavitt (1986, p. 51) reminds us, "Forceps could be an instrument of salvation for birthing women; it could also be the means by which women were reduced to post-partum invalidism," if used too soon so the tissues tear, providing a site for which bacteria can grow and lead to septicemia. Yet obstetrical textbooks at the turn of the century promoted aggressive intervention, instructing physicians to manage every stage of labor and birth with anesthetic and instruments.[5] By 1920, a reasonably well-informed doctor

> believed that "normal" deliveries, those without convulsions, deformed pelves, protracted and difficult labor, and threat of sepsis or tears in the woman's perineum, were so rare as to be virtually non-existent.... They concluded, therefore, that routine intervention should be made in every labor and delivery in order to prevent trouble" (Wertz & Wertz, 1989, p. 141).

The ironic outcome, sadly, was the increased morbidity and mortality associated with "the carelessness, the impatience, the scorn of proper antisepsis, and the numerous instances of clumsy, dangerous and unnecessary interference" by attendants at that time (Louden, 1992, p. 295).

Unfortunately, obstetrical intervention had taken hold before aseptic techniques were fully understood and accepted. DeLee (1916) in his textbook for nurses stressed the importance of cleanliness by recounting the story of the famous mid-nineteenth century Hungarian physician Ignatz Simmelweiss, who is considered the father of aseptic technique. Simmelweiss noticed that the clinic operated by midwives next to the hospital at which he practiced lost fewer than two of 1000 maternity patients while the hospital lost almost ten times that many. Upon investigation, Simmelweiss discovered that physicians in the hospital were likely to move from examining cadavers to maternity patients without washing their hands, or to examine one patient after another without washing their hands between exams. Midwives may not have been any cleaner, but they were less likely to carry contagious disease (Shorter, 1982), and more likely to encounter soap and water, at least in carrying on their routine household tasks.

The highest maternal mortality rates were found in maternity hospitals. Originally established in the late eighteenth century primarily to provide charity to poor, often unwed expectant women, they attest to the desperate circumstances of those women, for outbreaks of puerperal, or childbed, fever were known to regularly close the wards (Oakley, 1984). Maternal mortality rates recorded in 1867 indicated that 28 of each 1000 women succumbed to puerperal fever.[6] With so many poor and usually unhealthy women delivering together under one roof, disease and infection spread rampantly. Popular wisdom dictated that it would be far safer to return to the former practice of giving birth at home. Charity outpatient centers subsequently established for poor women to deliver in their own homes with the aid of midwives, in contrast, lost only 5 of 1000 women (Donnison, 1977).

That issues of safety were a topic circulating in scientific discourse is not surprising at a time when puerperal fever was a major cause of maternal death (Brown, 1923; Nicoli, 1929). The literature of the early twentieth century reveals that even though U.S. public health officials tended to support the training of midwives and improvement of midwifery services, finding it sufficient to reduce any problems (Holmes, 1908; Levy, 1923, 1929), American physicians endorsed the medical model and sought to upgrade medical education instead (Brown, 1923; Lobestine, 1922). European countries favored the former approach and have enjoyed marked improvement in both maternal and infant mortality using the midwifery model for most cases (Litoff, 1978). Indeed, following legislation mandating training and supervision of midwifery, midwives have become professionalized in European countries, where they routinely assist in the majority of births (Oakley & Houd, 1990; Shorter, 1982; Willett, 1981).

Yet the alarming mortality rates did not undermine the reputation of nineteenth and early twentieth century obstetricians, largely because of a successful public health campaign aimed at convincing the American public that these new methods and techniques were a *normal* and *necessary* part of childbirth care. Intervention was not framed as part of the problem, but rather as part of the solution (Shaw, 1974). In a deft political move, the larger scientific community, instead of condemning its own role in perpetuating unsanitary and alarmingly dangerous practices, found a scapegoat on which to blame the appalling mortality statistics – the unlicensed, uneducated, unsophisticated, and most of all, powerless midwife (Ehrenreich & English, 1979). Spicing the stew was "prejudice against the intelligence and capability of women, immigrants, black people, and poor people," groups most likely to be overrepresented within the ranks of midwives (Rooks, 1997, p. 24). Mortality will improve, they claimed, as soon as something is done about "the midwife problem" (Rucker, 1923), namely regulating them out of existence.

By the beginning of the twentieth century, physicians were serving the vast majority of middle- and upper-class childbearing women, leaving midwives to serve the poor. From the beginning, no strong disapproval existed for women working as midwives among the poor, as physicians were hitherto uninterested in serving indigent patients. Merry Weisner (1986) reports that medieval city councils in Europe regularly provided funds for midwives to serve the destitute. And in this country, Florence Nightingale in 1861 organized a school expressly for training midwives to serve needy women (Donnison, 1977).

Prior to 1900, midwives still attended approximately half of all births, the bulk of which were indigent patients that physicians disdained. Although the idea of using poor women as "teaching material" had been attempted in the past in charity hospitals, it had been abandoned due to high mortality (Oakley, 1984). However, by the beginning of the twentieth century, poor women had been rediscovered as the ideal and necessary resource to upgrade medical education. With general acceptance of aseptic techniques already in place, the profession was certain that other problems could be overcome with better obstetrical training. Once again, medical schools began to staff charity hospitals and "outdoor clinics" in order to teach students and experiment with new obstetrical techniques. Indigent women were assisted at no charge on the condition that students were able to participate or observe (Litoff, 1978).

Nancy Dye (1986, p. 554) provides an extensive historical examination of a turn of the century New York midwifery dispensary providing maternity services in exchange for empirical training. Dye pays particular attention to how the doctor-patient relationship became structured within these contexts. She discovered that the physician, who until then had been largely the obsequious servant of the elite, inverted the relationship when serving poor women. In these relationships, he (as most were male) was able to reserve for himself "unilateral authority." Poor women tended to be agreeable to these arrangements, but only when they perceived medical intervention as desirable. Frequently they hedged their bet by engaging at the same time a local midwife whose ministrations were familiar and preferred to the roomful of medical students who often busied themselves taking turns doing vaginal exams. Patients were often ordered by physicians to dismiss the midwife; those who refused were considered insubordinate and denied care. Dye showed that physicians whose professional identity had been thus offended would often leave the case, no matter how grave, whenever the woman refused to concede complete control to his authority. Training in charity hospitals and among the indigent continues to this day as an integral part of medical schooling. With the near elimination of the independent profession of midwifery in this country, women, especially poor women, were left few options for autonomy in birth.

THE DEMISE OF MIDWIFERY IN THE U.S. IN THE TWENTIETH CENTURY

While the public acceptance of the science of obstetrics continued on a sharp linear increase, the practice of midwifery descended on somewhat of an extinction curve during the first three decades of the twentieth century. Better general health prevailed throughout most of the population. The prevalence of rickets had diminished, and women were no longer wearing corsets; both of which had been tacit contributors to complications in childbearing (Donegan, 1978; Leavitt, 1986). Increased attention to hygiene and increasing use of drugs such as ether and chloroform provided the safety and pain relief women had so eagerly sought (Caton, 1999).

Eventually, as most women, even indigent women, were becoming swept up and included in the new definition of birth – the male-dominated, medicalized model of control of the childbearing woman – a cultural revolution in birthing was underway (Davis-Floyd, 1992; Howell-White, 1999; Rothman, 1989). When a professional role such as midwifery, imbued with a feminine gender identity, carrying the connotations associated with this identity, begins a gradual shift and then a complete gender reversal, what female association it carries falls away to be replaced by a male mode of operation. Assistance converts to dominance, and science, technology, and most importantly, *action*, are imposed. Or, as Wertz and Wertz (1989, p. 137) assert, "The medical posture became one of manipulation, intervention and active combat."

Though time and science have not yet been able to change the fact that women physically give birth to babies,[7] the masculine orientation in the medical model of birth is striking. Since males first appropriated this role, there has been a reconstruction of the activity such that the birth attendant not only appears to be the primary actor, but indeed *is*. The connotations in the word "delivery" are all innately interventionist. Birth becomes something *done* to women. Too often the modern attendant does not receive the child, but rather *seizes* it. While the dragon in the biblical *Book of Revelations*, bound as he was by his cultural context and ways of knowing, was content to stand before the woman and wait for her child to be born, the modern obstetrician lacks the dragon's constraints. With the woman in a completely passive position, reduced to "lumps of flesh from whom a baby is pulled," the physician takes the baby from her, literally, with forceps or by performing a caesarian section (Shaw, 1974, p. 74). The biblical notion of women of the active childbearing woman

> is a far cry from prenatal care that focuses primarily on the uterus and fetus, the possibility of pathology, and a sequence of tests and procedures; and on childbirth care that interferes with normal processes to such an extent that 30% of women cannot give birth on their own bur must be assisted by Caesarian section, forceps or vacuum equipment to pull the infant out of its mother (Rooks, 1997, p. 2).

Other gadgets and tools such as ultra-sound scanners, intravenous drips containing drugs which can either speed up and slow down the labor process according to the doctor's convenience, and fetal monitors proliferate, turning the birth into a high-tech medical event (Arms, 1975; Oakley, 1984). This trend toward obstetric intervention continues unabated. A recent report from the Bureau of Vital Statistics notes that while caesarean births have declined slightly (from 22.8 to 20.8% of births) in the last ten years of the twentieth century, the use of fetal monitors and ultrasound have increased, and the rate of labor induction has doubled. Now more than a third of all births are induced or stimulated (Curtin & Park, 1999).

These changes are reflected in the language of birth – granting agency to the doctor as "deliverer" permits and indeed normalizes aggressive intervention. As participants submit to and experience the way birth *is* handled, it becomes firmly entrenched in cultural assumptions about the way birth *should* be handled. The more the new assumptions gain currency, the more they permeate the culture, the more persons begin to lack alternative ways to think about them, the more the legal system begins to support them as necessary and useful, the more resistant they become to change (Todd, 1989). Thus, is the American medicalized model of birth anchored in our culture, our consciousness, and our language (Davis-Floyd, 1992; Mitford, 1992).

TWO DISTINCT IDEOLOGIES

Throughout this paper, I have been tracking the development of two separate ideologies of birth, the medical model and the midwifery model. It is easy to see at this juncture how each went careening off in different directions: The male-dominated medical model gained ascendancy, bolstered as it was by culture and structure and so embedded in our common language that it was difficult to even envision another approach. The midwifery model, its flimsy supports further undercut by medical regulation, its ideas and language archaic, was fated at best to lie dormant, at worst to be remembered as an historical artifact. With the advent of formal education, certification and a new developing technology, modern maternity, or obstetrics, became redefined by the development of a medicalized model of birth as a *delivery*, a doctor-controlled process to which women would at first eagerly, and eventually mindlessly, submit. Midwifery, in contrast, would become mired in serviceable, if dated, techniques which would for the most part rapidly fall out of fashion as scientific progress and its attendant promise of safe and painless birth became more alluring.

The disparity in the early training and methods between midwives and physicians was as marked as the disparity between the statuses that the two professions would each develop. Midwifery has not been the lucrative practice for women to the degree that obstetrics has been for male physicians, a fact that is still the case today with lay midwives forced to work underground and even licensed or certified nurse-midwives serving as low-paid doctor's assistants (Peterson, 1983; Smith, 1992). Their non-scientific demeanor in a growing scientific age and lack of education led midwives to seemingly pale in comparison to the paragons of knowledge and expertise that physicians came to represent, and for which they were so well rewarded (Howell-White, 1999).

For a span of several generations, long enough to erase any substantial imprint on the culture, midwifery, for both the attendants and the childbearing women, would remain the refuge of the remote, the alienated, the marginal, and the poor. Midwives still served rural women on horseback in Kentucky, for example, where childbirth assistance became more often a charitable than a business transaction, or Iowa where they often assisted women as an act of friendship (Peterson, 1983). Yet during this period of subordination, midwives developed an ideology even more woman-centered and non-interventionist, embracing the feminist precepts of empowerment and solidarity (Rooks, 1997; Rothman, 1989). Whether proactively political or merely self-protective, this ideology paradoxically developed within a tradition of practice rich in empirical wisdom but limited, if not totally blocked, by the derth of educational and employment opportunities for women in this field.

This matrix of differences in the development of the two ideologies of birth have each contributed to two different perceptions of childbirth that are reflected in the language as well as the practices of each group. Most midwives did not, and still do not, *deliver* but merely *catch the child*, reserving autonomy for the woman in a way that male practitioners do not. Donegan (1978) notes that early physicians scoffed at the midwives' use of this homespun expression, a phrase which to them merely displayed the midwives' ignorance, as they appropriated the term "deliver" to describe their involvement. However, this language use reflects the perception of birth as a natural woman-centered, *woman-powered* phenomenon that is best left undisturbed, a tradition that modern day advocates of midwifery share (Peterson, 1983; Rooks, 1997).

Man-midwives, on the other hand, represented scientific progress. Their profession was built upon interventionist strategies from which women's participation, both as attendants and as active agents in the birth process, was impeded. Their training was in intervention, and their focus was to approach the abnormal or pathological as the rule rather than the exception (Shaw, 1974). John Smith (1992, p. 137), a twentieth century obstetrician who has come to question his own involvement in this role, argues that male "boredom . . . with uncomplicated pregnancies may pose a hazard to those pregnancies" to the degree they are interfered with in order to speed events along and make them more challenging. Thus, particularly active language came into their vocabulary and into their perception of their role. As males also dominate cultural institutions, their language fell into common usage and their perception of birth became the common perception. Males in every capacity, whether as barber-surgeons, man-midwives, physicians or obstetricians, did, deliberately and *manfully*, act upon the bodies of women, to *deliver*, or save, them from their child – even when there was absolutely no need to do so. This image of savior or deliverer is so imprinted upon the sphere of male action that any male who usurps the doctor's role somehow comes to bask in its reflected glory. This is why we are so inordinately impressed with the John Rosenbergers of the world, the taxi-driver, and even the husband in the delivery room who cuts the umbilical cord. Shaw (1974, p. 100) remarks that it is not by accident that husbands were until quite recently barred from the delivery room. The doctor, she asserts, did not want to share the "starring role" with another male.

INSTITUTIONALIZING THE MEDICAL MODEL

Few would dispute that modern women willingly negotiated the deal. They bartered autonomy for comfort and perceived safety. Although fewer than 5% of American women gave birth in hospitals as late as 1900, by the 1920s more than half did, and by 1970, almost all did, and to this day still do (Curtin & Park, 1999). Early in the twentieth century, they were attracted to the hospital for a number of reasons. For one, it was promoted in the popular press as a cleaner, safer, and more comfortable place for a woman to give birth. But probably more importantly, only in hospitals were they able to receive a type of pain relief viewed as too risky and too difficult to administer at home, the anesthetic scopolamine, commonly known as "twilight sleep" (Wertz & Wertz, 1989). As long as home was the typical birthplace, physicians were loathe to administer this drug, despite shrill accusations that they were "callously indifferent" to their patients' pain (Caton, 1999, p. 141). Indeed, the clamor for this new anesthetic where a woman could "just go to sleep and wake up and find she'd become a mother" turned into a social crusade and became a plank on the platform during the first wave of feminism.

No matter that the "woman was separated from the people she loved; she was in an unfamiliar environment controlled by others; and she was unconscious during part of her labor and delivery. She was also without the fears and anxieties that had haunted generations of her foremothers," Leavitt (1986, p. 181) explains. In the beginning, that was enough. With twilight sleep, the laboring woman entered the hospital and was anaesthetized almost immediately with a combination of drugs which masked, but (and this she did not know) did not remove, her pain. Women under twilight sleep required more supervision as they were likely to scream and thrash about, and they had to be confined in special cribs to keep from hurting themselves. Twilight sleep patients required restraints and obstetrical intervention, establishing a number of management procedures such as delivery tables and stirrups that since have become institutionalized into the hospital routine. These drugs had a powerful amnesiac effect, so that when the women awoke, they remembered not a bit of their suffering (Caton, 1999). This was the "birth experience" women so eagerly sought to attain (Howell-White, 1999, p. 9). In their zeal to obliterate the unpleasant aspects of birth, women paradoxically managed to lose control of their bodies. The twilight sleep movement helped change both the location and the definition of the birthing experience and institutionalized a dominant role for physicians in the process (Leavitt, 1986).

The transfer of birth to the hospital intensified the idea that birth is a perilous event, reinforcing the reliance on highly trained professionals to safeguard one's well-being. The long term battle with germs could be better fought in the hospital, and in that location women could be subjected to a plethora of procedures such as shaving and enemas and sterile drapes intended to make her as sanitized as her environment. Finally, the permanence of the hospital permitted the emergence of technological innovations that could be called into service to supervise and micro-manage the birth process (Martin, 1987; Wertz & Wertz, 1989).

But more than anything else, the hospital undercut birth's social moorings and became a relatively isolated, and ultimately alienating experience. Leavitt (1986, p. 194) reminds us that hospitals could not provide the supportive environment that the community of women did in years past, and in fact "obliterated a millennia of women's own birthing traditions." Even after twilight sleep gave way to the spinal block, or epidural, in the 1940s, it was becoming increasingly clear that there was a profound difference between pain and suffering. Medicine was increasingly able to control pain, but its inability to control suffering caused faith in science to decrease (Caton, 1999).

One can be free of pain yet still experience psychological suffering from alienation. A woman can feel alienation in childbirth if there is an absence of social support in this time of travail, as was certainly the case in the early years of hospitalization when even expectant fathers were separated from their partners and confined to waiting rooms. The importance of social support during labor has been recognized and incorporated back into the medical model. Yet even with support, a woman can still feel alienated, in the Marxist sense, an alienation from the birth experience itself. This alienation cannot be remedied by the medical model because it is an outcome, or product, of the medical model. Marx viewed alienation in the broadest sense – as the deprivation of human needs, the giving up of one's self, or even as "making [an action] external to one's self" (Zeitlin, 1990, p. 89). In this last sense, the childbearing woman suffers alienation because her actions are perceived, or at least spoken of, as if they are external to herself. She is a passive participant in the experience. Her labor is no longer meaningful to her. She can no longer draw true self-actualization from childbirth, for self-actualization now belongs to someone else.

QUESTIONING THE MEDICAL MODEL

A slight stirring of a movement, but noticeable nonetheless, began in the middle of the twentieth century. Physicians and hospital administrators were suddenly confronted with women for whom mortality was no longer a concern and pain only an option who were now desiring to "experience" childbirth. These women were questioning the cold impersonality of the medical model of birth. Wertz and Wertz (1989, p. 173) assert that "hospital birth became a regime against which many women began a critical struggle, questioning the need for such extensive manipulation, questioning the safety of the procedures, and demanding that birth be an experience that permitted them a sense of self-fulfillment."

The first adjustment was "natural childbirth," a movement that arose in the 1950s, with the Lamaze movement following rapidly upon its heels. Ironically conceived by male obstetricians who had no lived understanding of birthing pain, each began with the premise that pain is merely psychological, indeed only the expression of fear, a fear that women are capable of controlling through conditioning. Proponents of natural childbirth claimed that as a woman learns to relax and overcome her fear, she will overcome her pain and a joyous birth experience will result (Dick Read, 1954). With Lamaz (1970), the conditioning is psychoprophylactic; Lamaze advocates contend that through breathing and other exercises, the laboring woman can block pain signals with powerful counter-signals.

Similar in concept, yet different in technique, the Dick Read method of natural childbirth and Lamaze recognized and attempted to jolt women from their growing passivity in the birthing role. And, while each method challenged the woman to educate herself and to control her own labor (Wertz & Wertz, 1986), they also imposed upon the woman a set of standards, arguably masculinized in their regimentation, by which to judge her progress. These methods also ushered in the practice of holding childbirth classes for both expectant parents, a custom which elevated the father's role from interested outsider to that of an integral member of the birthing team (Mitford, 1992). Since both methods require expectant mothers to have a labor coach (usually the father or, more recently, a professional coach called a "doula"), the natural childbirth movement has incorporated a source of social support for the childbearing woman. Empirical studies have shown that support has positive psychological and medical benefits (Caton, 1999). Though they did not wrest control of birth from doctors, and may have even ultimately decreased the woman's confidence in her own ability and increased her dependency on the staff (as the discussion below will show) these movements were a first step in rehumanizing birth (Wertz & Wertz, 1989).

Labor nurse Susan Diamond (1996) adds that the childbirth classes designed to prepare couples for natural childbirth may also introduce a source of conflict for the parents and the medical staff when the couple enters the hospital. While the purpose of the classes is to teach the couple what to expect so that they will be better prepared to deal with and control the experience, it is not in the interest of the staff or the institution "to encourage patients to be actively involved in their own treatment decisions . . . to explain each procedure, to ask her opinion, to keep her informed" (p. 66). Prepared parents, she insists, make the staff's job more difficult, and some are punished for this infraction. For example:

> When a [prepared patient] 'succumbs' to her pain and fear and begs for relief, the staff, quite often, relishes her 'failure' . . .. The antagonistic glee some doctors exhibit is appalling. *I knew she would be hollering for an epidural. These people think they know everything from their classes and then the real world hits them!* (emphasis in the original) Perfectly reasonable human beings . . . become almost sadistic in their vindictiveness. They want to see the patient's plans fail so they can say "I told you so." They want to swoop into the room with an epidural cart and *play the savior* (emphasis added), self-righteous about their years of experience with laboring mothers (p. 67).

Diamond further argues that no matter how well informed the patients may be, they are still at the mercy of the staff, who may resort to scare tactics about her or the baby's safety to get the mother to acquiesce to the procedures the expectant parents had preferred to avoid.

The difficulty lies in the rigidness of the medical model and its inability to absorb contradictory definitions of birth. "Concerns about the mothers' emotional needs, about a warm, loving, positive birth," she notes, "are always secondary to concerns about the pathological characteristics of the birth process" (Diamond, 1996, p. 67). Yet childbirth classes are not without benefit to the medical personnel, she reports, for they teach the parents what routines to expect, "which saves the staff some explaining" when they begin to use them (p. 68). Indeed, Davis-Floyd (1992, p. 184) suggests that prepared childbirth, rather than posing a threat to the medical model of birth, actually helps sustain it. Rather than "retain[ing] control over *birth*, . . . the method they are taught generally promises only that the laboring woman can retain control over her *behavior* (emphasis in original)." It provides anticipatory socialization, keeps the childbearing woman occupied in labor, and coopts the husband. "Mother, coached by father, behaves herself, while Doctor delivers the baby" quips Rothman (In: Davis-Floyd, 1992, p. 165).

CHALLENGING THE MEDICAL MODEL

While the natural or prepared childbirth movement altered neither the location of birth, the physician as attendant, nor the power differential of the participants, the home birth movement, which arose in the decade of the 1970s, presented a clear challenge to the developments in childbearing that had become normative by the second half of the twentieth century. Home birth proponents not only eschew the hospital as a location for birth, they also replace the physician with the midwife as attendant and "emphasize a redefinition of the client-patient relationship . . . retaining [for the childbearing woman] personal authority in decision making" (O'Connor, 1993, p. 149). In short, home birth enthusiasts completely reject the medical model. They view birth as natural and normal, not potentially pathological. Even in terms of risks, proponents of home birth tend to view the *hospital* as the most dangerous environment in which to give birth.

Though interest in home birth rose concomitant with the second women's movement, some, but not all, proponents of home birth are feminist. Bonnie O'Connor (1993) interviewed twelve couples who had babies at home and found that none considered themselves feminist. More frequently they were members of staunchly conservative religious groups, such as the Amish (also Williams, 1999). They had in common dissatisfaction with modern maternity and the way it is practiced, faulting in particular the invasive procedures and the physician's lack of empathy or even interest. Most intriguingly, O'Connor found that the illegal status of the midwives *enhanced* the perception of the quality of care. She notes:

> Several women reasoned that the midwives' legal status contributed positively to the safety of employing them as birth attendants. Awareness of their own liability, they felt, prompted the midwives to be very conservative in taking risks with a client's health or well being . . . In the same vein, privileged legal status was cited as a factor in making physicians cavalier toward their patients and in shielding their errors from scrutiny (p. 163).

This extreme philosophical inversion is espoused by the most minuscule proportion of the childbearing population. As O'Connor (1993) points out, estimates of completed home births were remarkably stable at around one percent of all births throughout the period between 1970 and 1990, a percentage that remains unchanged today (Curtin & Park, 1999). This small proportion could have been easily dismissed by the medical establishment, yet curiously was not. The home birth movement caused hospitals to begin wallpapering their delivery rooms and calling them alternative birth centers (Klee, 1986; Nelson, 1983). Home birth also brewed a storm of controversy in medical journals (see Acheson, Harris & Zyzanski, 1990; Pearse, 1979), possibly because this small, but vocal minority with its sharp critique of the medical model had something to say which *resonated* at some deep level with women. It made women cognizant that alternatives to the medical model exist, and it made at least some of them start questioning, at least in a small way, their assumptions.

Davis-Floyd (1992) studied 100 childbearing women, most of whom desired an ordinary hospital birth. Interestingly, Davis-Floyd noticed a pattern that developed among her subjects, a shift in thinking that occurred between their first and subsequent births. Around a third of the women reported being dissatisfied with their birthing experience. They resented the medical intervention, harbored feelings of anger surrounding the birth, and some developed severe post-partum depression. She noticed a strong shift in their values and beliefs that spilled over into other areas of their lives as they prepared for subsequent births. While most planned to use the hospital again, but next time as more assertive consumers, 8% planned to have their next child at home. She reports:

> I noticed that as they switched from hospital to home birth, they not only fired their obstetricians and searched for midwives, but also developed decided affinities for naturopaths, massage therapists, recycling, herbs and whole-wheat bread. It seemed that something farther-reaching than a simple change in birthplace was going on with these women. It seemed as if they were actually using their births as a means to change their personal belief systems (p. 293).

Similarly, Howell-White (1999) studied 200 childbearing women who were self-selected into one of three different medical treatment conditions: the standard hospital birth with an obstetrician, a certified nurse midwife (CNM) working in a hospital, or a CNM working in a out-of-hospital birthing center. All three treatment conditions were covered by a managed care plan, thus cost was no incentive in any choice. She found that when given a choice, almost half of the women chose

CNM's for their care. Those choosing obstetricians scored highest on concern about risk and potential complications, and those choosing CNM's scored highest on measures of egalitarian ideals. Intriguingly, Howell-White identified the same shift in belief systems following the birth as among Davis-Floyd's (1992) subjects. When reinterviewed following the birth, she found the proportion of patients willing to select a CNM for subsequent births greater than the proportion willing to select an obstetrician again (86 vs. 65%). She too reports that her subjects began to redefine their belief systems once having experienced the event. They found their births to be less dangerous than expected, and emotionally less gratifying than desired.

TAKING BACK MATERNITY

Within the last century of so, there has been a radical changing of the guard in terms who attends to the needs of childbearing women. For millennia, birth, as woman's exclusive domain, was woman-centered. But males came to appropriate it because management of birth provided a portal to professional practice in other areas of medicine, and they dominated and controlled it as they dominated and controlled all social institutions. Under male tutelage, midwifery became obstetrics, and its orientation became masculine. In the beginning, males were called upon to act aggressively in the most desperate of circumstances, and action became the predominant mode of operation regardless of circumstances. In time, maternity became male-centered, as males claimed for themselves the conspicuous and necessary role in the activity. This inversion of roles, with males as the active participants and women as the passive recipient of services, became normative and was reflected in the language used to describe birth, as women no longer "gave birth" to children, but were, somewhat gratefully, "delivered" of them instead.

As physical suffering was conquered, however, in its place rose a vague, almost ephemeral spiritual suffering. Missing from the masculinized medical model was emotional support, gratification, and a sense of accomplishment. Women began a quest for a meaningful birth experience and stumbled upon midwifery with its laissez-faire approach, sensitivity and constraint. In it they found the more natural, woman-centered model of childbearing. Fueled partly by the feminist movement with its insistence on women regaining control of their own bodies (Boston Women's Health Collective, 1979), but also in reaction to widespread dissatisfaction with the doctor's brusque and chauvinistic attitude (Smith, 1992; Zadoroznyj, 2001), childbearing women in increasing numbers were beginning to appreciate once again the midwife, whose forte is emotional support (Rushing,

1993), who *listens*, for whom "there is 'all the time in the world' " (Shaw, 1974, p. 136).

Howell-White (1999) suggests that we may be yet again in the process of cultural redefinition – shifting away from total reliance on the medical model for maternity. She predicts that we are moving closer to the European model of birth which combines elements of both the midwifery and medical models of birth. In most European countries, most maternity cases are attended by midwives working in hospitals, where women enjoy the unique social support typical of midwifery, and yet have access to emergency intervention if needed. Midwifery has become a dynamic profession in Europe because concern about infant and maternal mortality early in the twentieth century prompted decisions to provide governmental support to train and supervise midwives (Oakley & Houd, 1990). In this country, in contrast, the same impetus resulted in a sustained campaign to quash the practice. Thus, while midwifery in the U.S. is not as vibrant or broadly accepted as it is in Europe, its professionalization project is certainly underway and the profession is growing rapidly.

With professionalization, midwifery has become more mainstream. While some traditional midwives still practice in remote areas or among immigrant populations today, it is a mischaracterization of the profession as a whole to view modern day midwives as uneducated or merely empirically trained. There are now approximately 50 schools of midwifery, and these educational programs graduate around 400 new midwives each year. Most midwives are college educated, either before entry to midwifery training or while in the process of acquiring midwifery training, and many programs are now requiring master's degrees. Nor do many midwives attend births at home these days. In fact, the percentage of home births attended by midwives has dropped to less than 5% (Rooks, 1997). Instead, midwives routinely train and practice under the supervision of physicians in hospitals (Benoit et al., 2001).

The European model is already being realized in the U.S. by the growth of CNM practice in hospitals settings. While the number of births occurring in hospitals remains unchanged at 99% of all births, the proportion attended by physicians has dropped to 92%. Midwives accounted for 7% of all births in 1997, with almost all of the growth in CNM's (Curtin & Park, 1999). Since the midwifery model dovetails nicely with the tenets of low-cost, low-intervention health care provision favored by managed care providers, third party support, particularly managed care, may have had a role in shaping these trends (Rooks, 1997).

In the late 1990s, there were around 10,000 CNM's practicing within the United States. Although there were three times that number of obstetricians, midwives entered the twenty-first century comprising a full quarter of the practitioners dedicated to serving childbearing women (National Center for Health Statistics,

2001). If one considers the increasing numbers of women physicians who are choosing obstetrics as their specialty, childbirth assistance is rapidly losing its status as a male-dominated field, and may even become a female-dominated field in the future.

These very recent and exciting developments beg numerous questions for social scientists to explore. If women, as practitioners, regain control of obstetrics, what will happen to childbirth? Will it become re-femininized under female control just as it became masculined under male control? Or has its masculine orientation become indelibly imprinted with the medical model institutionalized in our structural arrangements, culture and language? Very likely maternity patients themselves will determine the answer to that question. Recent research conducted by Zadoroznyj (2001) identifies growing reflexive consumerism among maternity patients. She found among her subjects increasing involvement in managing many aspects of the birthing experience, but more than that, they were demanding "full recognition of the birthing woman's social personhood . . . [where] provider and patient are equals" (p. 137). Where early twentieth century women clamored for the medical model and an obliteration of the birthing experience, this research suggests that today's women are calling for an enhanced birthing experience and "open discussion and communication which takes into account women's feelings and wishes, and of course takes time" (Zadoroznyj, 2001, p. 137). Can the medical model "deliver" this? Perhaps, but to do so, its orientation must radically shift. To do so, it must become more like the midwifery model.

The midwifery model of birth is not about whether childbirth occurs in a hospital or in the home. It is not about whether males manage childbearing women or women do. The midwifery model is a philosophy, one with a unique language which describes a shared understanding about the primacy of the birth experience over the technological aspects of birth (O'Connor, 1993). Also understood is that the childbearing woman herself owns and accomplishes the birth. Both of these tenets are radical departures from the medical model, for neither emotionality nor deference are typical masculine approaches to any activity.

In this paper I have suggested that the masculinized language of birth has pushed women farther and farther away from the center of natal activity. As a consequence, too many women have come to view birth as an activity in which they merely participate, instead of an action that they *accomplish*. The solution may be to restore women's primacy in management of the activity, which is suddenly happening as more women begin reclaiming their roles as healers, either as midwives, physicians or obstetricians, and more patients seek their care. But one must be on guard lest the old routines get not replaced but reinforced, which is likely to happen if women healers think, speak and act like men. As George Bernard Shaw once sagely remarked, "It was clear to me that what women had to do was not repudiate their femininity, but to assert its social value; not to ape masculinity, but to demonstrate its insufficiency (cited in Key, 1975, p. 147)."

Hoffert (1995, p. 4), in her analysis of the speech of women activists in the earliest days of the women's rights movement, found that speech was "the single most important weapon" in that movement. More importantly, "the transformation of society that women's rights activists envisioned was expressed in words long before it began to take place in fact." Consider language reforms already in place, such as the use of "Ms," the elimination of the generic "he" in reference to all human beings, the suffix "-person" instead of "-man," the coinage of new expressions such as "server" or "attendant." When first proposed, many of these language changes were met with ridicule, but all were gradually adopted, and each has certainly raised the consciousness of speakers and listeners and may even have helped lessen the degree of sexism in society (Frank & Anshton, 1983).

Taking back maternity entails more than accepting concessions such as wall-papered delivery rooms (DeVries, 1980) and husbands as co-participants. These modifications merely mask the continued control over reproductive processes imposed by the male-dominated culture (Rothman, 1989). Reclaiming birth requires far more than a changing of the guard in terms of attendant, but rather a changing of a culture, including thought and the language used to express it. Twenty-first century women have rediscovered the ages-old wisdom of the humble midwife, and are appreciating her deference to, and respectfulness of, things female. But in order to truly reclaim ownership of birth, women must go one step further. They must self-consciously listen to their own speech and question the assumptions built into the words and expressions that all in this culture so carelessly use. If they do not restore female ownership of birth in language, regardless of the sex of the attendant, they will not be able to restore female ownership of birth in act, leaving the idea of childbearing women as active participants in birth to erode away completely.

NOTES

1. See, for example: "To Enoch was born Irad . . ." *Genesis* 4:18.
2. *Revelation* 12:4.
3. Shorter (1982) claims that some traditional midwives adopted from barber-surgeons hooks and crochets and performed embryotomies when faced with the same desperate circumstances, illustrating how "interventionist lore had filtered ineradicably into village culture" (p. 63). Interestingly, midwives were averse to the use of forceps.
4. Not until 1847 was the first woman, Elizabeth Blackwell, admitted to medical school.
5. Textbook author Joseph DeLee (1916, 1934), who aggressively promoted these policies, would later retract from this position, alarmed by the needless injury of mothers and their infants that resulted (Leavitt, 1988).

6. In contrast, maternal mortality rates were 8.3 per 100,000 in the U.S. in 1999 (National Center for Health Statistics, 2000).

7. Corea (1985) predicts that the goal of science is to eventually remove women from the process completely.

REFERENCES

Acheson, L., Harris, S., & Zyzanski, S. J. (1990). Patient selection and out-of-hospital births in one family practice. *Journal of Family Practice*, *31*(2), 125–136.

Arms, S. (1975). *Immaculate deception: A new look at childbirth in America*. Boston: Houghton-Mifflin.

Associate Press (2002). Community rallies around Millerburg midwife on trial. *News Journal*, March 13, 8A.

Benoit, C., Davis-Floyd, R., Teijlingen, E. R., Sandall, J., & Miller, J. F. (2001). Designing midwives: A comparison of educational models. In: R. G. DeVries, C. Benoit & E. R. Tiejlingen (Eds), *Birth by Design: Pregnancy, Maternity Care and Midwifery in North America and Europe*. New York: Routledge.

Brown, W. H. (1923). The trend in maternal and child hygiene. *American Journal of Public Health and the Nation's Health*, *13*, 636–638.

Caton, D. (1999). *What a blessing she had chloroform*. New Haven: Yale University Press.

Clark, V., Eschholz, P. A., & Rosa, A. (Eds) (1981). *Language* (3rd ed.). New York: St. Martin's Press.

Corea, G. (1985). *The mother machine: Reproductive technologies from artificial insemination to artificial wombs*. NY: Harper and Row.

Curtin, S. C., & Park, M. M. (1999). Trends in the attendant, place, and timing of births, and in the use of obstetric interventions: U.S., 1989–1997. *National Vital Statistics Reports*, *47*(27), http://www.cdc.gov/necdphp/drh/pdf/nvs47_27.pdf.

Davis-Floyd, R. E. (1992). *Birth as an American rite of passage*. Berkeley: University of California Press.

DeLee, J. B. (1916). *Obstetrics for nurses*. Philadelphia: Saunders.

DeLee, J. B. (1934). Obstetrics vs. Midwifery. *The Journal of the American Medical Association*, *103*(5), 307–311.

DeVries, R. G. (1980). The alternative birth center: Option or cooptation? *Women and Health*, *5*(3), 47–60.

Diamond, S. L. (1996). *Hard labor*. NY: Tom Doherty Association.

Dick Read, G. (1954). *Childbirth without fear*. London: Heinemann Publishing.

Donegan, J. B. (1978). *Women and men midwives: Medicine, morality and misogyny in early America*. Westport, CT: Greenwood Press.

Donnison, J. (1977). *Midwives and medical men: A history of interpersonal rivalries and women's rights*. NY: Schocken Books.

Dye, N. S. (1980). History of childbirth in America. *Signs*, *6*, 97–108.

Dye, N. S. (1986). Modern obstetrics and working-class women: The New York midwifery dispensary. *Journal of Social History*, *20*, 549–564.

Ehrenreich, B., & English, D. (1973a). *Witches, midwives, and nurses: A history of women healers*. Old Westbury, NY: Feminist Press.

Ehrenreich, B., & English, D. (1973b). *Complaints and disorders: The sexual politics of sickness*. Old Westbury, NY: Feminist Press.

Ehrenreich, B., & English, D. (1979). *For her own good: 150 years of expert's advice to women.* Garden City, NY: Doubleday Anchor Books.

Frank, F., & Anshen, F. (1983). *Language and the sexes*. Albany, NY: State University of New York Press.

Friedson, E. (1970). *Professional dominance: The social structure of medical care*. New York: Atherton Press.

Friedson, E. (1994). *Professionalism reborn: Theory, prophecy and policy*. Chicago: University of Chicago Press.

Giddens, T. (1986). Home delivery. *Anderson Independent Mail*, December 31.

Griffen, S. (1989). Split culture. In: J. Plant (Ed.), *Healing the Wounds*. Santa Cruz, CA: New Society Publishers.

Hoffert, S. D. (1995). *When hens crow*. Bloomington, IN: Indiana University Press.

Holmes, R. W. (1908). The midwives of Chicago. *Journal of the American Medical Association*, *17*, 1346–1350.

Howell-White, S. (1999). *Birth alternatives: How women select childbirth care*. Westport, CT: Greenwood Press.

Key, M. R. (1975). *Male/female language*. Metucken, NJ: Scarecrow Press.

Klee, L. (1986). Home away from home: The alternative birth center. *Social Science and Medicine*, *23*, 9–16.

Kitzinger, S. (2000). *Rediscovering birth*. New York: Pocket Books.

Lamaz, F. (1970). *Painless childbirth: The psychoprophylactic method*. New York: Henry Regnecy Company.

Larson, M. (1977). *The rise of professionalism*. Berkeley. University of California Press.

Leavitt, J. W. (1986). *Brought to bed: Childbearing in America, 1750–1950*. New York: Oxford University Press.

Leavitt, J. W. (1988). Joseph B. DeLee and the practice of preventative obstretrics. *American Journal of Public Health*, *78*(10), 1353–1361.

Levy, J. (1923). Maternal mortality and mortality in the first month of life in relation to attendant at birth. *American Journal of Public Health and the Nation's Health*, *13*, 88–95.

Levy, J. (1929). Maternal and infant mortality. *American Journal of Public Health and the Nation's Health*, *19*, 225–228.

Litoff, J. (1978). *American midwives: 1860 to the present*. Westport, CT: Greenwood Press.

Lobestine, R. W. (1922). Practical means of reducing maternal mortality. *American Journal of Public Health and the Nation's Health*, *12*, 39–44.

Louden, I. (1992). *Death in childbirth: An international study of maternal care and maternal mortality, 1800–1950*. Oxford: Clarendon Press.

Martin, E. (1987). *The woman in the body: A cultural analysis of reproduction*. Boston: Beacon Press.

McClain, C. S. (1987). Some social network differences between women choosing home and hospital birth. *Human Organization*, *46*(2), 146–152.

Mitford, J. (1992). *The American way of birth*. New York: Dutton.

Mueller, C. (1973). *The politics of communication*. New York: Oxford University Press.

National Center for Health Statistics (2001). *Health, U.S.: 2000*. Hyattsville, MD: Public Health Service.

Nelson, M. K. (1983). Working-class women, middle-class women, and models of childbirth. *Social Problems*, *30*, 284–297.

Nicoli, M. (1929). Maternity as a public health problem. *American Journal of Public Health and the Nation's Health*, *19*, 961–968.

Oakley, A. (1984). *The captured womb: A history of the care of pregnant women*. Oxford: Blackwell.

Oakley, A. (1993). *Essays on women, medicine, and health*. Edinburgh: Edinburgh University Press.

Oakley, A., & Houd, S. (1990). *Helpers in childbirth: Midwifery today*. New York: Hemisphere Publishing Corporation.

O'Connor, B. (1993). The home birth movement in the U.S. *Journal of Medicine and Philosophy*, *18*, 147–174.

Pearse, W. H. (1979). Home birth. *JAMA*, *241*(10), 1039–1040.

Peterson, K. J. (1983). Technology as a last resort in home birth: The work of lay midwives. *Social Problems*, *30*, 272–283.

Rooks, J. P. (1997). *Midwifery and childbirth in America*. Philadelphia: Temple University Press.

Rothman, B. K. (1989). *Recreating motherhood*. NY: Norton.

Rothstein, W. G. (1972). *American physicians in the nineteenth century: From sects to science*. Baltimore: Johns Hopkins University.

Rucker, M. P. (1923). The relation of the midwife to obstetric mortality, with especial reference to New Jersey. *American Journal of Public Health and the Nation's Health*, *13*, 816–822.

Rushing, B. (1993). Ideology and the reemergence of North American midwifery. *Work and Occupations*, *20*, 272–283.

Sacks, S. R., & Donnenfeld, P. B. (1984). Parental choice of alternative birth environments and attitude toward childrearing philosophy. *Journal of Marriage and Family* (May), 469–475.

Shaw, N. S. (1974). *Forced labor: Maternity care in the U.S.* New York: Pergamon Press.

Shorter, E. (1982). *A history of women's bodies*. New York: Basic Books.

Smith, J. M. (1992). *Women and doctors*. New York: Atlantic Monthly.

Starr, P. (1982). *The social transformation of American medicine*. New York: Basic Books.

Sullivan, D. A., & Weitz, R. (1984). Obstacles to a practice of licensed lay midwifery. *Social Science and Medicine*, *19*(1), 1189–1196.

Tew, M. (1990). *Safer childbirth? A critical history of maternity care*. London: Chapman and Hall.

Thorne, B., Kramarae, C., & Henley, N. (1983). *Language, gender and society*. Rowley, MA: Newbury House Publishers.

Todd, A. D. (1989). *Intimate adversaries: Cultural conflict between doctors and women patients*. Philadelphia: University of Pennsylvania Press.

Weisner, M. E. (1986). Early modern midwifery: A case study. In: B. Hanavalt (Ed.), *Women and Work in Preindustrial Europe*. Bloomington, IN: Indiana University Press.

Weitz, R., & Sullivan, D. A. (1984). Obstacles to the practice of licensed lay midwifery. *Social Science and Medicine*, *19*, 1189–1196.

Wertz, R. W., & Wertz, D. C. (1989). *Lying-in: A history of childbirth in America* (expanded edition). New Haven: Yale University Press.

Whyde, K. (1988). Midwifery: Defendant and law both going on trial. *Indianapolis Star*, April 24, F1.

Willett, M. K. (1981). Midwifery in seven European countries. *Journal of Nurse-Midwifery*, *26*(4), 28–33.

Williams, C. (1999). Personal communication.

Wilson, L. G. (1977). The couvade syndrome. *American Family Physician*, *15*(5), 157–160.

Zadoroznyj, M. (2001). Birth and the 'reflexive consumer': Trust, risk and medical dominance in obstetric encounters. *Journal of Sociology*, *37*(2), 117–139.

Zeitlin, I. (1990). *Ideology and the development of social theory* (4th ed.). Englewood Cliffs, NJ: Prentice-Hall.

HOW I BECAME A MIDWIFE: IDENTITY, BIOGRAPHICAL WORK, AND LEGITIMATION IN MIDWIVES' WORK NARRATIVES

Lara Foley

INTRODUCTION

This chapter is concerned with the varied legitimizing discourses used by midwives to frame their identities in relation to their work. This sociological issue is particularly important in the context of an occupation, such as this one, that exists at the border of competing service claims. Drawing on 26 in-depth interviews, I use narrative analysis to examine the stories that midwives tell about their work. Through these women's work narratives, I show the complex intersection of narrative, culture, institution, and biography (Chase, 1995, 2001; DeVault, 1999).

While each midwife brings biographical particulars to the interview, the story she tells unfolds within a specific historical, political, and social environment. The environment provides a communicative space in which the story can be told. This is not to say that an environment denies the artfulness of these respondents' narrative compositions; the environment does not totalize their stories, homogenizing beyond individual recognition. Rather, their varied skills at storytelling combine with the discursive mandates of medicalization, regulation, and professionalization,

Gender Perspectives on Reproduction and Sexuality
Advances in Gender Research, Volume 8, 87–128

ISSN: 1529-2126/doi:10.1016/S1529-2126(04)08004-X

on the one hand and the sentiments of traditional midwifery on the other, to produce narrative complexity.

IDENTITY WORK AND SOCIAL CONSTRUCTION OF SELF

Several key concepts surround the analysis of respondents' narratives. All of these bear on the relationship between personal narratives, identity, and broader social discourses. Scholars of narrative and the life course argue that the life story *is* identity (Faircloth, 1996; Foley & Faircloth, 2000; Gearing, 1999; Giddens, 1991; Gubrium & Holstein, 1995; Holstein & Gubrium, 2000a; McAdams, 1993). Throughout the life course, individuals craft and re-craft a life story, incorporating new events in a way that gives coherence and meaning to their experiences, constructing their identities. As Anthony Giddens (1991) argues:

> Self-identity is not a distinctive trait, or even a collection of traits, possessed by the individual. It is the self as reflexively understood in terms of her or his biography . . . The existential question of self-identity is bound up with the fragile nature of the biography which the individual "supplies" about herself. A person's identity is not to be found in behaviour, nor – important though it is – in the reaction of others, but in the capacity to keep a narrative going. The individual's biography, if she is to maintain regular interaction with others in the day-to-day world, cannot be wholly fictive. It must continually integrate events which occur in the external world, and sort them into the ongoing "story" about the self (pp. 53–54).

Holstein and Gubrium (2000a) assert that individuals engage in *biographical work* to assemble and manage consistency and continuity in the telling of a life story, "assuring that the past reasonably leads up to the present to form a lifeline" (p. 155). While some ethnographers and qualitative researchers are concerned with the "authentic voice" of the subject, an interpretive approach seeks to uncover how the seeming coherence of stories is accomplished in the telling (Gubrium & Holstein, 1998). Denzin (1996) describes this tension claiming, "the point to make is not whether biographical coherence is an illusion or reality. Rather, what must be established is *how* individuals give coherence to their lives when they write or talk self-autobiographies" (p. 62).

In *The Self We Live By*, Holstein and Gubrium (2000b) continue to flesh out the narrative construction of self. Arguing that people use biographical particulars as resources in self-construction, the authors expand and claim that these resources are "used circumstantially, identified and descriptively mobilized to become part of local selves-in-the-making" (p. 169). The self is not merely a reflection of how we think others perceive us; instead we are active creators of multiple social selves. Yet our stories of self must be believable and accountable in a particular local culture. Local understandings condition, but do not determine, how we present ourselves and which identities we choose to put forth.

LEGITIMIZING DISCOURSES AND NARRATIVE PRACTICE

From a postmodern perspective, it is important to note the decline of the legitimating power of grand narratives, such as the foundational position of science, while attending to local narratives of legitimation (Lyotard, 1984). Habermas (1975) speaks of legitimations as ideas produced by the political system to justify its continued existence. In describing systems of domination, Weber (1958, 1919) also explains that these systems make every effort to authenticate and encourage the belief in their legitimacy. Theoretically, we can think of legitimations beyond the political system as ideas produced by any system to support its own existence or belief in its own legitimacy. The midwives in this study engage various discourses to legitimize or justify their existence.

My research employs a social constructionist perspective, informed by both Foucauldian discourse analysis and ethnomethodology. Combining these two approaches allows for the examination of both the *hows* and the *whats* of the construction process. Foucauldian analysis points toward the *whats* of discourse. Ethnomethodology focuses on *how* things are practically articulated through talk and interaction (Garfinkel, 1967). I am especially concerned with what Foucault (1977) terms the "conditions of possibility" for reality construction. In other words, *what* interpretive resources are made available, what vocabulary is used, when a particular vocabulary is used, in what circumstances, to what audiences, and with what implications. But Foucault's perspective tends to overlook the artful side of discursive activity. I am also concerned with *how* the midwives use available interpretive resources as sense-making devices for constructing identities in relation to midwifery (Gubrium & Holstein, 1997; Miller, 1997), as these are articulated in relation to the conditions of possibility presented by the midwifery discourses in question.

The narrative environment in which my respondents interact consists of certain histories, politics, regulations, and social contexts that to some extent dictate what the respondents can tell. The environment is one that tends to homogenize the stories that are told, reproducing specific discourses in the process. These discourses provide the women with resources for the artful construction of self, which come forth in the interviews.

The chapter is organized the following way. First, I give a description of the respondents and discuss my research methods. Next, I highlight the narrative environment, from which the midwives can call upon legitimizing discourses. In the bulk of this chapter, I explore the work narratives of certified nurse-midwives and direct-entry midwives. The important questions here are: What kind of identity work are they engaged in as they talk about their work or about how they came to be involved in midwifery? What legitimizing discourses do they utilize as they tell their stories? Are there differences between LMs, CNMs, and empirically-trained midwives? Finally, I revisit debates in narrative analysis and discourse theory, raising questions of narrative and identity.

THE RESPONDENTS AND METHOD OF PROCEDURE

Midwifery is the ancient practice of women attending other women in childbirth. Although widely practiced throughout the world, a burgeoning medical profession nearly eliminated midwifery in the United States in the late 19th century. The current climate for midwifery nationwide is ambiguous. While nurse-midwives practice legally in every state, direct-entry midwifery is illegal in some states. However, midwives from around the country are organized and pushing for professional recognition, licensure, and legal standing.

In Florida, primarily two different types of midwives may legally engage in practice: direct-entry, licensed midwives (LM) and certified nurse-midwives (CNM). I interviewed 11 CNMs. Two were students, five were practicing, and four were retired. *Certified nurse-midwives* receive a bachelor's degree in nursing and a master's degree in midwifery. CNMs are typically trained in a hospital setting, and the majority practice in hospitals, although some practice in freestanding birth centers. In the State of Florida, CNMs are licensed as Advanced Registered Nurse Practitioners (ARNP). This provides them with the professional capacity to prescribe medicine and provide well-woman care, while working under the supervision of a physician. There are currently more than 500 CNMs registered in the State of Florida (American College of Nurse Midwives, 2000).

Twelve of my respondents are direct-entry midwives. Five are currently practicing, four are students, and three are retired. The term *direct-entry* is taken from the European model of midwifery in which one enters directly into midwifery practice without first becoming a nurse. In Florida, direct-entry midwives are licensed under the Midwifery Practice Act (Chap. 467 F. S.), and are called "licensed midwives" (LM). Since 1992, student midwives are required to participate in three years of intense academic and clinical training based on core competencies established by the Midwives Alliance of North America (MANA) and the American College of Nurse Midwives (ACNM). Licensed midwives may provide care for women with normal, low-risk pregnancies in a variety of settings, particularly in free-standing birth centers, and clients' homes. There are currently more than 80 LMs in the State of Florida (Midwives Alliance of North America, 1999b).

There were three women in this study whom I refer to as *empirically-trained* midwives. These women practiced midwifery in the underground movement of the 1970s and 1980s. Their training is more in line with a direct-entry model. The empirically-trained midwives that I interviewed for this project, for various reasons, chose not to become licensed, but continue to be vital participants in the midwifery community. I will use the term "empirical" when referring only to empirically-trained midwives and the term "direct-entry" when referring to both licensed midwives and empirically-trained midwives.

DATA COLLECTION AND ANALYSIS

I was a participant observer in the midwifery community in Florida from April 1999 until August 2001. During that time, I volunteered at a direct-entry midwifery school and eventually was hired by the school as the academic director and instructor for research methods. During this time, I participated in board meetings, a banquet planning committee, and a curriculum review committee. I also attended births at a birth center, participated in childbirth education classes, doula training, and a doula collective. A doula is someone who provides emotional and physical support for a laboring woman.

The data presented in this article was obtained from in-depth, qualitative interviews. Because of my involvement in the community, I consider my data collection and analysis to be ethnographically informed. I used a semi-structured interview guide. Questions were adapted depending on whether respondents were nurse, licensed, or empirical midwives. The interviews were usually conducted in participants' homes. Some were conducted in offices with various amounts of activity going on around us. The interviews lasted from one to three hours, were tape recorded, and later transcribed.

I began each interview by asking respondents to tell me the story of how they came to be involved with midwifery. In many cases, this question led to a long narrative incorporating their training and their practice of midwifery. This chapter focuses primarily on the midwives' responses to this initial question. The larger project also deals with questions about their training and practice, the relationship they have had with the medical community and whether this relationship has changed over time, and what they believe to be the general public's perception or understanding of midwifery.

In this study, as with most qualitative research, data collection and analysis took place simultaneously. As a framework for the project began to take shape, I carefully selected respondents who would provide data that could elaborate the framework. For example, I quickly realized, based on what I learned from the respondents, that I needed to be sure to interview nurse-midwives who follow more closely to a medical model as well as ones who do not. I also realized that I must interview women who practiced as unlicensed direct-entry midwives as well as those who have practiced or are practicing under the current laws. This approach is similar to that of the "theoretical sampling" of grounded theory (Charmaz, 1983; Glaser, 1978; Glaser & Strauss, 1967).

NARRATIVE ENVIRONMENT

The following section describes the narrative environment from which midwives in Florida may draw interpretive resources to make use of in telling their stories. Because my primary data are narrative accounts, my analysis does not focus on what midwives do, but rather on how they talk about what they do.

Historical Environment

Much has been written about the history of childbirth in the United States (see Arms, 1994; Chase & Rogers, 2001; Leavitt, 1986; Litoff, 1978; Mitford, 1992; Rothman, 1991, 1982; Sullivan & Weitz, 1988; Wertz & Wetz, 1989, 1977). Also, the history and development of both nurse-midwifery and direct-entry midwifery has been carefully and comprehensively documented by Judith Pence Rooks in *Midwifery and Childbirth in America* (1997). In this section, I outline broadly the history of childbirth and midwifery in the United States in order to give the reader a general sense of the historical context that has preceded the environment in which midwives currently practice. Because the midwives I interviewed have knowledge of this history, it can serve as a sense-making resource in their stories. Not only is this history available as a resource, it also makes up a piece of the framework from which midwives' work narratives can unfold.

Midwives have attended women in birth throughout time. Historically, most midwives learned their skills by observing more experienced midwives. In Europe, during medieval times, midwives attended women in birth and men were only called upon when it was necessary to perform surgery to save either the life of the mother or the child. With the invention of new tools, such as forceps, in the 17th century, medical men began to gain a technological advantage over midwives. This initiated the medicalization of childbirth (Rothman, 1991, 1982; Wertz & Wetz, 1989, 1977).

In the late 19th century, physicians began a campaign to eliminate the practice of midwifery, especially in areas where doctors were readily available to provide obstetric services. Physicians were attempting to promote pregnancy and birth as dangerous and complicated events that must be cared for by trained specialists. They accused midwives of undermining the progress of medical obstetrics. Two basic and conflicting solutions to the "midwife problem" were proposed. Private physicians and academic obstetricians wanted to bring midwifery under the control of doctors and to have the elimination of midwifery practice as an ultimate goal. A second solution to the "midwifery problem" was posed by public health leaders, especially in the South, who thought that it would be more beneficial to train and educate midwives since it would be impossible for doctors to provide medical care to all women. Southern midwives were providing services for poor, working class, rural, immigrant, and African American women, not the well paying clientele sought out by physicians (Rooks, 1997; Sullivan & Weitz, 1988). By 1935, midwives were only attending 12.5% of births nationwide. Further, by this time, 80% of all midwives were located in the rural south. The campaign to eliminate midwives had effectively worked (Sullivan & Weitz, 1988).

The first midwifery training program, established through public funding, began at Bellevue Hospital in New York in 1911. Advocates of midwifery training introduced the idea of the "nurse-midwife" as an alternative to the traditional midwife. In 1925, Mary Brekenridge brought nurse-midwives from England to the United States and established the Frontier Nursing Service (FNS) in rural Kentucky. The nurse-midwives traveled by horse-back to provide midwifery and nursing services to the surrounding areas. Through excellent record keeping, FNS was able to document its success. Maternal and infant mortality rates in the rural counties served had been among the highest in the country before their arrival. The services of FNS led to a dramatic drop in mortality rates (Rooks, 1997; Rothman, 1991, 1982; Wertz & Wetz, 1989, 1977). By 1945, five nurse-midwifery schools had been established in the United States. The graduates of these programs worked in rural areas or urban slums, serving poor families. It was not until 1955 that the first mainstream medical institution, the Columbia-Presbyterian-Sloan Hospital in New York City, accepted nurse-midwives (Rooks, 1997).

Hospital Practices and Consumer Movements

In the early part of the 20th century, an increasing number of births were taking place in hospitals. Because of this shift, certain practices, particular to medicine, came to be regarded as routine. Among other practices, these include the lithomy position, episiotomies, use of forceps, and "Twilight Sleep," a mixture of morphine for pain relief and scopolamine which served as an amnesiac (Caton, 1999; DeLee, 1940). Dr. Joseph DeLee, a leading obstetrician at the time, recommended the routine use of these practices, and his teachings became standardized in obstetrical practices well into the 1960s.

In the 1940s and 1950s a small natural childbirth movement began in the United States. Spurred by the teachings and writings of men such as Grantly Dick-Read, Robert Bradley, and Ferdinand Lamaze, childbirth education classes were established and women and their partners were taught new techniques of breathing to reduce pain. By 1960, 97% of births in the U.S. were hospital births (Rooks, 1997). The experiences of women in the hospital were not ideal. Increasing consumer criticism of the medical management of childbirth and the emergence of an alternative birth movement in the 1960s and 1970s coincided with the civil rights movement, the women's movement, various other consumer movements, the antiwar movement, and the health food movement (Daviss, 2001; Mathews & Zadak, 1991; Umansky, 1996). Importantly, it also coincided with the introduction of the birth control pill in 1960. Because women were having fewer children, particularly women in the middle-class, they were searching for a more rich and emotionally satisfying birth experience. As consumers, these middle-class women began to seek out midwives. This led to an important shift for a group who had previously served primarily poor and rural women.

In the early 1970s, some women took their criticism of medical management a step further and refused to birth in a hospital. They decided to birth at home by themselves. With other, like-minded women they began to study and learn about birth. They read medical texts, but also relied on "birth stories" as evidence of their authoritative knowledge surrounding birth. Birth stories are narratives of experience and birth outcomes that are shared with the community (Lay, 2000). This coincided with the publication of several texts, critical of the medical establishment and advocating that women take control of their bodies (i.e. *Our Bodies Our Selves*; *Immaculate Deception*; *The Birth Book*; *Spiritual Midwifery*). On the west coast, Raven Lang started the Santa Cruz Birth Center which provided prenatal and postnatal education for women planning home births. On the east coast, Ina May Gaskin initiated the midwifery practice on The Farm, a collective in Summertown, Tennessee. The lay midwives in each of these locations kept excellent records of their birth outcomes and were able to show that for normal, low-risk pregnancy, home birth was as safe as hospital birth.

During this period, midwives around the country were practicing illegally in an underground network and often feared legal action or the threat of it. The Santa Cruz midwives were the target of a sting operation in the early 1970s. The State

Board of Consumer Affairs sent a pregnant undercover agent to the birth center along with a confederate "husband." The midwives responded to this woman's call when she pretended to be in labor. When they arrived at her house, they were arrested for practicing medicine without a license (Rooks, 1997; Ventre et al., 1995). In the late 1970s several women in Florida were also under legal scrutiny. There were cases pending in Stewart, Tampa, Clearwater and Jacksonville. A woman with a large underground midwifery practice in Jacksonville had been charged with practicing medicine without a license. The women in all of these locations worked collaboratively and eventually, through a series of highly publicized court cases, were successful in changing Florida's midwifery laws.

POLITICAL AND LEGAL ENVIRONMENT

Certified Nurse-Midwives

The first professional organization for nurse-midwives was established in 1929. In the late 1940s, nurse-midwives were part of the National Organization for Public Health Nurses and later, in the 1950s, were part of both the National League of Nursing and the American Nurses' Association. Dissatisfied with their lack of visibility in these organizations, a group of 20 nurse-midwives formed the American College of Nurse Midwifery in 1955, and later merged with the American Association of Nurse Midwives to form The American College of Nurse Midwives (ACNM). The goals of the organization were to establish standards for education, to sponsor research, to develop services, and to participate in the International Confederation of Midwives (Rooks, 1997).

The ACNM has achieved much success as a political body. They have been effective in establishing training programs, in securing insurance and Medicaid reimbursements for nurse-midwives, in gaining hospital privileges for CNMs, and in obtaining prescriptive authority for CNMs in many states. ACNM is currently active in the debates surrounding the expansion of CNMs' scope of practice to include primary care provision and in debating whether or not CNMs should be allowed to perform abortions.

Nurse-midwives practice legally in every state in the United States. However, the laws that govern their practice vary considerably. Educational requirements, the credentialing process, the scope of practice, authority to prescribe medicine, and the extent of required collaboration with physicians are key elements of these various laws. In Florida, nurse-midwives are licensed as Advanced Registered Nurse Practitioners. They are governed by the Department of Health, Board of Nursing, and practice under the Nurse Practice Act (Chap. 464, F. S.). Since

1988, Florida's nurse-midwives have had the authority to write prescriptions. They practice under a joint practice protocol, signed by both the nurse-midwife and a physician. In Florida, state law requires insurance companies to reimburse for nurse-midwifery services, and Medicaid must reimburse nurse-midwives at 80% of the physician rate (ACNM, 2000).

Direct-Entry Midwives

In 1981, the ACNM's national convention included discussion as to whether they should expand membership to include direct-entry midwives. ACNM and the American College of Obstetricians and Gynecologists (ACOG) were looking for ways to communicate with direct-entry midwives, but there was no national organization that represented this group. The president of ACNM at the time, Sister Angela Murdaugh, convened a group of direct-entry midwives from around the country. This meeting led to the formation of the Midwives Alliance of North America (MANA) in 1982.

The Midwives Alliance of North America (1999a) currently is working toward several political goals. They seek access to affordable, community-based midwifery care for all women. Although they acknowledge all midwives, MANA supports the development of examinations and certification processes. Barring certification, they encourage midwives to use informed consent with their clients. Another goal of MANA is to decriminalize midwifery practice in places where it has been criminalized. Finally, MANA continues to seek insurance and Medicaid reimbursement for direct-entry midwives in states that have not already obtained this.

The legal status of direct-entry midwifery varies by state. It is illegal in eight states and Washington, DC. In seven states, it is legal by statute, but licensure is unavailable. Direct-entry midwifery is not clearly legal or illegal in seven states. In 13 states, it is legal but not regulated. And in 15 states, including Florida, it is legal and regulated through either licensure, certification, registration, or documentation (Midwives Alliance of North America, 1999c; Rooks, 1997). Because midwives in many states are pushing for legislation to legitimate their work, and states where direct-entry midwifery is legal and regulated are often threatened with deregulation, the above categories shift and change.

Florida's midwifery law was in flux throughout the 1980s. A law passed in 1982 recognized the right of parents to choose the manner, cost, and setting for their child's birth. A Lay Midwifery Advisory Committee was established within the Department of Health and Rehabilitative Services (DHRS). Under this law, DHRS licensed midwives based on examination. To be eligible, one must be a high school graduate, in good health, and have completed an approved midwifery education program. An approved midwifery education program at the time was required to be associated with a state-accredited educational institution and provide three years of course work and clinical training. In 1984, two schools that met these requirements opened in Florida. However, in that same year, the 1982 law was reviewed and amended to limit licensing of midwives to those already enrolled in school. In 1990, Florida was suffering a crisis in maternity care and infant mortality. More people were using CNMs, but there were not enough CNMs to meet the demand. This led to a reinstatement of the 1982 law with increased standards for education. Under the leadership of Governor Lawton Chiles, the Midwifery Practice Act passed in 1992 (Chap. 467, F. S.; Rooks, 1997).

BROADER CULTURAL DISCOURSES

Feminism

There are several feminist discourses available that midwives can and do use to make sense of their work. Two that the participants in this study often evoked are a feminist evaluation of health care and a feminist critique of the medical model of birth.

In May 1969, a workshop entitled "Women and their Bodies" held at a women's liberation conference in New England sparked a heated discussion about the patronizing treatment many of the participants had received from male doctors. The events of this workshop eventually led to the formation of the Boston Women's Health Book Collective which published *Our Bodies, Ourselves* first in 1970, then later editions, with the most recent published in 1998. The book marked the beginning of a second wave of activism focusing on women's health. A broad-based women's health movement beginning in the 1970s and continuing to the present day intersected with movements for better birth control, better birthing options, and abortion rights. One aspect of this movement involved the formation of autonomous women's health centers and clinics which sought to empower women to know their bodies. Another aspect has focused on bringing a feminist perspective to health education and policy. And a third aspect of a broadly constructed women's health movement has sought to increase the numbers of women represented in health professions (Clarke & Olesen, 1999).

Part of the feminist critique of health care in general has been a criticism of the medicalization of childbirth (Davis-Floyd, 1992; Rothman, 1991, 1982). One of the most striking differences between the medical or technocratic model and a midwifery model of care is how the subject (woman) is constituted. In a medical model, pregnancy is seen as pathological and the woman is seen as a patient in need of care. Consequently it is the doctor who delivers the baby. This is quite different from a midwifery model in which pregnancy is seen as a normal condition and the woman is the doer, the giver of birth. Further, the medical model relies on technology and medical interventions during birth. A midwifery model sees these as useful in high risk cases, but an unnecessary part of normal birth. Armstrong and Feldman (1990) suggest that society's increasing dependence on technology has prevented many women from being able to view birth as a natural process, and from being able to think of themselves as naturally equipped to handle this process. They argue that women willingly accept unnecessary and uncomfortable procedures with the hopes and expectations that technology will deliver a perfect baby.

Education and Professionalization

Midwives are divided over the issue of education. There has been an historical conflict between American College of Nurse Midwives and Midwives Alliance of North America over the most appropriate educational route for midwives (Tritten & Southern, 1998). Davis-Floyd (1998a, b) outlines and evaluates several different types of midwifery training. At one end of the spectrum are formal university programs, and at the other are apprenticeship and self-study. Middle range education programs include distance-learning, university-affiliated programs, college-based direct-entry programs, and private midwifery schools. Most of these types of programs to some degree combine didactic learning and experiential learning (Benoit et al., 2001).

ACNM strongly advocates formal university training and has moved toward requiring a bachelor's degree and even a master's degree, although they have very recently taken the position that one's bachelor's degree does not necessarily have to be in nursing. An evaluation of the first direct-entry program accredited by the ACNM shows clearly that students without a nursing background achieve the same standards of academic excellence and clinical competency as students who are nurses (Fullerton et al., 2000). MANA, on the other hand, insists that a university degree is not necessary for becoming a midwife, and recognizes the value of apprenticeship and self-study as legitimate forms of learning.

The upside to standardized education in midwifery includes recognition, legitimacy, access to government funding, and the possibility of training larger numbers of midwives (Davis-Floyd, 1998b; Myers-Ciecko, 1999; Osborn & Esty, 1998). A downside to mandated standardized education is that it serves as an important means of social control (DeVries, 1996). For many traditional midwives and advocates of an apprenticeship model, there is also concern that standardized education is increasingly moving in the direction of the medical model and that it will lead to the diminishing of the autonomy and independence of midwifery practice.

Alternative Medicine

The midwives, particularly the licensed and empirical midwives, in this study frequently invoked a discourse of alternative medicine, including massage therapy, herbalism, and acupuncture, to give meaning to the work they do as midwives. While a western biomedical model and an eastern holistic model often overlap to some degree in practice, theoretically they are oppositional models. A biomedical model focuses on disease rather than prevention, treats mind and body separately, and relies heavily on technology and invasive practices (Loustaunau & Sobo, 1997; Payer, 1996, 1988; Todd, 1999). A holistic model views the person as a whole being situated in a social environment. Medicine is generally preventative and minimally invasive, a physical and emotional balance is sought, and patients are seen as active participants in their own healing (Goldstein, 1999; LaPointe, 2000).

WORK NARRATIVES

This section explores the work narratives of midwives. First, I look at the narratives of entry into the work of midwifery from both CNMs and direct-entry midwives respectively. Next, I examine the narratives of future expectations. I also include a section in which midwives narratively struggle with the terms (job, calling, career) they most closely identify with in relation to their work. Finally, I conclude with some remarks about narrative analysis.

When analyzing the paths taken by midwives into their profession, the narratives of nurse-midwives differ in a patterned way from the narratives of licensed and empirical midwives. I began each interview with the question, "Can you tell me the story of how you came to be a midwife?" Because certified nurse-midwives must first be nurses, the stories of these women tend to have a very different starting point than the stories of other types of midwives. In other words, CNMs typically (eight out of eleven) begin their stories with nursing school or practice. Other studies suggest that, increasingly, CNMs claim "midwife" as their primary professional identity (Davis-Floyd, 1998a; Scroggin, 1996). Davis-Floyd (1998a) exclaims that " 'I am not a nurse, I am a midwife!' is a statement I have heard countless times in my interviews" (p. 83).

Unlike CNMs, licensed and empirical midwives evoke a variety of starting points, the most common being the birth of their own children. Others begin their stories in the context of childhood, medical backgrounds, including alternative medicine, legal battles, and counterculture. While the narratives have a distinct starting point, the stories midwives tell about the paths leading up to their practice are sometimes short and succinct and sometimes long and winding, interwoven with stories of childhood, families, and life experiences.

In the following narratives we will see midwives engaged in biographical work, that is, constructing who and what they are as midwives in relation to their lives as a whole (Gearing, 1999; Gubrium & Holstein, 1995; Holstein & Gubrium, 2000a; Marvasti, 1998; Ronai & Cross, 1998). Providing information relevant to the topic at hand, respondents select, interpret, reinterpret, and contextualize aspects of their biography to make sense of and give meaning to the work they have done, are doing, and will do in the future. Through the telling of their stories, midwives "shape, support, and strengthen professional identity" (van der Hulst et al., 2001, p. 166).

Entry Narratives of Certified Nurse-Midwives

Scholars of work and occupations have long been interested in how and why people choose to enter certain occupations and professions (Brewis & Linstead, 2000; Chumdler & Ford, 1998; Glen, 1981). It has been suggested that for women, career choices are influenced by the socioeconomic status of the family, mother's occupation, academic achievement, age, attitude toward marriage, and social and religious attitudes (Gagne & Poirier, 1985). Gender differences in occupational choice are also thought to exist, with women, more than men, attributing importance to intrinsic, altruistic and social rewards (Marini et al., 1996; Mottaz, 1986). In this study I am interested in the paths these women took to the occupation of midwifery as revealed in narrative understanding. In the following excerpts, we will hear their narratives of entry. What comes forth is a more complex picture than a mere listing of variable conditions would suggest.

Through the Door of Nursing

When asked to tell how they came to be midwives, eight out of eleven nurse-midwives begin their stories by identifying themselves as nurses. Beyond that point, they draw upon a variety of resources, including education, family, and prior hospital experiences to further describe their paths to the profession. Melanie, a

CNM working in a birth center setting, begins her story at a point where she had "gotten out of nursing." Listen as she narrates her path to becoming a midwife:

> I had gotten out of nursing, I had worked in psych nursing and I had gotten out, and my husband and I were working at a bar and restaurant we'd helped some friends start. And I had two children at the time and the second birth had been, although no bad results for either of us, had been pretty much botched by hospital routine and I had a lot of lingering kinds of feelings about that, that I couldn't really place. And then the book *Immaculate Deception* came out and a friend gave it to me and it really just kind of gave me a focus of why I had felt upset with that birth and what I could do. That I could make it different for other women and that was basically when I knew I wanted to be a midwife (Melanie, CNM).

While she establishes nursing as a framework for her story, she quickly shifts to a negative hospital birth experience and a subsequent book that helped to make sense of that experience. The book helps her make sense of her experience and thus serves to legitimate her experience. Further, the experience and book together legitimate her decision to become a midwife and "make it different for other women." Biographical particulars clearly mediate her story to construct the account as her own.

I then asked Melanie how she went from knowing she wanted to be a midwife to actually becoming one.

Melanie: Well, I went back into nursing, I decided that since I was a nurse I was going to go the certified nurse-midwifery route. I definitely believed in education and I didn't want to just go apprentice with somebody.

Lara: And that was the only other option at the time?

Melanie: That was the only other option at the time, and also I needed to go to a master's program because there was one were I lived and I couldn't really easily move my family or leave them; I had young children. Because I had probably wanted to go to the Frontier School of Nursing, where you didn't need to have a degree, at that time. But I went back to school and started nursing again and went back to school to get my bachelor's degree and did it kind of part-time, weekends, evenings, that kind of thing for a few years, then applied to midwifery school (Melanie, CNM).

Here, Melanie returns to her initial framing of the story by "going back into nursing." She invokes education to legitimate her decision. At the time, nurse-midwifery was the only route that offered a formal education. After deciding to pursue a degree in nurse-midwifery, Melanie then references her family situation – "I couldn't really easily move my family or leave them" – to give further meaning to the particular path she chose. Interestingly, Melanie is one of the few CNMs who cited family concerns in relation to her decision-making process. This is consistent with much literature on work and family that suggests that women take family into consideration when making career decisions (Bielby & Bielby, 1992; Frame & Shehan, 1994; Gerson, 1987; Hardill et al., 1997; Sidel, 1990). What is interesting is that so few others mentioned family in the context of how they came to be a midwife. A few women cited family as reasons for changing direction in their career. For example, it was difficult to be "on-call" while raising children. They also cited family in the context of where they see themselves in the future, possibly cutting back hours in order to stay home and raise a family.

For Andrea, a student nurse-midwife, nursing is also the starting point of her story. She cites collaborative efforts between nurses, medical students, and doctors, but she ultimately rejects a medical model of birth in favor of "the natural, compassionate art of nursing." She chooses midwifery training as consistent with the type of care she wants to provide:

> I decided to go back to school for midwifery after working as a labor and delivery nurse in a teaching hospital for about three years. I was 25 and was ready for a change of pace in nursing. I always knew throughout nursing school that I wanted to work in obstetrics, and while working at this teaching hospital, I realized I knew the same, if not more, than the resident doctors practicing there. Each July, the new first-year residents arrived and basically they really knew very little about labor and delivery, and it was up to the nurse to kind of lead them along as to what to do. I also loved learning from the attending MDs and chief residents about different procedures and techniques. I found that I was at a point in my life, totally independent and single, where I was ready for a change and welcomed the challenge of moving up in my field. I chose midwifery, as opposed to going to medical school, because I did not wish to give up the nursing component of care. The natural, compassionate art of nursing is, in my opinion, essential to assisting women with labor and birth (Andrea, CNM student).

Books, Birth, and Better Care

Samantha stands out among nurse-midwives in this study because, in the context of how she became a midwife, she does not identify at any point as a nurse (although she does in other contexts). For her, her own birth, a book, and feminist ideals influenced her decision, while creating a biographically specific work narrative:

> Well it was, I had a child and I just thought it was the coolest thing that ever happened to me. And it was very, very marvelous. And so, then I started reading more books about childbirth and as I read more about different options, I was real young, the first child I had, I was 19. But I started reading all these books and read about midwifery and, you know, I started reading more about feminist approaches to taking charge of your own healthcare. I think that the book that inspired me was *Immaculate Deception*. So I decided with my next child that I wanted a midwife. There were no midwives. I was in Virginia, in Roanoke, Virginia and this was in 1978. And there were no midwives at all. All I could find was a small group of people who were like gonna do their own babies at home by themselves and I didn't feel comfortable with that. So I decided there needed to be midwives and started going into midwifery then. But it was mostly

> the birth of my child. I just thought this is like an incredible miracle and I want to be around this (Samantha, CNM).

Samantha first identifies as a birthing woman. Next, she shifts into a story of being a consumer of alternative knowledge, reading books and ideas about feminist health care. She cites a lack of available services and a discomfort with unassisted home births, the only alternative at the time, as a reason for choosing to go into midwifery. She finishes her narrative by returning to the birth of her own child – "this is like an incredible miracle and I want to be around this" – to make sense of her decision to become a midwife.

Stacey, like Melanie in the beginning of this section, had a negative hospital experience and "wanted to provide care to women so that someone else didn't have to suffer the humiliation I endured." Also, like Melanie and like Samantha above, Stacey refers to a book she read as being instrumental in her decision to become a midwife. The book she mentions is one that several of the women in this study referred to as "the midwife's bible":

> I was 18, in my freshman year of college and had some serious gynecological issues arise. I got some good references from a friend, but I also went to the library and found a copy of *Spiritual Midwifery*. As corny as it sounds, it was like a light went off in my head. I knew right away I wanted to go to nursing school and pursue this route. The gynecological issues were handled poorly from the doctor who treated me and I wanted to provide care to women so that someone else didn't have to suffer the humiliation I endured. I got better care from nurses and nurse practitioners than from an MD (Stacey, CNM).

After describing her desire to help other women avoid experiencing what she did, Stacey makes a distinction between the care she received from nurses and from a doctor, with the nursing care being superior in her opinion. This lays the groundwork for her eventual identity as a nurse, and more specifically a nurse interested in labor and delivery and maternal and infant health:

> In nursing school, the only thing I ever liked was my labor and delivery rotation. Upon graduation, I immediately became employed at [local hospital] in the labor and delivery ward. I had to rethink my plans only once. I actually have my master's degree in women's health because I had a new baby and was recently divorced, and I knew I wouldn't be able to take the necessary call needed for the midwifery program. Now my kids are older, my parents live next door, and I live with a wonderful man who is very supportive. My current employer approached me about returning to school for this certificate, so I jumped on the opportunity (Stacey, CNM).

Stacey, again like Melanie at the beginning of the section, cites family responsibilities to make sense of the career path she chose. While she may have wanted to go directly into midwifery, as a single mom she was not able to "take the necessary call needed for the midwifery program." Now, in the midst of pursuing a midwifery certificate, she once again refers to family, but in a different context.

Where family once prohibited her from pursuing midwifery, her current family arrangement makes it possible for her to do so.

Casey, another CNM, is no longer "catching babies," but works providing well-woman care in a couple of different settings. She, too, starts her story by referring to a book. The book she came across resonated with "how I knew I'd have a baby; it was home and it was natural." From understanding how she would want her own birth to happen, she moves to the thought that "this would even be neat to do":

> Well really, I was a, I had a friend who was pregnant in Austin, Texas, probably back in the 70s and she was showing me this book called *The Birth Book* by Raven Lang and it just captured me. I remember looking through it and I thought, "This is really how I know I'd have a baby, it was home and it was natural." And then I thought, "I would, this would even be neat to do" (Casey, CNM).

We can then hear Casey thinking "about going back to nursing school to become a midwife," but her plans were delayed by her own pregnancy. In her search for a midwife for her own birth, she joined a group of midwives practicing underground. The group she refers to includes several midwives in this study, some of whom eventually became licensed midwives and some who stopped practicing when the laws changed. Casey is one of the few women in this group who chose the nurse-midwife route:

> And at that time I just had a bachelor's in social sciences and many years past. And then I, I don't really remember really thinking, I thought about going back to nursing school to become a midwife and then I got pregnant and started looking for a midwife myself, and then got connected to some midwives here in town, because we had just moved here. And then as soon as I met them, I said I want to do what you do and they said, well you can come with us to prenatals. So, there were a group of midwives in the, this was in 1980, and they would weekly do prenatal care in somebody's house. And I guess I kind of joined with them and started just going to prenatal care and home births. At the same time I went back to nursing school with that in mind of doing nurse-midwifery though. I think I just intuitively knew that would, for me, give me more opportunity than doing licensed, there wasn't licensed at the time, but lay midwifery. I wanted, I guess do a more conventional approach because I thought it would make sense in the end (Casey, CNM).

In her discussion of working with a group of midwives, Casey tentatively claims a collective identity, "and I guess I kind of joined with them and started just going to prenatal care and home births." She then quickly mentions that she went back to nursing school at the same time because it would give her "more opportunity." In the time period that Casey refers to, nurse-midwifery was the only legally sanctioned midwifery option. Today, licensed midwifery is a legal and viable option for women who want to practice midwifery. Casey told me at another point in our interview that, even today, she "walks the fence," explaining that she and a handful of other nurse-midwives still work very closely and share similar ideas about birth with the licensed midwives. She aligns her identity with both licensed midwives and nurse-midwives, but not with either entirely.

Entry Narratives of Direct-Entry Midwives

While most of the nurse-midwives began their narratives identifying as nurses, the direct-entry midwives had a variety of starting points to their stories, including their own birth experiences, childhood memories, participation in countercultural movements, legal barriers or challenges, and an interest or background in medicine, including alternative medicine. While the narratives of entry told by the CNMs were usually quite succinct, asking direct-entry midwives the question "How did you come to be a midwife?" often elicited narratives that filled seven or eight pages.

This section, like the last one, looks at the paths these women took to the occupation of midwifery. Here, though, we will hear entry narratives from licensed and empirical midwives. The complexity of these narratives is evidenced in the variety of narrative resources from which they draw, including their own birth experiences, childhood memories, prior medical experience, alternative medicine, legal battles and countercultural involvement.

Birth Experiences

The most common theme to arise in the narratives of direct-entry midwives was their own birth experience. In response to the question, "How did you come to be a midwife," 10 out of 15 women referred to their births. Of the five who did not refer to their own birth experience, two do not have children and two had their children after they had already decided to pursue midwifery. Often, at gatherings of direct-entry midwives, a typical round of introductions sounds something like, "Hi, my name is Jane Doe, I'm a licensed midwife, mother of three, two of those born at home"; "Hi, I'm Nicky, I'm a doula. I have two children, one a hospital birth and one a home birth." Thus, these women, in their introductions, immediately establish a maternal identity in connection with their work. After observing this type of introduction several times, I thought it was important to ask those midwives who have not given birth how this influenced their work. One response was that male gynecologists, who deliver most of the babies in the United States, have also never given birth. Stella, a direct-entry student claims that she "[has] more experience with babies than some first time parents. So, I think that comes through, I'm told I have a very maternal personality."

Sandra, a practicing LM, offers a more extended explanation:

> After I have a baby, some people will give me credentials automatically because I have a baby, but I think it will also make a difference for me that, which is odd because you know what, one child is not the world of experience in terms of having a child, you know there's so, so many experiences, but nonetheless it's an experience. And so, you know I think that I will also feel more confident about what I know because I'll know it from a personal place (Sandra, LM).

Laura, a licensed midwife working at a birth center, begins her story by describing her experience as a young woman, new to the United States, and unfamiliar with the health care system:

> I grew up in [European country] and came over to America when I was young, 21, promptly got married, got pregnant shortly afterwards, moved to a rural area of Florida, and being a very well-brought up, conscientious young woman, knew that you should get early prenatal care. So, I went down to the local health department and presented myself with my accent, terminal case of naivety, and said to them, "Good morning, I'd like to register with a midwife, I'd like a home delivery please, and I'd like to see about getting prenatal care." And the lovely women in the health department just fell about laughing and called everybody else up and had me repeat myself several times, so they could hear my adorable little accent, and then broke the news to me that there were no midwives in this area of Florida and that we don't do it like that here honey. You come to the health department for your care and then you go deliver at the teaching hospital. That didn't sound like a terrific idea, but it's what I had to work with (Laura, LM).

Laura's story needs to be understood in a particular cultural context. In many European countries, midwifery and home birth have long been legitimate practices. By referencing her upbringing, she supports and legitimizes her desire to have midwifery care at home, even in the face of laughter by the workers at the health department. However, while becoming a midwife would have been easier for Laura in Europe, she tells us that she would have been a "very different midwife when I came out of it, and I don't think I would have appreciated it." The path she did take was harder:

> And looking back, I mean I grew up in [European country]. If I'd known what I wanted to do when I graduated from high school, I could have walked right into midwifery training in [European country], no problem. The government would have paid my tuition, paid for my books, and paid me a living allowance. How much easier would this have been? You know, I threw [newspapers] for a year and a half at 3:30 in the morning so that I could afford to go to school, so I could pay for daycare for my kids so I could go to school. You know, the other route would have been much easier, but I would have been a very different midwife when I came out of it, and I don't think I would have appreciated it. And I certainly wouldn't have learned the patience I've learned doing it this way (Laura, LM).

Discouraged by local birth practices and by the lack of midwives in Florida, Laura continues her story:

> So, I was about three months pregnant at the time, so I started care like that and started asking questions about what kind of care I could expect in a hospital and was really not happy with

> the answers I was getting. So, then I started reading everything I could get my hands on about midwifery, midwifery in Florida, went to the local lawyer's office and the copy of the Florida statutes and found out how you could become a midwife in Florida. And as the result of that search decided that that was what I wanted to do. The things that I was uncomfortable about with the hospital at that time, which is about now 25 years ago, were things like being strapped down for delivery, in the operating room, nobody was allowed to be with you, you were shaved, you had an enema, you got an episiotomy, the baby had to go to the nursery for 24 hours, there was just no options on any of it. So, we wound up actually staying at home and delivering our baby ourselves. In retrospect, not probably the brightest thing to do. And that was probably the first real step in my journey (Laura, LM).

Citing dissatisfaction with hospital practices at the time, Laura began to read and seek information on midwifery, specifically how to become a midwife in Florida. It was through this process that she decided "that's what I wanted to do." But, she cites her actual birth at home as the "first real step in my journey." While Laura begins her narrative with a story about her own pregnancy and birth experience, she continues, as we will see later, by retrospectively recalling childhood memories of birth.

Like Laura, Sheila begins her story with her own birth experience, but unlike Laura, Sheila's multiple births are the focus of her story and run throughout the narrative:

> Well, I had my first child 27 years ago. So, in the process of becoming pregnant and realizing that I didn't want to go to a hospital, I became aware of, that I wanted to do it at home mainly, and that I would like to have assistance and I didn't particularly care if it was physician, if it was a midwife, that would be fine. We were in Canada, it was in a very rural area and I didn't know of anybody. And there was a doctor practicing in the little town, but I didn't speak to him right away about coming out to the home. So, I had heard about the midwives on the Farm in Tennessee and actually right around that time received a booklet in the mail about the Farm and about the midwives. And the last few pages of the book was about midwifery which was exciting because I thought, oh this is exactly what I am doing, I wish I had somebody like that around here. So, they didn't have midwives in the area that we were in Canada (Sheila, empirical).

Sheila did have a home birth, assisted by a doctor and his wife who was a nurse, but did not get the type of support she was looking for "emotionally or spiritually." This experience sparked her interest in midwifery, but it would be a few more years before she knew she wanted to practice midwifery. She continues her story:

> And other friends in the area started getting pregnant and you know the idea of going to assist with somebody else was formulating, and didn't actually get to do that at that particular time until a few years later. So, it was basically just a process of learning about pregnancy, and discovering the process for myself that I felt like I just started learning about things that really interested me and were really important to women and to myself and that there wasn't a lot of that kind of awareness going on. It was beginning. So it was just kind of getting interested and learning about it. Then I had another son up there and he was born in the hospital because I had rubella, so we weren't sure what his condition would be and until my third child who was born

> in the Farm, with the Farm midwives then I really decided this is, you know I want to do this, I want to apprentice (Sheila, empirical).

Sheila's story takes us from Canada with one home birth, one hospital birth, and an interest in midwifery, to Tennessee where she birthed on the Farm, "with the Farm midwives" and decided "I want to do this, I want to apprentice." Later we will hear Sheila talk more about The Farm and the importance to her of being in a countercultural, intentional community.

Unlike Laura and Sheila above, Dawn does not begin her story with her own birth experience, but rather with her desire to go to medical school. After an early disappointment with the experience of working in an obstetrician's office, Dawn continues her story:

> So, I just kind of chunked the whole school thing and didn't know what I wanted to do with my life and met my husband, got married, got pregnant, and had a baby. And that first baby that I had, you know I always knew, I had this thing about hospitals, so I didn't want to be in hospitals, so I looked for or sought out a place where I could birth out of hospital with the assistance of midwives. My dad comes from a family of 16, they were all born at home, so I sought out a midwifery practice and found one. And after I birthed with the midwife for the first time, I knew hey this is what I want to do, this is exactly, probably half way through my labor, through my 24-hour labor, when she didn't leave my side for one minute, and rubbed exactly the spot that I wanted rubbed for 23 hours. Yeah, I knew, I knew then, it was real clear, that's the kind of care I wanted to give related to birth, vs. the you know the medical type, OB/GYN type. So, that's when I knew (Dawn, LM).

Dawn tells us that during her labor with her first child, as she was receiving care and attention from a midwife, she knew "this is what I want to do." She makes a distinction between "medical type" of care and the type of care she received – "she didn't leave my side for one minute, and rubbed exactly the spot that I wanted, rubbed for twenty-three hours" – and realized she wanted to give. While others have expressed a similar preference for a midwifery model of care, Dawn's decision must be seen in the context of her initial desire to be an obstetrician/gynecologist. The event she cites as changing her mind was while working for a prominent obstetrician in town, "we would come in many mornings and find him passed out in the chairs in his office." So, in addition to seeing a difference in a midwifery model of care and a medical model of care, Dawn was also turned off from medicine because of the long hours, presumably spent away from family, that she observed in her former job. She always knew she "wanted to have a family . . . So, you know it just wasn't for me."

While each of the stories above tell of home births or midwife-attended births, several of the direct-entry midwives in this study did have at least one birth in a hospital. Lisa had a "really great experience." Christy's first hospital birth was an "okay birth," and after her second hospital birth she met a nurse-midwife who spent a lot of time talking with me and she was just really cool. And I was like, this person's great, she's talking to me, she's not talking at me, it's just a whole different way of interacting. Carrie had a complicated pregnancy and negative experiences with the hospital staff during her first birth. Her second birth was in a hospital, attended by a midwife and it was "different in the fact that I had support."

Childhood Memories

The second most common theme in the entry narratives of direct-entry midwives involves childhood memories. For two women, their immediate response to the question of how they came to be midwives involved stories of childhood. For three other women, childhood memories were told retrospectively. In other words, after deciding to pursue midwifery, they thought back to childhood experiences that now make more sense to them in light of their occupational choice.

Carrie and Helen both begin their stories with a tale of childhood. Both express an early interest in birth. For Carrie, the desire to become a midwife re-emerges with the birth of her first child:

> Well, it's a long story, but I'll make it short. When I was five-ish, around that age, I saw a TV birth, woman screaming, doctor comes in and catches the baby, and I said I wanted to be a baby doctor. Later found out that you know that's a pediatrician. Then my mom had three children. Single child, only child until I was nine. My brother was born a year later, my sister a year later, my other sister. So, that peaked my interest. But even when the second one was born, I still didn't know how because I didn't go to the birth, wasn't involved in sibling classes, just her belly got big and she had a baby. And I was about 10 and every pregnant woman I saw, when's your baby due?" All that silly stuff. Then with my own children, my first one brought it up again, that this is what I wanted to do. And at that time it was, what I want to do eventually, I want to be a midwife (Carrie, LM).

While Helen expresses an early interest in birth, she claims that her interest in midwifery in particular developed in early high school and was further legitimated by reading an article in a magazine about the midwives on the Farm.

> Well, I was always fascinated with and extremely attracted to babies and pregnancy and birth. I was the oldest of all the grandchildren, so about every three years there was a baby born in my immediate family, if not my siblings, my cousins. And my mother, labored at home with my little sister when I was six. And she wanted to have an unplanned home birth because her family didn't support her. So, her intention was to have this unplanned home birth, but my father found out she was in labor, so he carried her off at the last minute. But, that would have been my first birth which turned out to be a footling breech. But she flew right out, so it would have been an uncomplicated footling breech. But anyway, so I think I figured out about early high school years that I was interested in midwifery specifically. I used to get *Parent* magazine, yeah strange. And they had an article on the Farm, and that's where I found out about the Farm. But I had already known about midwifery and already wanted to be a midwife (Helen, empirical).

Retrospective Childhood Memories

After beginning their stories in other ways, three women also recalled childhood memories. Stella's decision to become a midwife was precipitated by an unanticipated need to change careers. As she thinks back over the circumstances that led to her life change, she also recalls her childhood. She remembers being "inspired through my mom's stories of, she had nine children and eight of them lived into adulthood, she was actually pregnant 13 times." All of Stella's mom's births were natural births. Once Stella really understood what that meant, she "caught at a very early age the reverence for motherhood through her. When I finally realized as a child where those children actually come from, I was like astonished and I always honored my mom on her birthday."

Carol begins her narrative by letting us know that while she will pursue a somewhat linear narrative, her decision to become a midwife was not quite so clear cut. She says, "well, I think directly, because now that I look back on it there was a lot of indirect things that I never put together until after I was about 30 years old." She went to high school, then to college, pursued a degree in medical technology, and then went to work in a series of hospital laboratories. When she "look[s] back," this is what she recalls of her childhood:

> But now, like I said, indirectly when I look back and I think I was the oldest of five kids, so my mom had lots of babies, I'm from a big Italian family, lots of kids. I was a weird kind of a kid that when families were getting together and there were these big reunions and gatherings with gazillions of cousins and everything, I wanted to stay inside with the ladies and hear about babies and look at the babies and play with the babies. So that was an early, early indication of, I would rather have done that than played outside (Carole, LM).

Earlier we heard Laura's story of her own birth experience. Like Carole and Stella, Laura also "look[s] back" to childhood:

> When I look back at my childhood I can see other things that I go, oh gosh, I should have got it then. Oh, I should have worked out, that's why I enjoyed that job. When I was two my sister was born at home in [European country]. And I have, my earliest memory that I have is the standing out by the bedroom door at my grandparents' house with my father behind me, with our ears glued to the door, waiting to hear people cry. And then, I don't remember walking through the door, but I remember being told that if I sat all the way up on the bed, with my feet up and my back on the wall and was very, very careful I could hold the baby, and then being given my sister to hold. When I told my mother about this, she couldn't, couldn't believe that I remembered it, because I was so young. Totally confirmed everything, I mean I knew which room it was, where the bed was, which was not normal. And then she added, oh yeah we called you two in before the placenta was even delivered, the baby wasn't even cleaned up, she was just wrapped in the first towel. And you and your dad were allowed in to see her and then you had to go out while the midwife finished up (Laura, LM).

After relating this memory of childhood, Laura concludes "it all fit in after I decided that's what I wanted to do." From a very early age, Laura invokes experiential knowledge as legitimation for her decision to become a midwife:

> So, that was kind of, you don't mess with those impressions when you're two. You know, I knew with absolute certainty that babies could be born safely at home, without needing any kind of intellectual proof. I knew it from that experience . . . So, it kind of, it all fit in after I decided that's what I wanted to do (Laura, LM).

Countercultural Movements and Legal Barriers

Several women describe their participation in the counterculture as significant in their decision to pursue midwifery. I use the term "counterculture" very broadly to include communal living, the alternative birth movement, the hippie movement, and underground midwifery practice. Five of the midwives in this study, including one certified nurse-midwife, reported being involved in at least one of these activities. Many of the same women who entered midwifery through the counterculture were also participants in the legal battles to make direct-entry midwifery legal in Florida.

Sheila reports her desire to live in a communal setting, and suggests that midwifery was the "by-product" of this living arrangement:

> I felt like I wanted to try to live in an intentional community like the Farm. And I felt like it would be really good for being a new family and having a lot of agreement about raising children and just about how you want to live. So, that's why we went and the by-product was the midwifery (Sheila, empirical).

After moving to Florida, Sheila became involved with a group of women who "formed a loose network cooperative and started doing prenatal care together for women and started to do births together." She took a course in emergency medicine, "because I felt like if we're not going to be on the Farm or practicing and working where there are EMT's and doctors then I want to learn emergency medicine." This group of women practiced together, underground, for about six to eight years, until the law changed. Once the law changed, Sheila opted against becoming licensed and stopped practicing midwifery because the risks under the new law were too high. Practicing midwifery without a license went from being a misdemeanor to being a felony.

Jeanne, like Sheila, describes a communal living environment in which attending births happened primarily out of need:

> Well, back in the, I guess it was the mid-70s, people in my community lived, a lot of people in my community lived communally and where they did a lot of cooperative ventures together

> like food co-ops and child care and schools and that sort of thing. And so, once in a while when our friends would get pregnant, the women would band together and do births together. And the women who had the most experience either with having babies or having been to births would kind of take more of the leadership roles. But we didn't really have a midwife. And so, over the course of about 10 years, I go to maybe six or seven births. A little average of one birth a year would just so happen to come my way. And it wasn't that I was practicing midwifery or even considered myself a midwife, or really even knew what midwifery was, it was just part of what we all did with each other. And so, in the course of doing that we would learn, we would explore and learn from different books and different people. Of course, Ina May's book *Spiritual Midwifery* was our bible. And basically we didn't have much interaction with uh, what you would call the dominant culture and we just did what we wanted to do and we didn't expect anybody to help us and so we just helped ourselves. And that's basically how I got any experience at all with midwifery (Jeanne, LM).

In the community in which Jeanne lived, because they "didn't have much interaction with what you would call the dominant culture," attending births became a necessity. Jeanne was one of the women in the community who was called upon to take on this role even though as she insists, "I didn't consider myself a midwife, or really even [know] what midwifery was, it was just part of what we all did with each other." So, here Jeanne establishes a collective identity as a community member rather than an individual identity as a midwife.

Gina also did not start out with the intention of being a midwife. Rather, she claims, "it was a series of circumstances and the subculture that I was growing up in that led me to this." Gina was influenced by the alternative birth movement and several books that emerged out of that period, including *Immaculate Deception* and *Spiritual Midwifery*. She claims that knowing she did not want to have her baby in a hospital "probably went along with just the whole hippie movement of that time. I mean we were all like back to land, back to nature, using, studying about herbs, it was all part of the picture." Because Gina had her baby at home without assistance, many women in her community who wanted to do the same thing called on her for support and assistance, and she responded to this. But, she claims, "it really just started with just girlfriend helping girlfriend more than oh I think I want to be a midwife and I'm gonna go to school for this." Gina and a couple of other women in her community formed a study group and, with the assistance of a nurse-midwife, a chiropractor with midwifery training, and other nurses and doctors in the community, learned about birth. Some women who had been trained as midwives on the Farm moved to Gina's community, and together they attended births and supported each other for several years. But, like Jeanne, Gina states, "we didn't use the word midwife, we just said that we were birth attendants and we made it very clear to people about what we could or could not do."

One woman in this study ended up in Florida participating in the alternative birth movement after having been involved in the women's health movement in the northeast. She practiced midwifery in the underground until she was able to become licensed by suing the Department of Health and Rehabilitative Services. After that personal victory, she became active in attempting to change Florida's midwifery laws. Again, these efforts were successful and in 1982 the Midwifery Practice Act was established in Florida, which required three years of formal education. Another woman in this study was influential in establishing one of the first schools for direct-entry midwifery after the new law. In 1984, the law was reviewed based on a "sunset" provision. Based on this review, licensure was limited to those already enrolled in school. Several women, including three of my respondents, hoped to become licensed under the 1982 law, but all "missed the window of opportunity." Two of these women both had babies during this time and as a result missed the chance to become licensed. One of these became actively involved in changing Florida's midwifery laws. Once that was achieved in 1992, she was very influential in opening a school for direct-entry midwifery.

Medical Background

Four of the direct-entry respondents had some kind of medical background prior to entering midwifery. We have already heard from Carole, who began her professional life as a medical technician working in hospital laboratories. We have also heard part of Dawn's story who had hoped to enter medical school until she recognized that she wanted to provide a different type of care and realized that the hours of work and time away from family were "not for her."

The two other women who had prior medical training or experience were a nurse and a physician's assistant. The nurse was working at a birth center in the early 1980s, providing labor support and teaching childbirth education classes. The volume at this birth center was high, and there was only one CNM providing care. A doctor convinced this woman to become licensed as a midwife under a law established in the early 1930s. At the time, a doctor signed a document declaring a midwife competent after attending a relatively small number of births in the doctor's presence. The midwife also had to take a test which this respondent called "sort of a joke." Another respondent began her professional life as a physician's assistant (PA) and was disturbed by the hospital practices she encountered during her obstetrics rotation. After moving to Florida, she began working with others who were involved in home birth. The doctor she was working with eventually left the state, and left her without legal means for delivering babies since PAs must work under the supervision of a physician. She attempted to become licensed as a midwife under the same 1930s law that the nurse, described above, had been licensed under, but initially her application was declined by the Department of Health and Rehabilitative Services (DHRS). She sued the DHRS, won, and continued working for legal midwifery reform.

Alternative Medicine and Doula Practice

Sandra, Nadine and Carrie each cited an interest in some type of alternative medicine as being influential in their decision to pursue midwifery. After leaving a career in public policy work, Sandra spent time traveling, taking classes in storytelling, painting, and weaving, and eventually became interested in the conscious death movement. She says:

> I pretty much went from reading about death to reading about birth and the issues were just so parallel in terms of, so-called patient rights, but really human rights, you know, in terms of having it be a dignified experience . . . After I read about the conscious death movement a bit, I went on to reading *Spiritual Midwifery* and based on that decided that I wanted to be a midwife (Sandra, LM).

Nadine had always had an interest in alternative medicine and massage therapy. In college, she became a women's studies major. For her, midwifery was "like putting together my interest in alternative medicine with my interest in women's issues." Carrie, after deciding to pursue midwifery, first became licensed as a massage therapist, hoping to make enough money to pay for midwifery school. She had learned of a direct-entry midwifery school from an acupuncturist for whom she worked as a nanny. Unable to support herself through massage therapy, she turned to doula practice.

Carrie was one of five women who referred to their experience as a doula, prior to becoming a midwife. Barbara provided labor support services at a birth center before becoming licensed as a midwife. Carole began teaching childbirth education classes in the hospitals in which she worked as a medical technician. The students in her classes often asked her to be with them at their births. After doing that for awhile, Carole learned about doula certification and became one of the first doulas certified by Doulas of North America. Sandra spent more than two years as "what most people call a doula, but I call a labor support person," before pursuing midwifery. Finally, Lisa spent more than 15 years informally providing labor support for friends and family before becoming formally trained as a doula and opening a doula business with a partner. Unfortunately, even with a grant from Healthy Start, Lisa and her business partner were unable to make even enough money to cover the costs of their business.

In the context of entering the profession, direct-entry and nurse midwives have different stories to tell. This difference can be explained in part by the structural differences in education and practice of these two groups. All of the nurse-midwives I interviewed entered from the established and legitimized occupation of nursing into an already legitimized occupation of nurse-midwifery. The more senior among the licensed midwives on the other hand had to struggle to legalize their occupation. The two groups also have a different relationship to the medical establishment, with nurse-midwives being firmly established in the "medical team," and licensed midwives being independent practitioners. Therefore, it also makes sense that licensed midwives might enter midwifery through various forms of alternative medicine, while nurse-midwives generally would not. Despite the structural differences of these two occupations, in the next two sections, we will see more similarities in work narratives than differences.

THE FUTURE

I asked each of the respondents where they saw themselves in five to 10 years. The following responses come from four women who are still actively practicing midwifery, and one woman who has "retired" from practices, but continues to teach and be involved in the midwifery community. Andrea, who above said that when deciding to become a midwife "found that I was at a point in my life, totally independent and single, where I was ready for a change," now cites eventual family responsibilities as a reason for expecting to "choose a less rigorous schedule" in the future:

> I do think I'll be doing this in five to 10 years, though I may choose a less rigorous schedule or perhaps be working part-time. I am getting married in May 2000 and plan to stay home as much as possible to raise my family. I plan to stay abreast of the latest in obstetrics and midwifery so as to not let go of it completely and find it difficult to re-enter after being away for awhile. I also wonder where nurse-midwifery will be in five to 10 years. With managed care taking over, its fate could go either way. Though we are more cost effective and yield higher patient satisfaction, we must practice under a physician thus adding additional cost to a practice (Andrea, CNM).

After suggesting that she may choose part-time work in the future, she shifts from a discussion of the personal to a discussion of health care issues, connecting biographical particulars to broader narratives. Wondering not only what she will be doing in five to 10 years, but also what the state of midwifery will be at that time, she calls upon cost effectiveness and patient satisfaction to legitimate the practice and profession of midwifery. Yet, the downside is that nurse-midwives are not independent practitioners, and because they must be under the supervision of a physician, the cost increases. Andrea's concerns with the ambiguous state of midwifery in the context of managed care are in-line with others in her field (Williams, 1999). So, while Andrea portrays her future decision to work part-time and raise a family as being under her control, she has very little control over the future of the profession in general, making this less her own story than the story of women in her circumstances.

At the time of the interview, Samantha was working in two different settings, both part-time. She hopes that in the future she will be doing full-time work. In describing this desire, she struggles with the pros and cons of both full-time and part-time work:

> I'm looking for something, well I'm open to something a little more full time now. I like my job except that there's no continuity of care. Like I see, when I go to the same health department I see the same women, but I don't deliver people that I know. And I've found it more rewarding to have a job where I would do their prenatal care and do the delivery to the same person. It's hard to get a job like that where you don't work too much. Like, it seems like you either have a job with really great rapport with your patients and you work *all the time*, or you have a job where you really don't have a lot of continuity but you have great schedules. My job I had in [neighboring town] was kind of somewhere in the middle. And the job I have now, I have less continuity than I'd like to. I'm open to finding something different (Samantha, CNM).

The issue Samantha struggles with is an interesting one. Continuity of care is something that is very important in a midwifery model of care. Samantha aligns herself with this philosophy: "I've found it more rewarding to have a job where I would do their prenatal care and do the delivery to the same person." However, she also alludes to the fact that she does not want to work "all the time." Following this discussion, Samantha adds, "In 10 years I might want to not do deliveries anymore. Just because, you know, two o'clock in the morning gets old." Time becomes an overarching theme in Samantha's narrative, but yet there is a tension between personal time and level and quality of care she provides for her patients.

Like Andrea, Sandra also mentions starting her own family in the future and the impact that might have on her practice. She also ponders other factors:

> Yes, I do, I do. I think I will be doing it in five years, and I think I will be doing it in eight years. In 10 years, I'm not sure, it really depends on, it depends on how, how much support I'm able to build for myself in my community of midwives, in my colleague world. And it depends on, I don't know, it depends on family life, you know we'd like to have kids, I don't know you know what kind of impact that will have on the practice. I can imagine that in 10 years, I'd either want like a serious sabbatical (both laugh) or I'd want to shift a little bit. So, yeah, I don't know (Sandra, LM).

While she sees herself continuing to practice in the immediate future, thinking about 10 years from now, Sandra recognizes the need for support and establishing herself in a community of midwives. The ability to build this community and support will depend in large part on the state of direct-entry midwifery education and practice over the next few years.

Laura also expects to continue her practice for quite a few years, yet being in a very different place in her life, older with grown children and grandchildren, than Sandra she draws upon different narrative resources to make sense of her long-range plans.

> Five years definitely, 10 years most likely. Although gosh, it's taking longer to recover from staying up all night than it used to. And I really do have to get back to yoga classes soon so I can sit in all those weird positions and not be stiff afterwards. You know, there's definitely things that get harder as you get older. You know, I'm 47 now, so I figure I've got a good few years left. Some of the old granny midwives just worked until they were way up in years, up in their 60s and 70s and some of them only gave up reluctantly when their sight started to fail them and they started feeling like they were no longer safe practitioners that they should be (Laura, LM).

Laura cites age as a potential factor in her decision to continue practicing, "there's definitely things that get harder as you get older." But she also draws on the historical resource of the "granny midwife," to make sense of the fact that she continues to practice, despite "it's taking longer to recover from staying up all night than it used to."

Jeanne is no longer actively practicing midwifery, but continues to teach and expects to continue this for some time. Here she explains why:

> I expect that I'll be doing more teaching. I think that now, at my age and with my experience, and with the way things are going, and I'm very encouraged that there are so many young women that are interested in midwifery, because back when we were interested, there weren't. And for many years we didn't have any interest. So, part of me is glad to see that. Although, I don't know, don't always see the young women that are interested in midwifery going into it for what I would call the right reasons. A lot of women go into it because they think it's a good career opportunity or they think that they're gonna make money on it, or they think it sounds groovy or whatever. I don't really see it so much as a spiritual calling as it was for us. So much, I do see some women that have that relationship to it. But it's becoming more and more professionalized and more and more mainstream, which in some ways is good and in some ways isn't. So, I feel like I need to stay actively involved in teaching so that I can be a link between the modern midwife and the traditional midwife, because I think that's very important and I don't think there's very many midwives out there that actually have a grip on what the traditional midwife is about (Jeanne, LM).

Jeanne engages in identity work based on generations. Social movement scholars write extensively about political generations, suggesting that they share a collective identity and their collective experiences become a lens through which to interpret future experiences. Earlier we heard Jeanne discuss how her start in midwifery was firmly embedded in a countercultural context. Here she distinguishes between women of her generation coming to midwifery as part of a spiritual calling and young women entering midwifery today for professional reasons. She cites her role as a teacher as important in order to be a "link between the modern midwife and the traditional midwife."

While we saw a distinct difference between licensed midwives and certified nurse-midwives in the context of entering the profession, when talk turns to future work identities, there is less of a clear cut distinction between the two. Thus, it becomes important to pay attention to the narrative resources that link the identities of these midwives to broader cultural discourses such as family, education, time, and larger health care issues.

CAREER? JOB? SERVICE? CALLING?

Initially, I was using the term "career narratives" when speaking with potential respondents. Among direct-entry midwives, in particular, I began to hear a strong resistance to the term "career." This distancing from the concept of career has also been noted by Garey (1999) in interviews with nurses in the context of "weaving work and motherhood." Slater (1976, 1970) described this same phenomenon, arguing that the term career was associated with men, created by and for men and connoting a demanding, rigorous, all-encompassing occupational path. He emphasized that women want their work to be "meaningful and stimulating activity," full of "excitement, challenge, [and] social satisfaction" (p. 78). Garey (1999) laments that this gendered distinction has seemingly not been erased in the 20-plus years since Slater's description. While direct-entry midwives resisted the term career, nurse-midwives had more ambiguous feelings about it, a seemingly minor terminological distinction that speaks loads of narrative difference. When phrasing my question, I listed a number of terms, including "career," "profession," "job," and "calling," and asked which term best fit how they see the work they do. Samantha responded this way:

> I don't really care. But I've heard it called a calling and certainly you could, with the same degree of education, you could make more money and work less hours doing other things. You have to love it to do it. But, I don't care what you call it (Samantha, CNM).

While her response, "I don't care," demonstrates an ambivalence about terms, she cites education, money, and hours as potential ways to define work.

As the following exchange shows, Bridget distances herself from the concept of career, identifying instead as a woman's advocate. She links career with a "corporate ladder" and suggests that by stepping down from a director position, she is not entirely focused on "climbing":

Lara: If you had to choose between some of these words I'm about to say or another word? Profession, career, occupation, job, calling . . .

Bridget: I don't know what you mean exactly by profession because I think that is a big category. But I really look at myself as a woman's advocate.

Lara: I had been using the term "career" when I talked to people and there were some people who didn't really like that word. So, I've just been interested in how people . . .

Bridget: No. I guess that because to me a career connotes climbing the corporate ladder and that's not, I've been a director of a program, of this program and I'm no longer a director, so that it's really, what is it that you want to do. And I don't believe that's within a career, at least my impression of what a career means (Bridget, CNM).

While Samantha was ambivalent and Bridget was resistant to the term career, Tracey tentatively embraced it, but ultimately felt that there was no one single word that could sum up the work that midwives do:

> Definitely not a job, definitely not a job in the usual sense of that word. I suppose career is maybe palatable in terms of something I've done to make a living and I've worked at it and had to increase, had to have educational goals to achieve, so I guess in that sense it's a career. Profession, I feel very strongly and proud of nurse-midwifery as a profession and feel that that is what midwifery should be. I know there are those who disagree. But I feel there has to be, there should be that component there. I would probably, if there was some word that would say kind of a calling plus a career plus profession all rolled up in one word, that would probably be, I don't really take offense at the other words, just they don't quite . . . (Tracey, CNM).

Taken together, the hesitation in fully embracing a professional identifier such as career, or a non-professional appellation such as job, harkens back to the complexity noted at the start of this chapter. Across the board, these women's narrative positioning is not squarely settled at either end of the professional/job spectrum, but exists, in their work narratives, in dynamic relation with the broader work narratives that surround midwifery.

The idea that midwifery is a "calling" is often suggested by direct-entry midwives. Even for those women who do not necessarily feel it is a calling, this concept is made available by the larger community as a narrative resource to describe the work of being a midwife. Sandra begins her answer with a reference to the idea of a calling:

> Ya know, some people talk about feeling a calling, I can't say that I ever felt, ya know I didn't grow up in a Christian household, so it's not like I resonate with that word anyway. It's not like I had some kind of experience ever of like, oh now I *feel* called to do this. But, in some ways I find that word appropriate in that it, it's so definitely far from a nine to five routine, where you are essentially responsible for, you know where there may be a lot of stress but essentially what you produce is of no particular import (laughs), it's so not a job. Calling does the job for talking about what it is, in that it respects that it's something that comes from your heart. So, I don't know what I would call it, I guess I don't have a word. Profession is too, I just object to that in all kinds of ways, and same with career. It has a very like you know kind of tracking kind of feel to it (Sandra, LM).

Sandra distances herself from the religious connotations of the term "calling," but later redefines the concept as "something that comes from your heart."

Sandra rejects both the term career and the term profession. Stella, on the other hand, begins by calling what she does a "service," but quickly embraces the term profession:

> I see it as a service. I know that's like not very glamorous and, but I see it as a service. I also have to look at it as a profession. Because, I'm being, you know the state is, the taxpayer is paying for my tuition. I'm being vocationally rehabilitated and so, I don't see myself as, I mean I see myself as a worker or a, I don't know how to explain it. I just see it as a profession that is in its infancy and I've always tried to keep my professional life and my personal life like separate, and those ethics that I have aren't working in this arena. You can't, I mean I'm not gonna move in with my clients, but I have to meld it somehow, I have to, because you're in a very intimate relationship with them and so, and it's very hard to concept that I'm getting paid for this kind of intimacy. . . . So, I don't have any problems with calling it a job or profession or service and I'm proud of it. I'm proud to say that's what I do for a living. It's taken me a while to say it (Stella, LM).

While Stella is comfortable with a variety of terms to describe what she does, she problematizes the concept of separating personal and professional life. She mentions the intimate nature of her work and her struggle to comprehend that she is "getting paid for this kind of intimacy."

When phrasing this question to Christy, I said, "I've heard calling, career, how would you characterize, in that sense of work, what you do?" She, like Tracey, the CNM in the last section, says, "well, I mean it's all those things I guess, to me." She continues, expanding and contextualizing the definition of her work:

> I mean it's, sometimes it's a job even. I mean when I'm on the phone with the insurance companies, it's a job. When I'm watching that woman and I'm just amazed at how she's progressing and how things are going and I'm watching all that, it's more like a calling or a passion (Christy, LM).

Christy distinguishes between the different roles she plays in her work. Her definition of what she does depends on the aspect of work in which she is engaged. She continues, struggling, like Stella above, with the issue of separating personal and professional life:

> I mean I've, I feel so fortunate to have found this because I've always wanted that whatever work I do in my life would be meaningful and to come from something I believe in and am passionate about and not to feel too much like work. And that's what this is. But I know there's people who, well it has to be a calling, or it has to be this. Well, it has to be whatever you need it to be. I don't think, I think you could probably be a really good midwife and consider it your job. And maybe for you and the person that you are you need that little bit of distance from it to call it a job. It demands a lot of you, it demands a lot of you emotionally, it demands a lot of you in a lot of ways. And maybe some people's way of coping with it is to consider it a job and think of it more in that respect you know. But, I mean I think the cool thing about midwifery

> and what makes it an art is that you bring who you are to it so much that we have to allow for all ways of dealing. I think there can definitely be problems come about by people thinking of it only as a job. That may have its ramifications and repercussions, but so can someone who's so embedded, and their whole life is so embedded in it that who they are is so tied up in it and they don't have anything outside of that, you know what I mean? So, I mean, I think you call it whatever you want to call it. I mean there are people who come, you know they're doing the Lord's work when they're doing midwifery. You know, I feel like I'm doing feminist work, you know when I'm doing midwifery. There's space for all of them. I mean there's Christian midwives, and then there's pagan midwives (Christy, LM).

Christy suggests that midwifery should be "whatever you need it to be." She also recognizes that it is different things for different people. At the same time that she claims a feminist identity in her work, she also recognizes that some people are "doing the Lord's work when they're doing midwifery." Feminism can be used to legitimize the work as can religion.

We have heard narratives of entry from both certified nurse-midwives and direct-entry midwives. While the nurse-midwives tend to initiate this narrative at the point of nursing school or practice and with the identity of nurse, direct-entry midwives invoke a variety of entry points, and thus a variety of identities. The most common identity invoked by direct-entry midwives in their entry narratives is that of mother. However, alluding to one's own birth and maternal identity is often only a starting point. These narratives tend to be a complex web of childhood memories, legal battles, countercultural involvement, and interest or background in medicine or alternative medicine.

As far as the futures that these women see for themselves, nurse-midwives and licensed midwives both cite personal factors, such as age and family situations, as well as "state of the profession," factors as being determinants of whether they will continue practicing or working in the same manner as they are now. Also, as far as the preferred terminology for the work they do, there is overlap between nurse-midwives and direct-entry midwives, with direct-entry midwives being only slightly more resistant to the term career.

Clearly, their stories complicate related work identities by incorporating both biographical particulars and midwife-specific discourses of legitimation, something which a narrative approach brings to the fore. These women are not merely "catching babies," but construct the activity from the standpoint of diverse senses of who and what they are and what this means. The idea of "the" midwife, as distinguished as that term is legally, still does not bring forth the narrative differences in place. Further, because of the structural differences between licensed midwives and certified nurse-midwives one might expect their work narratives to be distinctly different, however this seems to be the case only in the context of entering the profession. When speaking of the future or of the type of work they do there are more similarities than differences. Similarly, because of the structural differences in relationship to the medical establishment, one might expect licensed midwives to be more likely to distance themselves from medicine and certified nurse-midwives to be more likely to embrace it. However, I have argued elsewhere (Foley & Faircloth, 2003) that this is not true, but rather that both groups draw upon the same narrative resource of medicine and use that resource in various ways depending on the context.

LANGUAGE, METHOD AND RAPPORT

There is a certain elasticity to the stories these midwives tell. But, that does not mean that "anything goes." Rather, the elasticity is delimited by available discourses or occupational structures. In this chapter we saw midwives from different occupational paths each at a different point in the process of professionalization. Where each stood in relation to professionalization gave rise to a particular narrative form. So, in this case, the structure of the occupations and the discourses available to each shape the stories they tell. Direct-entry midwives, with a few exceptions, have not been trained as nurses and thus do not have a nursing discourse available to them.

One dilemma I encountered in my research was the differing types of narratives produced by nurse-midwives and direct-entry midwives. Nurse-midwives, with a few exceptions, seemed to deliver relatively straight-forward, succinct, linear narratives about their life and work. Direct-entry midwives, on the other hand, often told long, complex, semi-linear stories. These stories were much more conducive to the elements of narrative analysis, with narrative resources, narrative frameworks, narrative linkages, and horizons of meaning being more readily identifiable.

Whether they consider their work a job, profession, career, calling or something else, the clearest difference in the narratives of nurse-midwives and direct-entry midwives is that most of the nurse-midwives begin their stories with nursing school or nursing practice, while the direct-entry midwives have a variety of starting points and tell a more complex story of how they entered the profession. In many ways, it makes sense that nurse-midwives would begin their stories with a nurse identity. One must be a nurse before becoming a nurse-midwife. I shared this aspect of data analysis with two different groups of direct-entry midwives (senior students and members of the school's board of directors). Both theorized that nurse-midwifery is more thoroughly "professionalized" and, for nurse-midwives, midwifery is a form of advanced practice nursing. One board member suggested that as direct-entry midwifery becomes increasingly professionalized similar narratives will emerge from direct-entry midwives. Chances are that if I asked these same nurse-midwives to tell me the story of how they came to be nurses, I would hear very different stories.

In thinking through this dilemma, I speculate that the training that each type of midwife receives influences the way she tells stories about her work. Helen, an empirically-trained midwife observed, "I think where you're trained and how you're trained makes a huge difference on how you practice and where you're comfortable practicing and how you perceive birth." I would add to Helen's observation that where and how one is trained also "makes a huge difference" on how one narrates her work. In other words, nurse-midwives are trained in a university setting, presumably learning that research must follow a deductive, scientific method. Direct-entry midwives have either been trained by apprenticeship or formal education. However, at least in my research context, the formal education of direct-entry midwives has only recently begun to incorporate research methods into the curriculum. As academic director of the school, I have been instrumental in that process and have introduced inductive and interpretive approaches to research methods along with more traditional deductive approaches.

Bruner (1986, 1996) suggests two different ways of thinking used to make sense of our worlds: paradigmatic and narrative. Paradigmatic thought, claims Bruner, is promoted in science and philosophy and honored in formal education, and "leads to good theory, tight analysis, logical proof, and empirical discovery guided by reasoned hypothesis" (1986, p. 98). Narrative thought, he argues, is the mode of thinking used in literature and in life and "deals with the vicissitudes of human intention" and "leads instead to good stories, gripping drama, believable historical accounts" (1986, p. 98). This distinction fits well with the differences I observed in the narratives of nurse-midwives and direct-entry midwives. I am not certain if the explanation for this difference involves the content of the research or the very process of research itself. In other words, if I were to interview nurse-midwives about some other aspect of their lives, something other than their training and work, would they produce different kinds of narratives? Or perhaps, by presenting myself as a researcher, they assume a deductive research process. This is a strong possibility. The question, "What is your hypothesis?" was asked of me prior to the interview by almost every nurse-midwife respondent. Direct-entry midwives were curious about my project but did not use the language of scientific research to question me.

This dilemma exists in different ways for other groups as well. A colleague, who is interviewing adolescent males, and I have discussed this issue at length. For him the problem seems to be a developmental one, with adolescents being relatively narratively unsophisticated. Many scholars discuss narrative competence in the context of human development (Berman, 1994; McAdams, 1988, 1993, 1996;

Randall, 1995) arguing that it is not until late adolescence that we develop the ability to become "biographers of self" (McAdams, 1988). Building on Gardner's (1993) theory of *multiple* intelligences (linguistic, musical, logical-mathematical, bodily-kinesthetic, spatial, interpersonal and intrapersonal) and on Goleman's (1995) idea of "emotional intelligence," Randall (1999) discusses the concept of "narrative intelligence," as "the capacity to formulate a story . . . [and] the capacity to follow a story" (p. 13). Randall (1999) considers narrative intelligence in the context of aging. As we age, our lives become more complicated and "our life-plot thickens" (p. 20) and eventually begins to "narrow" as we approach the end of our lives.

These dilemmas raise interesting questions about narrative practice and narrative analysis with various groups or populations of respondents. Whether we are dealing with people in distinct developmental ages or stages or whether we are dealing with people who have been differently trained or come from atypical backgrounds, we must take into account that different narrative forms will likely emerge.

REFERENCES

American College of Nurse Midwives (2000). *Certified nurse midwives in Florida*. Retrieved April 20, 2000. http://www.acnm.org/press/florida.htm.

Armstrong, P., & Feldman. S. (1990). *A wise birth*. New York: Morrow.

Benoit, C., Davis-Floyd, R., van Teijlingen, E. R., Sandall, J., & Miller, J. F. (2001). Designing midwives: A comparison of educational models. In: R. DeVries, C. Benoit, E. R. van Teijlingen & S. Wrede (Eds), *Birth by Design: Pregnancy, Maternity Care, and Midwifery in North American and Europe* (pp. 139–165). New York: Routledge.

Berman, H. J. (1994). *Interpreting the aging self: Personal journals of later life*. New York: Springer.

Bielby, W. T., & Bielby, D. D. (1992). I will follow him: Family ties, gender-role beliefs, and reluctance to relocate for a better job. *American Journal of Sociology*, *97*(5), 1241–1267.

Boston Women's Health Book Collective (1998). *Our bodies, ourselves for the new century: A book by and for women*. New York: Simon & Schuster.

Brewis, J., & Linstead, S. (2000). The worst thing is the screwing (2): Context and career in sex work. *Gender Work and Organization*, *7*(3), 168–180.

Bruner, J. S. (1986). *Actual minds, possible worlds*. Cambridge, MA: Harvard University Press.

Bruner, J. S. (1996). *The culture of education*. Cambridge, MA: Harvard University Press.

Caton, D. (1999). *What a blessing she had chloroform: The medical and social response to the pain of childbirth from 1800 to the present*. New Haven: Yale University Press.

Charmaz, K. (1983). The grounded theory method: An explication and interpretation. In: R. Emerson (Ed.), *Contemporary Field Research: A Collection of Readings* (pp. 109–126). Prospect Heights, IL: Waveland Press.

Chase, S. E. (1995). *Ambiguous empowerment: The work narratives of women school superintendents*. Amherst: University of Massachusetts Press.

Chase, S. E. (2001). Universities as discursive environments for sexual identity construction. In: J. F. Gubrium & J. A. Holstein (Eds), *Institutional Selves: Troubled Identities in a Postmodern World* (pp. 142–157). New York: Oxford University Press.

Chase, S. E., & Rogers, M. F. (2001). *Mothers and children: Feminist analyses and personal narratives*. New Brunswick, NJ: Rutgers University Press.

Chumdler, N. R., & Ford, T. E. (1998). The orientation of health professional students towards the care of older adults: The case of podiatry. *Health, 2*(3), 259–281.

Clarke, A. E., & Olesen, V. L. (1999). Revising, diffracting, acting. In: A. E. Clarke & V. L. Olesen (Eds), *Revisioning Women, Health, and Healing: Feminist, Cultural, and Technoscience Perspectives* (pp. 3–48). New York: Routledge.

Daviss, B. A. (2001). Reforming birth and (re)making midwifery in North America. In: R. DeVries, C. Benoit, E. R. van Teijlingen & S. Wrede (Eds), *Birth By Design: Pregnancy, Maternity Care, and Midwifery in North America and Europe* (pp. 70–86). New York: Routledge.

Davis-Floyd, R. (1992). *Birth as an American right of passage*. Berkeley: University of California Press.

Davis-Floyd, R. (1998a). The ups, downs and interlinkages of nurse- and direct-entry midwifery: Status, practice and education. In: J. Tritten & J. Southern (Eds), *Paths to Becoming a Midwife* (pp. 67–118). Eugene, OR: Midwifery Today.

Davis-Floyd, R. (1998b). Types of midwifery training: An anthropological overview. In: J. Tritten & J. Southern (Eds), *Paths to Becoming a Midwife* (pp. 119–133). Eugene, OR: Midwifery Today.

DeLee, J. B. (1940). *The principles and practice of obstetrics*. Philadelphia: W. B. Saunders.

Denzin, N. K. (1996). *Interpretive biography*. Newbury Park, CA: Sage.

DeVault, M. (1999). *Liberating method: Feminism and social research*. Philadelphia: Temple University Press.

DeVries, R. G. (1996). *Making midwives legal: Childbirth, medicine, and the law* (2nd ed.). Columbus: Ohio State University Press.

Faircloth, C. A. (1996). Reconstructing a life: Claiming themes of gay men in a heterosexist culture. In: G. Miller & J. A. Holstein (Eds), *Perspectives on Social Problems* (Vol. 8, pp. 135–153). Stamford, CT: JAI Press.

Foley, L., & Faircloth, C. A. (2000). The parenting self: Narrative resources and identity work in parents' stories. In: G. Miller & J. A. Holstein (Eds), *Perspectives on Social Problems* (Vol. 12, pp. 235–254). Stamford, CT: JAI Press.

Foley, L., & Faircloth, C. A. (2003). Medicine as discursive resource: Legitimation in the work narratives of midwives. *Sociology of Health and Illness, 25*(2), 165–184.

Foucault, M. (1977). *Discipline and punish: The birth of the prison*. Translated by A. M. Sheridan Smith. New York: Vintage Books.

Frame, M. W., & Shehan, C. L. (1994). Work and well-being in the two-person career: Relocation stress and coping among clergy husbands. *Family Relations, 43*(2), 196–205.

Fullerton, J. T., Shah, M. A., Schechter, S., & Muller, J. H. (2000). Integrating qualified nurses and non-nurses in midwifery education: The two-year experience of an ACNM doa accredited program. *Journal of Midwifery and Women's Health, 45*(1), 45–54.

Gagne, E., & Poirier, P. (1985). Interpretation of women's career choices from a sociological perspective. *The Journal of Educational Thought, 19*(3), 238–250.

Gardner, H. (1993). *Multiple intelligences: The theory in practice*. New York: Basic Books.

Garey, A. I. (1999). *Weaving work and motherhood*. Philadelphia: Temple University Press.

Garfinkel, H. (1967). *Studies in ethnomethodology*. Englewood Cliffs, NJ: Prentice-Hall.

Gearing, B. (1999). Narratives of identity among former professional footballers in the United Kingdom. *Journal of Aging Studies, 13*(1), 43–58.

Gerson, K. (1987). How women choose between employment and family: A developmental perspective. In: N. Gertsel & H. Gross (Eds), *Families and Work* (pp. 270–288). Philadelphia: Temple University Press.

Giddens, A. (1991). *Modernity and self-identity: Self and society in the late modern age*. Cambridge: Polity Press.

Glaser, B. G. (1978). *Theoretical sensitivity*. Mill Valley, CA: Sociology Press.

Glaser, B. G., & Strauss, A. L. (1967). *The discovery of grounded theory: Strategies for qualitative research*. New York: Aldine de Gruyter.

Glen, E. N. (1981). Occupational ghettoization: Japanese American women and domestic service, 1905–1970. *Ethnicity, 8*(4), 352–386.

Goldstein, M. S. (1999). *Alternative health care: Medicine, miracle, or mirage*? Philadelphia: Temple University Press.

Goleman, D. (1995). *Emotional intelligence*. New York: Bantam.

Gubrium, J. F., & Holstein, J. A. (1995). Life course malleability: Biographical work and deprivatization. *Sociological Inquiry, 65*(2), 207–223.

Gubrium, J. F., & Holstein, J. A (1997). *The new language of qualitative method*. New York: Oxford.

Gubrium, J. F., & Holstein, J. A. (1998). Narrative practice and the coherence of personal stories. *Sociological Quarterly, 39*(1), 63–187.

Habermas, J. (1975). *Legitimation crisis*. Boston: Beacon Press.

Hardill, I., Green, A., Dudleston, A., & Owen, D. (1997). Who decides what? Decision making in dual-career households. *Work, Employment and Society, 11*(2), 313–326.

Holstein, J. A., & Gubrium, J. F. (2000a). *Constructing the life course* (2nd ed.). New York: General Hall.

Holstein, J. A., & Gubrium, J. F. (2000b). *The self we live by: Narrative identity in a postmodern world*. New York: Oxford.

LaPointe, E. (2000). Ideological and structural constraints in holistic health care: Massage therapy as a case study. Paper presented at the Society for the Study of Social Problems in Washington, DC.

Lay, M. M. (2000). *The rhetoric of midwifery: Gender, knowledge, and power*. New Brunswick, NJ: Rutgers University Press.

Leavitt, J. W. (1986). *Brought to bed: Childbearing in America 1750–1950*. New York: Oxford University Press.

Litoff, J. B. (1978). *American midwives: 1860 to the present*. Westport, CT: Greenwood Press.

Loustaunau, M. O., & Sobo, E. J. (1997). *The cultural context of health, illness, and medicine*. Westport, CT: Bergin & Garvey.

Lyotard, J.-F. (1984). *The postmodern condition: A report on knowledge*. Translated by Geoff Bennington & Brian Massumi. Minneapolis: University of Minnesota Press.

Marini, M. M., Fan, P. L., Finley, E., & Beutel, A. M. (1996). Gender and job values. *Sociology of Education, 69*(1), 49–65.

Marvasti, A. (1998). Homelessness as narrative redemption. In: G. Miller & J. A. Holstein (Eds), *Perspectives on Social Problems* (Vol. 10, pp. 167–182). Stamford, CT: JAI Press.

Mathews, J. J., & Zadak, K. (1991). The alternative birth movement in the United States: History and current status. *Women and Health, 17*, 39–558.

McAdams, D. (1988). *Power, intimacy, and the life story: Personal inquiries into identity*. New York: Guilford.

McAdams, D. (1993). *The stories we live by: Personal myths and the making of the self*. New York: Morrow.

McAdams, D. (1996). Narrating the self in adulthood. In: J. E. Birren, G. M. Kenyon, J. E. Ruth, J. J. F. Schroots & T. Svensson (Eds), *Aging and Biography: Explorations in Adult Development* (pp. 131–148). New York: Springer.

Midwives Alliance of North America (1999a). Position statements. Retrieved April 20, 2000. http://www.mana.org/positions.html.

Midwives Alliance of North America (1999b). State board chart. Retrieved April 20, 2000.http://www.mana.org/stateboardcht.html.

Midwives Alliance of North America (1999c). State-by-state chart of legal status of direct-entry midwives. Retrieved April 20, 2000. http://www.mana.org/statechart.html.

Miller, G. (1997). Toward ethnographies of institutional discourse: Proposals and suggestions. In: G. Miller & R. Dingwall (Eds), *Context and Method in Qualitative Research* (pp. 24–44). Thousand Oaks, CA: Sage.

Mitford, J. (1992). *American way of birth*. New York: Dutton.

Mottaz, C. J. (1986). Gender differences in work satisfaction, work-related rewards and values, and the determinants of work satisfaction. *Human Relations*, *39*(4), 359–377.

Myers-Ciecko, J. A. (1999). Evolution and current status of direct-entry midwifery education, regulation, and practice in the United States, with examples from Washington State. *Journal of Nurse-Midwifery*, *44*(4), 384–393.

Osborn, A., & Esty, L. (1998). Standardized education: Does it prepare better midwives? In: J. Tritten & J. Southern (Eds), *Paths to Becoming a Midwife: Getting an Education* (pp. 23–24). Eugene, OR: Midwifery Today.

Payer, L. (1996, 1988). *Medicine and culture*. New York: Henry Holt and Company.

Randall, W. L. (1995). *The stories we are: An essay on self-creation*. Toronto: University of Toronto Press.

Randall, W. L. (1999). Narrative intelligence and the novelty of our lives. *Journal of Aging Studies*, *13*(1), 11–28.

Ronai, C. R., & Cross, R. (1998). Dancing with identity: Narrative resistance of male and female stripteasers. *Deviant Behavior*, *19*(2), 99–199.

Rooks, J. P. (1997). *Midwifery & childbirth in America*. Philadelphia: Temple University Press.

Rothman, B. K. (1991, 1982). *In labor: Women and power in the birthplace*. New York: W. W. Norton & Company.

Scroggin, J. (1996). How nurse-midwives define themselves in relation to nursing, medicine, and midwifery. *Journal of Nurse-Midwifery*, *41*(1), 36–42.

Sidel, R. (1990). *On her own: Growing up in the shadow of the American dream*. New York: Viking.

Slater, P. (1976; 1970). *The pursuit of loneliness: American culture at the breaking point* (Revised Edition). Boston: Beacon Books.

Sullivan, D. A., & Weitz, R. (1988). *Labor pains: Modern midwives and home birth*. New Haven: Yale University Press.

Todd, A. D. (1999). Robust resistance. In: K. Charmaz & D. A. Paterniti (Eds), *Health, Illness, and Healing* (pp. 337–346). Los Angeles: Roxbury Publishing Company.

Tritten, J., & Southern, J. (Eds) (1998). *Paths to becoming a midwives: Getting an education*. Eugene, OR: Midwifery Today.

Umansky, L. (1996). *Motherhood reconceived: Feminism and the legacies of the sixties*. New York: New York University Press.

Ventre, F., Spindel, P. G., & Bowland, K. (1995). The transition from lay midwife to certified nurse-midwife in the United States. *Journal of Nurse-Midwifery*, *40*(5), 428–437.

Weber, M. (1958, 1919). Politics as a vocation. In: H. H. Gerth & C. W. Mills (Eds), *From Max Weber: Essays in Sociology* (pp. 77–128). New York: Oxford.

Wertz, R. W., & Wetz, D. C. (1989, 1977). *Lying-in: A history of childbirth in America*. New Haven: Yale University Press.

Williams, D. R. (1999). Preserving midwifery in a managed care environment. *Journal of Nurse-Midwifery*, *44*(4), 375–381.

MENSTRUAL EXTRACTION, ABORTION, AND THE POLITICAL CONTEXT OF FEMINIST SELF-HELP

Denise A. Copelton

INTRODUCTION

In 1920 Margaret Sanger called voluntary motherhood "the key to the temple of liberty" and noted that women were "rising in fundamental revolt" to claim their right to determine their own reproductive fate (Rothman, 2000, p. 73). Decades later Barbara Katz Rothman reflected on the social, political and legal changes produced by reproductive-rights feminists since that time. She wrote:

> So the reproductive-rights feminists of the 1970s won, and abortion is available – just as the reproductive-rights feminists of the 1920s won, and contraception is available. But in another sense, we did not win. We did not win, could not win, because Sanger was right. What we really wanted was the fundamental revolt, the "key to the temple of liberty." A doctor's fitting for a diaphragm, or a clinic appointment for an abortion, is not the revolution. It is not even a woman-centered approach to reproduction (2000, p. 79).

This article is about a woman-centered approach to abortion and reproductive health more generally – gynecological self-help and home abortion.

Gynecological self-help constituted the basis of the women's health movement in the 1970s and included such things as small group discussions about women's bodies, cervical self-exam, diagnosis and treatment of minor gynecological problems, and menstrual extraction. Early scholarly work on the movement pointed to the importance of self-help healthcare (Bart, 1981; Marieskind, 1975;

Gender Perspectives on Reproduction and Sexuality
Advances in Gender Research, Volume 8, 129–164

ISSN: 1529-2126/doi:10.1016/S1529-2126(04)08005-1

Ruzek, 1978, 1981), but more recent work tends to focus on feminist health centers and other institutions with less focus on lay provision of services (Joffe, 1986; Morgen, 1990; Simonds, 1996). This shift in the academic literature may be a product of the institutionalization of the movement overall and a reflection of the staying power of bureaucratic organizations compared with loosely affiliated small groups engaged in direct service. However, self-help continues to play an important role in the women's health movement and despite its decreased visibility, self-help periodically resurfaces at key political moments. This article documents one such moment – the politically conservative, anti-feminist, and anti-choice late 1980s and early 1990s – a time when women's access to abortion was increasingly restricted across the nation. In particular, it examines the re-emergence of self-help gynecology and menstrual extraction in response to political threats to legalized abortion. I document the connections between this larger political context and participants' self-help activity by uncovering the meaning women attached to their participation in a home abortion self-help group. I provide evidence that the self-help roots of the women's health movement persist despite decreased visibility and argue that the feminist self-help health group highlighted here embodies the radical potential of self-help more generally.

METHODS

Data sources for this study include historical documents taken from the published newsletters of various women's liberation organizations, feminist health centers, and other groups active in the women's health movement. I also reviewed articles on menstrual extraction published in feminist and academic journals and conducted an extensive search of newspapers and other popular media for evidence and accounts of menstrual extraction and other lay abortion techniques in use during the late 1980s and early 1990s.

I conducted in-depth, semi-structured interviews with two members of a feminist self-help health group (Jennifer & Gail[1]) that operated in the early 1990s in an Eastern city I call Metrotown. Phone interviews were conducted with each of the women in November of 1998. Open-ended questionnaires were distributed in December of 1999 and follow-up phone interviews conducted in February 2000. My original goal in interviewing members was to uncover the meanings the women attached to their participation in the group. What motivated them to participate in a feminist self-help health group? How was participation in the group related to their own identities as feminists? How did their participation reflect larger political concerns? How did abortion generally, and menstrual extraction more specifically, fit into the larger concerns of the group? I was also interested in documenting characteristics of the feminist self-help health group itself. What were the original goals of the group and how did these change over time? What type of organizational structure was put in place to achieve those goals? Did the organizational structure change over time to reflect changing organizational goals?

Because of the limited number of interviewees, I cannot and do not claim that the remarks and experiences of these women are representative of women in other feminist self-help health groups. The particular self-help practice I was interested in studying, namely menstrual extraction, limited the availability of research subjects. Groups practicing menstrual extraction rarely make this practice known to outsiders because of the nature of the activity itself. Because menstrual extraction [ME] borders uncomfortably between self-care and home abortion, women practicing the technique often do not want to advertise this fact, let alone speak to an outsider such as myself, for fear of police infiltration. Both women I interviewed expressed concern about infiltration and potential arrest for practicing medicine without a license. Because the group had disbanded several years prior to the interviews, the interviews are subject to recall bias. However, the retrospective design helped to alleviate some of the problems of researching an illicit activity. The subjects were willing to discuss their experiences precisely because they were framed as past experiences rather than on-going activities. While membership in the group fluctuated over time, both of the women I interviewed were active for the duration of the group's existence and thus their experiences span the three phases through which the group passed: feminist self-help health group; abortion referral group; and feminist support group.

Methodological limitations notwithstanding, the qualitative data generated from this study provide a vivid illustration of how participants imbue their activities with political meaning and significance and provide a detailed portrait of the changing nature of the group over time. The interviews shed light on some of the problems and tensions inherent in the practice of ME as both a practical and a political act, findings that would not have been forthcoming from the historical research alone. In detailing the experiences of the group, I attempt to allow the women to speak for themselves as much as possible.

The women in the feminist self-help health group on which this study centers tended to be heterosexual, white, middle-class, and highly educated, characteristics typical of women involved in the early phases of the women's health movement (Ruzek, 1978). They ranged in age from their early twenties to mid-forties. Some of the women were mothers, some worked in the health care professions and others were students. They shared a desire for woman-centered health care and sought what they perceived as "natural" remedies and contraceptives. For instance, women within the group tended to reject hormonal-based contraceptives and tended instead to use barrier methods. This was consistent with their desire for more natural or at least non-medical health care. This also helps to explain how the group was able to practice menstrual extraction specifically as a home abortion technique. The higher failure rates of barrier as compared to hormonal birth control methods, paired with the group's preference for barrier methods, resulted in several unintended pregnancies. These and other women's unintended pregnancies offered ample opportunity for the women in the group to learn menstrual extraction as a lay abortion method.

SELF-HELP AND MUTUAL AID

The concept of self-help has gained tremendous popularity among both health-care consumers as well as providers (Katz, 1981, 1993; Katz & Bender, 1990). The term self-help, however, is often applied to a variety of different types of groups, some of which are explicitly feminist but many of which are not. A few words of clarification are thus in order.

What is Self-Help?

The concept of self-help is not new. As Katz (1981, 1993) argues, self-help has its roots in the mutual aid societies, trade unions, and friendly societies of 17th and 18th century England. When the mutual aid and friendly societies were transplanted to the American colonies, they were supported by working class identification and ethnic identification among new immigrants. Throughout the 19th century, trade unions played an important role in promoting the ethos of self-help in America through such activities as collective bargaining for better wages and working conditions and in their support of health insurance and pension plans (Katz, 1993; Katz & Bender, 1990). Various immigrant groups also established mutual aid societies that promulgated an ethos of self-help by offering housing, sickness and death benefits, and burial insurance to their members. But as immigrants became assimilated and working class families moved into the middle class, the mutual aid societies that served them weakened. In their place, a new breed of self-help groups emerged, particularly in the post-World War II period (Katz, 1993; Katz & Bender, 1990). These new groups retained the earlier focus on mutual aid, but added to this a new middle-class emphasis on personal fulfillment and empowerment.

Self-help groups today take many forms and focus on a variety of issues. They consist of large national organizations such as Alcoholics Anonymous to smaller local groups focusing on the unmet needs of particular segments of the population. An example of the latter would include dissertation-support groups at universities, and gay, lesbian, and bisexual support groups. Some groups adhere to a 12-step program, while others are less formally structured. Most are initiated by lay-persons or persons without any formal education or training (Katz & Bender, 1990). Disease-related groups, like Alzheimer's support groups, are often organized by family members of afflicted persons. In other cases, individuals sharing a common experience that lacks a formal disease designation may form their own groups and advocate for formal medical recognition of their affliction. Mothers suffering the baby-blues or post-partum depression are one such example (Taylor, 1996). Yet, some so-called self-help groups are organized by physicians or other professionals. These groups are much less critical of the business-as-usual definitions prevailing in a given arena (medical, psychological, etc.) and may be created with the explicit purpose of converting "troublesome" patients or clients into "good" ones, where these designations are defined by the professionals themselves. Such groups may exist as yet another means for monitoring patients and encouraging them to comply with the medical model (Zimmerman, 1987).

Despite the large number and divergent focus of self-help groups today, from Al-Anon to post-partum depression groups, Verta Taylor (1996) emphasizes the characteristics that most self-help groups share. These include: mobilization around a common experience, a focus on experiential knowledge, embracing mutual support, and an emphasis on societal change.

First, self-help groups "mobilize around some *shared experience*, characteristic, or problem that so resonates with participants' sense of 'who they are' that it becomes a basis for building solidarity with others" (Taylor, 1996, p. 19; emphasis in original). Self-help eschews professional knowledge and instead prioritizes experiential knowledge, though experiential knowledge does not necessarily conflict with professional knowledge. Self-help groups embrace the concept of mutual support and cooperation in problem-solving and endeavor to effect positive social change. While individual change may be an important goal of self-help groups, Taylor argues persuasively that self-help groups share the goals of other more conventional social movements.

> To the extent that self-help groups call attention to problems not being met by existing institutions, propose alternative conceptions of problems, support changes in the self-concepts and social identities of their members, and exert pressure on professional and public agencies to allocate resources for new solutions to problems, there can be little doubt that self-help promotes not only personal but *societal change* (Taylor, 1996, p. 20; emphasis in original).

Thus, self-help groups take many forms and focus on a wide variety of issues, but they all have the same basic foundational principles, particularly mutual support for a given experience or problem.

What's Feminist About Self-Help?

Self-help played a pivotal role in second-wave feminist organizing (Ferree & Hess, 2000; Gartner, 1990). Gartner maintains that "one of the most important expressions of self-help is found in the feminist perspective" (1990, p. 36). Self-help groups encompass the consciousness raising (CR) groups that fed feminist activism in the 1960s and 1970s. Gartner classifies women's self-help groups according to their dominant concern: women as mothers, women as workers, women as wives, women and health, and women and mental health. With regard to women and health, she explains, "While other self-help activities focus on a particular condition, the women's health movement encompasses the full range of concerns regarding women's bodies, bodily processes, and related health care" (Gartner, 1990, p. 41).

Not all self-help organizations are feminist organizations, however, even those that cater to the particular needs of women. Martin defines a feminist organization broadly as "any relatively enduring (exists for more than a few sessions or meetings) group of people that is structured to pursue goals that are collectively defined," (Martin, 1990, p. 185) that is "pro-woman, political, and socially transformational" (Martin, 1990, p. 184). Martin also identifies five dimensions that qualify an organization as feminist. The first dimension is endorsement of a feminist ideology, which can take the form of either an official or unofficial endorsement. Second, feminist organizations emphasize feminist values such as caring, cooperation and support. The third and fourth dimensions are related in that the third is the pursuit of feminist goals, and the fourth is the production of feminist outcomes. Finally, feminist organizations may also include those organizations founded as part of the women's movement. The women's self-help health groups founded during the 1960s and 1970s or later including the Feminist Women's Health Centers and self-help gynecology groups such as the Metrotown group exhibit all five of these dimensions.

THE WOMEN'S HEALTH MOVEMENT

The women's health movement in the United States coincided with and in many ways grew out of the women's liberation movement of the late 1960s and 1970s as noted above (Dreifus, 1977; Marieskind, 1975, 1977; Ruzek, 1978, 1980; Zimmerman, 1987). While the women's health movement consisted of many diverse groups, they shared a common and general goal – "improved health care for all women and an end to sexism in the health system" (Marieskind, 1975, p. 219). Activists in the women's health movement felt that medicine in general and physicians in particular mystified women's bodies. "So mystified and medicalized had their sexual organs become, that few women had ever seen them for themselves, or even wished to do so" (Ferree & Hess, 2000, p. 107). If physicians shared information about women's bodies at all, they did so in complicated scientific terms, thereby rendering such information inaccessible to those lacking formal training (i.e. most women). This lack of information paired with the power imbalances built into the doctor-patient relationship prevented women from becoming active health care consumers and relegated women to a passive role in encounters with physicians. Women's health activists held that women's treatment as patients by (male) physicians both reflected and reinforced unequal gender arrangements in U.S. society (Marieskind & Ehrenreich, 1975; Ruzek, 1978; Zimmerman, 1987).

According to Zimmerman (1987), the specific goals of feminist self-help gynecology are threefold: to encourage women's active participation in their own healthcare, to gain knowledge about women's bodies and health through research and writing, and to provide health care services directly to women. In her discussion of the activities and goals of the women's health movement Marieskind (1975, p. 220) also includes raising individuals' consciousness about gender and health-related matters, and changing existing health care institutions to better suit the needs of women and other groups.

Sheryl Ruzek (1978) credits Carol Downer with inventing self-help gynecology at the Everywoman bookstore in Los Angeles in 1971. "After exhausting 'book learning,' Carol Downer, a member of the group, urged empirical observation. That evening, Downer inserted a speculum into her vagina and invited other women present to observe her cervix" (Ruzek, 1978, p. 53). For many women, cervical self-exam and other self-help health activities served as an initiation into the women's health movement and into the women's liberation movement more generally. Cervical self-exam has even figured prominently in some women's studies courses. These activities provided the basis of the movement's critique of the mystification of women's bodies and the monopoly of knowledge by physicians. Self-help gynecology functioned as both a consciousness-raising technique and a means of providing health services directly to women within the group (Lanzerotti, 1992; Ruzek, 1978; Zimmerman, 1987). Groups progressed from self-exam to the diagnosis and treatment of gynecological infections, checking IUD placement, performing breast examinations, and recognizing the early signs of pregnancy (Federation, 1994; Lanzerotti, 1992; Ruzek, 1978). But as Ruzek notes, "Self-help gynecology is not simply 'do-it-yourself doctoring.' It involves conceptualizing health and illness in a fundamentally different manner... Women involved in self-help conceptualize routine health care as an ongoing process which eliminates or minimizes distinctions between providers and receivers, experts and lay persons" (1981, p. 564).

Zimmerman (1987) argues that the women's health movement has utilized two key organizational structures to realize its overarching goal of improved healthcare for women: political action organizations and self-help groups. Political action organizations are those which are "mainly concerned with effecting political, legal, and institutional changes through activities such as public information campaigns, lobbying, community organizing, and mobilization" and contemporary examples of these include the National Women's Health Network and the Black Women's Health Network (Zimmerman, 1987, p. 460). Self-help groups include a much more diffuse collection of activities and organizations than do political action organizations. Zimmerman describes feminist self-help health groups as:

> any gathering of women who share common experiences, health care information, and skills. Usually these groups are small, with half a dozen to a dozen participants . . . The immediate purpose of the self-help group is for women to learn about themselves through mutual discussion and sharing information, including personal experiences (1987, p. 455).

In their comprehensive history of the New Feminist Movement in the U.S., Ferree and Hess (2000, p. 102) distinguish among three different organizational types that emerged in the 1970s – direct action/self-help, educational/political, and cultural/entrepreneurial – and discuss women's health movement organizations as a primary example of direct action/self-help. While Ferree and Hess note that these different organizational types often function in supportive ways, they stop short of claiming that organizations may exemplify two or more types. The goals of the women's health movement and the groups that comprise it actually span all three organizational types. Collectives such as Jane engaged in direct action by providing abortion services directly to women. In providing direct services to women, feminist-owned and operated health centers, though typically not-for-profit, may also be seen as an example of an entrepreneurial organization. Organizations such as NARAL (first, the National Association for the Repeal of Abortion laws, later the National Abortion Rights Action League, and still later the National Abortion and Reproductive Rights Action League) acted in the political arena by pushing for the repeal of statutes prohibiting abortion and, after 1973, by protecting women's right to an abortion and lobbying around other reproductive issues. In short, the organizations that comprise the women's health movement are multi-faceted and diverse and therefore elude neat classification.

ABORTION AND FEMINIST SELF-HELP GYNECOLOGY

In the late 1960s and early 1970s, a major concern for both the women's liberation movement and the women's health movement was the repeal and/or revision of existing statutes prohibiting abortion (Marieskind, 1975; Ruzek, 1978; Zimmerman, 1987). Both movements held that the prohibition of abortion, combined with a general lack of accessible information about women's bodies, prevented women from becoming equal participants with men in many areas of social life. Women's liberation thus entailed access not only to safe, legal, and effective contraceptives, but also to safe, legal, and effective abortion.

For some women active in the movement, the legal prohibition of abortion necessitated women taking matters into their own hands. While some groups of women organized underground abortion referral networks, others became providers themselves. Underground abortion services such as the Jane Collective proved to some that abortion was a relatively easy procedure that need not be conducted by physicians in order for it to be safe (Bart, 1981; Just call 'Jane', 1990; Kaplan, 1995). Moreover, feminist self-help health activists maintained that it was not the criminal status of abortion that made it dangerous, as the success of the Jane Collective proved. Rather, it was the rampant profiteering in clandestine abortions and the hurried and uncaring manner in which these were frequently provided that led to the unsterile and dangerous conditions that characterized many back-alley abortions (Bart, 1981; Kaplan, 1995).

Menstrual extraction (ME) offered an attractive alternative to back-alley abortions prior to the 1973 constitutional affirmation of a woman's right to terminate an unwanted pregnancy. ME consists of manually extracting the contents of the uterus at about the time of the month when a woman would normally expect her menstrual period to begin or up until approximately eight weeks from the first day of the last menstrual period (LMP) (An Abortion How-To, 1979; Chalker & Downer, 1992; Federation, 1981; Rothman, 1978; Ruzek, 1978). ME has been used by women wanting to avoid their menstrual periods, as well as by women believing themselves to be in the very early stage of a pregnancy since the process of extracting the menstrual flow also extracts any fetal tissue present in the uterus (Chalker & Downer, 1992; Federation, 1981; Rothman, 1978; Ruzek, 1978).

ME advocates have been careful to note the key differences between ME and Early Uterine Evacuation (EUE), a medical procedure used in early termination abortion. Another similar procedure known as Menstrual Regulation (MR) has been used in many industrializing countries which have legal prohibitions against abortion, but which allow the use of emmenagogues prior to quickening. MR has been used successfully in countries such as Bangladesh to reduce the mortality and morbidity associated with illegal abortion (Dixon-Mueller, 1988). Though technically similar, the difference between these procedures and menstrual extraction lies not so much in the procedure itself, but in the context in which it occurs. ME is performed within advanced self-help health groups and unlike

EUE and other early surgical abortion methods in which a physician, abortionist, or other health care worker maintains control over the procedure, with ME "the woman having her flow extracted controls all aspects of the procedure" (Federation, 1981, p. 121). ME's focus on minimizing power differentials between providers and receivers stands in direct contrast to EUE and MR, indeed to all forms of medicalized abortion, where physicians and health care workers are clearly in control.

In 1971, self-helper Lorraine Rothman invented and patented the Del-Em, the standard device used in menstrual extraction (Ruzek, 1978). "A simpler version of the more cumbersome and expensive vacuum aspiration equipment that was being used by physicians for early abortions in the late 1960s" (Ruzek, 1978, p. 55), the Del-Em can be assembled with items located in the home and in medical supply stores, and at one time, could be purchased as a kit from the Federation of Feminist Women's Health Centers (Uzelac, 1989). The equipment consists of the following: a Mason jar, a 50 c.c. syringe, a one-way bypass valve (to create a vacuum and prevent air from entering the uterus), plastic tubing (aquarium tubing is frequently used), a rubber stopper, a speculum, and a small flexible cannula (An Abortion How-To, 1979; Chalker & Downer, 1992; Federation, 1981; Rothman, 1978; Ruzek, 1978). Because the cannula used is small and pliable, ME does not require anesthesia or cervical dilation, making it easier to insert and less likely to result in uterine perforation.

The menstrual extraction process involves several steps. The following is a description of a "typical" ME. Before any ME process is begun, and to determine whether ME is a viable option, the group must determine the approximate length of pregnancy. ME is appropriate for use as a lay abortion method only for very early pregnancies (usually defined as up to eight weeks past the last menstrual period or LMP), though groups may differ in their determination of a cut-off or point at which an ME would not be initiated. A pamphlet distributed by Anonymous Queers warns, "If you think you might be more than eight weeks pregnant, *do not* proceed with this method" (1992, n.p.). The first step in the overall process, then, requires experienced group members to check the size and shape of the uterus to determine the stage of a woman's pregnancy. If the group determines that the pregnancy is within an acceptable range, then the process can begin.

In the next step, the woman undergoing the extraction or another group member inserts a speculum. Stressing that women should play an active role in their own healthcare, some groups prefer that the woman undergoing the extraction insert the speculum herself. Another group member then inserts the cannula through the cervix and into the uterus. The syringe, which is connected to the cannula by the aquarium tubing, is used to suction out the contents of the uterus and the

Mason jar serves as a collection unit. As with the insertion of the speculum, the woman herself or another member may control the suction. Some groups have a strong ideological preference for the former, emphasizing the importance of the woman herself controlling the procedure and claiming that this arrangement allows her to adjust the speed of the procedure according to her own tolerance for pain and cramping. Another group member moves the cannula back and forth in the uterus as the suction is created. After the extraction, group members examine the contents of the uterus for chorionic villi to determine if the procedure extracted the fetal tissue. If none is detected, but a pregnancy was suspected, the group may repeat the procedure (Chalker & Downer, 1992; Federation, 1981; Rothman, 1978).

ME advocates maintain that the procedure is safe when performed by a knowledgeable and advanced self-help group. Advocates are quick to point out that their safety records compare favorably with those of first-trimester clinic abortions, though others disagree with this assessment. "The primary reason for this excellent safety record is the rigorous selection process any group doing menstrual extraction follows and the care with which the procedure is carried out" (Federation, 1981, p. 122). I address criticisms of ME in a later section.

When the landmark Supreme Court decision, *Roe v. Wade*, legalized abortion in 1973, many previously underground feminist abortion services began operating as legitimate businesses by forming feminist health centers and clinics. Others, like the Jane Collective and groups practicing ME, simply disbanded feeling that their services were no longer required. As one columnist wrote, "most menstrual extraction practitioners hung up their speculums" (Japenga, 1991, p. 56).

FEMINIST SELF-HELP AND ABORTION POLICY IN THE LATE 1980s

Most work on feminist self-help health focuses on institutionalized forms such as the Boston Women's Health Book Collective, the Federation of Feminist Women's Health Centers, and other feminist health clinics rather than on the more diffuse and transitory self-help groups (Joffe, 1986; Morgen, 1990; Ruzek, 1978; Simonds, 1996; Taylor, 1996; Zimmerman, 1987). Sheryl Ruzek (1978) provides one of the earliest and perhaps most significant works on the women's health movement. Published in 1978, it is limited only by its very timeliness. While it provides a detailed analysis of the movement through the 1970s, it cannot account for shifts in the movement over time. Other scholarly work on the movement has focused on feminist health clinics and abortion clinics. For instance, Wendy Simonds (1996) examines the ideology and practice of a feminist abortion clinic, documenting the contradictions sometimes inherent in the two. In a similar vein, Sandra Morgen (1990) investigates a feminist health center, scrutinizing the tension between individualism and collectivism. Carole Joffe (1986) details the experiences of front-line workers in a non-feminist family planning clinic affiliated with a national family planning agency.

The focus on institutionalized forms of self-help is in part a reflection of the difficulty in documenting the more temporary forms of feminist self-help health groups. It is also a product of the shifting character of the movement and is indicative of the changing meaning of self-help more generally. For instance, Zimmerman (1987) notes the decline in popularity of feminist self-help health groups by the early 1980s, while Taylor (1996) observes changes in self-help groups through the 1990s. Zimmerman (1987) offers several explanations for the decline of self-help within the women's health movement in particular. First, self-help has been coopted by mainstream medicine through its promotion of health education, preventive medicine, and individual responsibility in health. Ruzek (1980) notes that cooptation has been a common response to self-help activities that do not severely threaten physician dominance. While other aspects of feminist healthcare may have been coopted, the feminist practice of menstrual extraction, with its focus on leveling hierarchical relationships between providers and receivers of care, is too disruptive of existing power relationships for it to be incorporated into male-stream medical practice. Physicians have generally not been interested in empowering women in the way that feminist self-help gynecology aims to do. Thus, medical institutions have incorporated an ethos of individual responsibility in health care while stopping short of empowering women to be self-sufficient in matters of health and illness.

Another contributing factor to the decline of feminist self-help gynecology centers on its practical limitations. Zimmerman notes that "self-help is tedious, time-consuming, and requires a high degree of personal commitment" (Zimmerman, 1987, p. 459), characteristics that may limit the appeal of self-help to diverse groups of women.

During the course of her fieldwork at a feminist abortion clinic during the 1990s, sociologist Wendy Simonds participated in a self-exam training session. She describes this experience as follows:

> Self-exam no longer initiates women into a new movement; like a sit-in or a candle-light vigil, it feels like a ritual performance undertaken to revive a tradition, a way of connecting with the not-so-distant feminist past (1996, p. 41).

Though rituals or vigils may be empowering in their own right, for Simonds, self-exam did not serve the same functions as it did for earlier feminists. Self-exam was not a means of realizing larger political ends. It was spiritual, but not political. It "no longer initiates women" into the larger feminist health movement. Simonds' point is well-taken – cervical self-exam and gynecological self-help more generally have different meanings in different social and historical contexts. Simonds' encounter with cervical self-exam was during a feminist abortion clinic training session, and in such a setting self-exam may seem superfluous because of the immediate availability of feminist health care. Self-exam may be more necessary and thus, more empowering in the context of limited information about women's bodies, the outright absence of caring and adequate medical services for women (including abortion), or in the context of political threats to the availability of such services. For many women involved in gynecological self-help in the late 1980s and early 1990s, the practice was indeed empowering and not merely a "ritual performance" precisely because the political climate was so threatening.

The initial successes of the pro-choice movement spawned a strong counter-movement (Luker, 1984). This pro-life or anti-choice movement gained momentum throughout the 1980s with two successive anti-abortion presidents, Ronald Reagan and George Bush. In their comprehensive history of the feminist movement, Ferree and Hess label the period 1983–1992 one of " 'defensive consolidation' because much of the movement's efforts were directed at defending feminist perspectives and programs, and because such efforts required more extensive consolidation among feminist organizations" (2000, p. 159). The 1980s witnessed the passage of legislation intended to restrict women's access to legal abortion services. For instance, Missouri enacted legislation that prohibits the use of public facilities and personnel for elective abortions. The law also requires physicians to perform fetal viability tests when a woman is believed to be twenty or more weeks pregnant. The challenge to the Missouri law eventually made its way to the U.S. Supreme Court in 1989 in *Webster v. Reproductive Health Services*. Given the anti-abortion political climate, the *Webster* decision had the potential to reverse *Roe* all together (Harrison & Gilbert, 1993a; Key United States Supreme Court Abortion and Privacy Cases, 1990; NARAL, 1999). Many pro-choice and family planning organizations feared the worst. The Missouri law was upheld and the then National Abortion Rights Action League reported that, "for the first time in sixteen years since *Roe v. Wade*, only a minority of the Justices – four Justices – voted to reaffirm *Roe*" (NARAL, 1999). In 1992 in *Planned Parenthood of Southeastern Pennsylvania v. Casey*, the Supreme Court upheld a provision of a Pennsylvania law that mandates that physicians "counsel" patients on alternatives to abortion, including presenting pictures of fetuses at various stages of development to women undergoing such counseling, in order to discourage women from pursuing abortions. The Court also upheld those sections of the Pennsylvania law that place a 24-hour waiting period on all abortions performed in that state and require minors to obtain parental consent for an abortion (Harrison & Gilbert, 1993b; NARAL, 1999). In the *Casey* decision, four Supreme Court Justices voted to overturn *Roe* completely (NARAL, 1999). Needless to say, many pro-choice organizations and advocates were outraged.

For many women participating in gynecological self-help in the late 1980s and early 1990s, self-help was not an end in and of itself as it might have been for Simonds. Rather, gynecological self-help was a means to directly challenge the increasingly anti-feminist, anti-abortion climate. In such a climate, self-exam and the acquisition of the knowledge and skills needed to perform menstrual extraction were political acts as the experiences of the self-help group I highlight in the following sections demonstrate.

THE RE-EMERGENCE OF MENSTRUAL EXTRACTION

Menstrual extraction resurfaced in the late 1980s and early 1990s at precisely the same time that legal threats to abortion became louder and stronger (Bauerlein, 1992; Boston Women's Health Book Collective, 1991; Foreman, 1991a, b; Fried, 1991; Gehorsam, 1992b; Japenga, 1991; Kolata, 1989; Planning for the day, 1992; Punnett, 1990; Salstrom, 1992; Shepos-Salvatore, 1992; Toufexis, 1989). While it is difficult to establish how widespread menstrual extraction and self-help gynecology were during this time period, accounts in the mainstream as well as the feminist press do indicate that these groups spanned across the United States. Articles appearing in popular newspapers and magazines verify that ME was practiced in Atlanta, GA; San Diego, Hillcrest, Los Angeles, and LaJolla, CA; Cleveland and Toledo, OH; Washington, DC; Dallas, TX; Minneapolis, MN; New York City; and Boston. An article in the *Atlanta Constitution* reported that women connected with the Feminist Women's Health Center in Atlanta had begun practicing the technique there. The spokeswoman for the Center indicated that "the home abortion movement has attracted a small but growing supply of recruits since the U.S. Supreme Court rendered its *Webster* decision in 1989" (Gehorsam, 1992a, p. D1). In many cases the groups on which these articles focused had their roots in a feminist health center in the area. In other cases, groups formed after members of the Federation of Feminist Women's Health Centers visited their city and demonstrated the technique.

A key moment in the re-emergence of ME occurred with the production and distribution of the videotape, *No Going Back* in 1989. Directed by Carol Downer and distributed by the Federation of Feminist Women's Health Centers, the 28-minute video contains footage of actual menstrual extraction procedures along with discussion of the pro-choice/pro-life debate (Fenly, 1989; Fried, 1991; Japenga, 1991; O'Brien, 1989). Videos were originally packaged and sold with the Del-Em as ME kits. Complete kits sold for $89.95 in 1989, but sales were halted that year when the California Department of Health Services warned the Federation that sales were in violation of medical-device licensing laws. Thereafter, the video was sold separately for $25 (Fenly, 1989). Downer and other members of the Federation of Feminist Women's Health Centers also toured the country, giving presentations to various feminist organizations to promote ME and the video (Japenga, 1991; Uzelac, 1989).

Another key moment was the 1992 publication of Rebecca Chalker and Carol Downer's *A Woman's Book of Choices* which included a detailed description of the menstrual extraction procedure. A 1981 publication, *A New View of a Woman's Body* by the Federation of Feminist Women's Health Centers, also detailed the procedure but did not spark the same reaction as Chalker and Downer's 1992 book (Fried, 1991; Kaufmann, 1992). This is perhaps because legal abortion was not threatened in 1981 to the extent that it was in 1992.

During the April 1992 largely NOW-organized (National Organization for Women) pro-choice March on Washington, members of the organization Anonymous Queers[2] distributed fliers describing menstrual extraction and promoting its use as an alternative to women's dependency on physicians and clinic abortions. Embodying the radical potential of self-help, the group wrote, "Letting go of the belief that we need doctors to perform abortions will set us free" (Anonymous Queers, 1992, n.p.). While the group's presence at the march illustrated their support for abortion rights, a central feature of their pamphlet was a critique of mainstream pro-choice organizations. They called leaders of institutions such as NOW and Planned Parenthood "cowardly" for not engaging in more direct action in the form of civil disobedience. They urged protesters at the march to "look around at this demonstration. Imagine that all the women here know how to perform menstrual extractions. In that light things look quite a bit different, right?" (1992, n.p.). Thus, Anonymous Queers and other advocates of ME argued that the practice of ME was liberating and empowering in ways that the medical model of abortion was not. ME offered an alternative to abortions that depended on legal and medical institutions for their legitimacy. ME-induced abortions were therefore a powerful source of female empowerment and offered a first-line of defense against a political climate increasingly hostile to feminist concerns. ME represented a necessary corrective to male-dominated and male-centered legal and medical institutions that falsely claimed to represent the interests of women. In the late 1980s and early 1990s ME symbolized Sanger's "fundamental revolt," the "key to the temple of liberty" that promised a woman-centered approach to reproductive health and freedom.

THE PREVALENCE OF MENSTRUAL EXTRACTION

In a 1989 article, Shireen Miles, then associate director of the Federation of Feminist Women's Health Centers claimed that ME had been performed approximately 20,000 times in the U.S. (Fenly, 1989). In a 1989 article in the *St. Petersburg Times*, Carol Downer estimated that the number of MEs performed in the U.S. since the 1970s was close to 10,000 (Uzelac, 1989, p. 3A). She is again cited in a 1991 article in the *Washington Post* as putting that number around 20,000 (Trueheart, 1991, p. C7). While all sources point to a rise in the use of ME since the *Webster* decision, it is doubtful that the number of MEs performed between 1989 and 1991 would equal the number performed between the early 1970s when the procedure was first popularized and 1989, as Downer's estimates indicate. The variation in the estimates of ME is more likely a reflection of the difficulty of quantifying the prevalence of a clandestine procedure.

Another indication of the popularity of the technique during this time period is the inclusion of ME on the programs of two key women's conferences. In 1992, menstrual extraction was included on the programs of NOW's annual conference and the Black Women's Health Project's annual Wellness Conference (Women turn to self-help, 1992, p. C13).

CRITICS OF MENSTRUAL EXTRACTION

In October 1991, the *Washington Post* ran an article on menstrual extraction calling ME advocates "proselytizers" and pointing out the possible dangers of ME (Trueheart, 1991). Criticisms of ME were particularly forthcoming after the production of *No Going Back*. For instance, O'Brien (1989, p. L01) calls ME "a very bad idea," and *Newsweek* openly declares, "Coat hanger abortions may be a thing of the past, but the modern abortion-at-home equivalents don't look any better" (Do-It-Yourself Abortion, 1989, p. 25). The *Newsweek* article is instructive in that the author groups menstrual extraction together with a wide variety of dangerous at-home abortion techniques in his or her condemnation of "do-it-yourself abortions." These include such things as the use of cocaine and crack cocaine; ingesting large amounts of vitamin C, ginger and motherwart; and the use of implements such as coat-hangers. This reflects a popular stereotype that equates all abortions not conducted by physicians with dangerous back-alley abortions performed by butchers or quacks. Similarly, in a curious statement that links the rise of ME with the rise of the pro-life movement, one apparently pro-choice commentator states, "Now thanks to pro-lifers, we have a new breed of back-alley providers in training: women learning the menstrual extraction procedure in self-defense" (Dorrough, 1992, p. 3D). Calling ME advocates "back-alley providers" clearly connects the practice with other unsafe procedures. Critics of menstrual extraction come from all sides of the abortion debate and include groups and individuals that consider themselves pro-life and pro-choice, as well as feminist and non-feminist (Foreman, 1991a, b; Hamm, 1989).

Pro-Life Criticism

Pro-life or anti-choice groups denounced the practice of menstrual extraction while simultaneously claiming that it was not a serious threat to their movement. Pro-life groups were particularly strong during the late 1980s and early 1990s, buoyed by a rising tide of conservative politics (e.g. the Reagan era). Though short of their overall goal of overturning *Roe v. Wade*, pro-life groups were making gains nonetheless, as state after state enacted restrictive laws regulating abortion. Some pro-life groups interpreted the rise of ME as a sign of the very success of their movement. Randall Terry of Operation Rescue stated, "If women are killing their children at home, then it shows the abortion industry is on the ropes" (Gehorsam, 1992a, p. D1). It is important to note the illogic of their position. Since ME is a potential method of abortion, and because most pro-life groups oppose all abortion largely on moral grounds, pro-life groups *should have been concerned* with ME. Because of their overall strength, however, pro-life groups *did not have to be* overly concerned with ME. Still others active in the anti-abortion movement maintained that ME was a tactic used by pro-choice advocates to gain media attention and to sway popular opinion. The former President of the National Right to Life Committee claimed, "This menstrual extraction is completely some kind of PR gimmick to scare people and get some response. It is a bit of propaganda" (Japenga, 1991, p. 56).

Pro-Choice Criticism

Pro-choice doctors and groups such as the Planned Parenthood Federation of America (PPFA), the National Abortion Federation (NAF), NARAL, and the American College of Obstetricians and Gynecologists (ACOG) also denounced menstrual extraction on the grounds that the procedure was unsterile and unsafe and represented a return to clandestine back-alley abortions such as those associated with the pre-*Roe v. Wade* era (Japenga, 1991; Salstrom, 1992; Toufexis, 1989).

Several commentators equated menstrual extraction with home dentistry, drawing a parallel between the absurdity, pain, and danger of filling cavities at home and performing abortions at home. For instance, the President of the New Jersey Obstetrics and Gynecology Society claimed, "To me, it's almost like filling your own cavities: it can be done, but it's more painful. When you try to do your own medicine, it's like making your own parachute. It's just not smart" (O'Brien, 1989, p. L01). After making a similar analogy between home abortion and home dentistry, the Missouri board president of NARAL went on to support the widespread contention among ME advocates that the political climate was so hostile to abortion that "within the next two years, *Roe vs. Wade* will either be completely overturned or so severely gutted as to be completely ineffectual" (McGuire, 1992, p. 1E). Thus, while pro-choice physicians and groups may have been opposed to women "seizing the means of reproduction" (Bart, 1981), many agreed with ME advocates' grim assessment of the future of legal abortion.

Other pro-choice groups opposed ME on the grounds that their first priority should be ensuring that abortion remained legal. Thus, they opposed ME out of fears that endorsing it would detract from their efforts within the legal system (Hamm, 1989). Whatever the argument, it stands to reason that ME must have been practiced by more than a scattering of groups for such influential pro-choice organizations to make public statements denouncing it.

Feminist Criticism

Feminists have not been silent in their opposition to ME either. As early as 1971, Ellen Frankfurt warned about possible infection and wondered about the long-term effects of monthly menstrual extraction, sharing many of the concerns expressed by physicians (Frankfurt, 1972). In 1982 the feminist newsletter *Off Our Backs* published a critical review of *A New View of A Woman's Body*. The author interviews menstrual extraction pioneers Carol Downer and Lorraine Rothman, criticizing them for minimizing the risks associated with ME and for failing to collect more accurate statistics on the safety of the procedure (Fugh-Berman, 1982). Similarly, an article in *WomenWise* focused on the dangers of the procedure and repeated the oft-cited warnings of physicians. The following is characteristic of the variety of concerns expressed: "the doctors we spoke to felt it's easier to miss the pregnancy with such an early procedure, and it's very difficult to see the pregnancy tissue after the procedure to verify its success" (Hendrick & Hayes, 1994, p. 8). Clearly, the radical potential of ME – the fact that it is controlled by women and not doctors – is entirely overlooked by these authors who ironically accept the concerns of physicians wholesale.

In most cases, the problems identified by feminists as well as by pro-choice groups usually revolve around the fact that ME is a lay procedure, and as such, has not been studied scientifically. The problem for these critics appears to be that ME has not been institutionalized into male-stream medicine. ME is not acceptable because it has not been validated by scientifically rigorous clinical trials and is performed outside of the medical system. In their earlier and successful drive to legalize abortion, pro-choice groups and reproductive-rights feminists have so demonized non-medicalized abortion by equating it with back-alley, dirty, and dangerous techniques, that pro-choice groups are unwilling or unable to consider that safe abortion does not necessarily equal medicalized abortion.

By the term medicalized abortion, I do not mean medical abortion as distinguished from surgical abortion. The term medical abortion generally refers to an abortion induced by medical or pharmacological means; that is, with drugs. Forms of medical abortion include methotrexate and mifepristone induced abortions. Surgical abortion refers to the termination of a pregnancy through surgery. Medicalized abortion, on the other hand, includes both medical/pharmacological abortion and surgical abortion when these are performed by a physician or conducted within mainstream medical practice. Non-medicalized abortion, therefore, occurs through any means (pharmacological or surgical) *outside of medical institutions, organizations and practices*. Rothman explains medicalized abortion most astutely. "As experience and as institution, abortion is medicalized, constructed as a medical event, under medical control, and with the culture of medicine providing the meanings, defining women's experiences. Abortion occurs in clinics, in settings removed from women's lives, by people removed from women's lives" (2000, p. 76). A non-medicalized understanding and practice of abortion would return abortion to settings of women's choosing, would be under the control of the women and other members of her life, would be understood not as a medical event, but an event in which women themselves provide the meanings and define their own experiences. The practice and institution of abortion would therefore necessarily be woman-controlled and woman-centered and inherently feminist. ME abortions more closely approach this ideal than do clinic abortions.

Pro-choice institutions and individuals are critical of non-medicalized abortion, and ME more specifically, in part, because the success of ME as an early abortion technique diminishes the effectiveness of their most powerful argument for protecting the legal status of medical abortion. In an anti-choice climate, the one politically untouchable argument available to pro-choice groups is the issue of health and safety. If arguments concerning women's rights are superceded by arguments concerning fetal rights as was increasingly the case throughout the 1980s and 1990s, then pro-choice groups could still rely on health and safety as their ultimate trump card. Rather than pressing for abortion as an issue revolving around women's self-determination and equal participation in social life, which can be refuted by claims to fetal rights, abortion can be supported as a woman's health issue. The latter is much more difficult to refute. Yet, if abortion can be performed safely outside of the legal and medical context, then the validity of the health and safety argument is seriously diminished.

Furthermore, to divorce abortion from the medical system as ME does, is to divorce it from the prestige of the institution of medicine. As long as abortion is performed by doctors it can be linked to scientific legitimacy. Similarly, when clitoral manipulation was prescribed and performed by physicians as it was in the nineteenth century, it carried more legitimacy than when carried out by women themselves in the comfort of their own homes as it is currently (Maines, 1999). The former was understood as treatment, the latter as irresponsible sexual indulgence. The same assessment could easily be made with regard to medicalized and non-medicalized forms of abortion. Despite a general distaste for abortion (Imber, 1986), medical practitioners and organizations may also be reticent to disengage from the practice all together since it would weaken medicine's monopoly on women's reproductive health matters. Thus, while an ACOG spokesperson indicated that ME is "not effective," she went on to assert, "But if it is used, it should be performed by a *physician*" (Uzelac, 1989, p. 3A; emphasis added).

Thus, whether the early lessons provided by the Jane Collective and menstrual extraction practitioners were forgotten or conveniently overlooked in more recent and politically-charged times is not entirely clear. It is important to note that while the official position on ME taken by pro-choice organizations has been negative, supporters of these organizations may hold contrary views.

Responding to the Critics

According to ME advocates, the fact that ME has not been institutionalized into male-stream medicine is precisely why it is such an indispensable procedure in the quest for women's liberation. In defense of ME, reporter Ann Japenga asserts,

> Menstrual extraction is being taught in anticipation of a time when safe, clinical abortions will not be available. So the more apt questions would be: How does menstrual extraction rank against alternatives such as self-induced abortions using caustic substances and sharp objects? How does it compare to abortions performed by unskilled laypeople for profit? (Japenga, 1991, p. 56).

Moreover, advocates claim that the notion of a "do-it-yourself" abortion stands in direct contradiction to how the procedure should and indeed *must* be performed. That is, ME advocates maintain that ME has always been intended as a self-help technique that must be conducted by an experienced group, *not* by individual women (An Abortion How-To, 1979; Brody, Grusky & Logan, 1982; Chalker & Downer, 1992; Federation, 1981; Rothman, 1978; Ruzek, 1978; Salstrom, 1992). They maintain that it would be physically difficult and certainly dangerous for a woman to attempt to perform ME on herself. For instance, the Federation of Feminist Women's Health Centers wrote, "the isolated woman, who generally has little or no familiarity with her own body, is risking the dangers commonly associated with self-abortion" (1981, p.122). Thus, advocates hold that the concept of "do-it-yourself" abortion is inaccurate, reflecting a misunderstanding of the social context and practical limitations of the procedure. Nevertheless, the debate over ME is certainly far from over and feminists, physicians, and family planning, pro-life, and pro-choice organizations alike will continue to be divided on the issue.

THE METROTOWN FEMINIST SELF-HELP HEALTH GROUP

"The Basics" and Beyond

The Metrotown self-help group originally formed in 1991 largely through the efforts of two women, Margaret and Jennifer. Jennifer was 29 and a nursing student when she co-founded the feminist self-help health group that later developed into a home abortion referral group. She explained:

> Margaret was in a group in California and had trained at [a feminist health clinic] before she moved to Metrotown for nursing school. We became friends and she wanted to start a group in Metrotown. From comments I had made she suspected I would be interested. So we developed a core group of people and had them ask three other people.

The group formed as a feminist self-help health group with the goals of learning about their bodies, alternative and self-care, and menstrual extraction. Gail, another original member, explained the overarching goal of the group "[We wanted] to gain more self-knowledge of our bodies."

Some members of the group, like Margaret, had previous experience with feminist self-help. Gail, too, had been exposed to self-help some time earlier, though she had never been an active participant in a self-help group. Gail explained that she first became interested in self-help and menstrual extraction as a teenager when she experienced an unplanned pregnancy:

> I had already had one D&C and wanted to avoid another such experience. My boyfriend was friends with some women who had done self-help in the late sixties and still continued to practice a bit. We tried a home ME, unsuccessful due to my retroverted uterus. [But] I was impressed by the notion that one could do this at home, [though] I didn't pursue it at the time.

Margaret and Gail were the only two members with any background or experience with self-help and ME. For other members of the group, their first introduction to self-help gynecology was in the Metrotown group.

Meeting monthly in members' homes, they developed a steady membership of approximately eight women. As Jennifer explained however, "Membership shifted over time, with new people coming in. We may have got to about twelve at one point." The group started by reading books such as *Our Bodies, Ourselves* and *How to Stay Out of the Gynecologist's Office* and organized study groups on various topics such as premenstrual syndrome (PMS) and herbal medicine. They progressed to cervical self-exam and began diagnosing minor gynecological problems like yeast infections, and experimenting with herbal and other home treatments. Thus, the group began by participating in activities typical of other feminist self-help health groups throughout the women's health movement. As Jennifer aptly explained, "We did the basics."

The original aims of the group went beyond what some might consider "the basics," however. Both Gail and Jennifer explained that they also explicitly intended to learn and practice home abortion techniques such as menstrual extraction, practices often limited to the most advanced self-help groups. Jennifer explained that one of the group's major goals was "for each of us to learn procedures including ME that we could then teach to others and perform on others." Jennifer is clear that their intent was not just to learn the procedure themselves, but to actively share their knowledge and skills with other women through both performing ME and teaching others how to do so. This goal of promoting ME through teaching is tied to the group's estimation of the climate surrounding legal abortion at the time. The *Webster* and *Casey* decisions, the appointment of anti-choice judges to various courts, and an anti-choice President (i.e. Ronald Reagan) were all mentioned as significant factors motivating the group to learn and actively teach ME. Gail explained,

> [I wanted] to be prepared should legal access to abortion become threatened. I was motivated in large part by the climate around abortion rights at the time. *Webster* had just been decided and access to abortion was looking potentially shaky in the not too distant future.

The group learned about the pre-*Roe* underground abortion collective Jane and decided that they too might need to take matters into their own hands. If courts were restricting access to legal abortion, the group felt it was their duty as feminists to minimize the impact this would have on women's control of their reproductive destiny.

> It was possible we might have to go underground within the next few years, and I wanted to be ready to make that choice if it came to that (Jennifer).

Comments by both Jennifer and Gail reveal that the group believed that abortion rights would continue to be severely restricted, if not completely erased, in the near future. Both envisioned a time when abortion would be illegal. Learning and teaching ME in the self-help group thus functioned as a kind of apprenticeship, a training period in preparation for the day when abortion services would be forced "underground." While *Roe* was never completely overturned, members nevertheless *believed* that it would be. They thus felt justified in preparing for what they saw as the impending criminalization of abortion.

Jennifer is acutely aware of the fact that outsiders might view her and the group's activities and motives as radical or extreme. She defends her own and the group's rationale. "I know it might sound overly dramatic looking back, but nearly every month another court ruled for restricting access to abortion and the political climate was very hostile." In such a hostile environment, the group believed their actions were both rational and just.

THE ABORTION REFERRAL GROUP

The opportunity to learn home abortion techniques came fairly quickly. Jennifer remembers, "Pretty soon after we started, someone got pregnant. We were itching to learn [menstrual extraction] and we had a willing candidate." She explained that the group started to perform ME specifically as a home abortion method, not merely as a period extraction device, but added, "I think we might have tried one or two non-pregnants as practice." For the Metrotown group, the point of learning ME was never merely to allow members to avoid their menstrual periods. The "one or two non-pregnants" served as safe practice material, but the understanding was always that these were practice for completing ME on pregnant women. Thus, the goal always revolved around performing home abortions. Jennifer remarked that they did not have an opportunity to perform many procedures on non-pregnant women because the group "quickly had all the pregnants we could handle."

Both Jennifer and Gail explained that the group became "really busy for about six to eight months" (Gail) when they started a home abortion referral group. The term referral group is a bit misleading in that they were not referring women to abortion providers or to other groups doing menstrual extraction. Rather, they were taking referrals from another feminist self-help group in Metrotown and performing ME for outsiders. "We ended up hooking up with another group in Metrotown for abortions. We started a home abortion referral group which people had the option to join" (Jennifer).

Women both inside and outside the Metrotown group sought menstrual extraction abortions for a variety of reasons. Some women had previous clinic abortions and were critical of its institutional setting and practice. Gail described her own experience with an incomplete clinic abortion that resulted in a repeat procedure. "The lack of support was the hardest. I was alone and didn't know enough to understand that the continued bleeding was a problem." Two things are notable in her description. First, Gail links a general "lack of support" with her lack of knowledge of abortion and her inability to recognize complications, despite her brief prior experience with ME as described earlier. Second, Gail complains of being "alone" at the clinic. She elaborated, "The part that bothered me the most was being alone before, during [the procedure], and especially during recovery." Though a physician and nurse were with her during the procedure, Gail stresses her feelings of isolation. Sitting by herself in the recovery room and later at home, it is clear that she was unaccompanied by friends or other loved ones. Thus, her experience of clinic abortion cannot be separated from the larger personal contours of her life, but it also cannot be divorced from the institutional setting in which it occurred. The lack of support she experienced may also be due in part to the lack of counseling provided to her at the clinic. While most clinics maintain that they do indeed provide sufficient counseling and education to women seeking services, these may be limited to distributing written materials on follow-up care, without adequate explanation. This may be especially true in fast-paced clinics with a heavy client load that streamline the procedure in order to efficiently process the large number of patients. Gail likened her experience with clinic abortion to industrial assembly-line production. She explained, "I also hate being on the conveyor belt of clinic procedures – 'Do this now; now come here; now do this.' " Clearly, she disliked the lack of personal attention given to her as a patient and the lack of supportive education and counseling this entailed. She also disliked the way clinic staff barked orders at her and prevented her from becoming an active participant in her own care.

Thus, women had sufficient reason to prefer home abortion with ME over clinic abortion, the only other safe abortion alternative open to them. ME offered a more appealing alternative to Gail and other women with prior experience with clinic abortion. Nevertheless, the abortion referral group presented several logistical challenges related to the groups' fears of infiltration and arrest, follow-up care (particularly for incomplete abortions), and unrealistic expectations of the women seeking abortions.

The Local Practice of ME

The procedure that the group followed closely mirrored the descriptions of ME found elsewhere, with a few notable exceptions. Gail explained, "We would size the uterus, place a speculum, wash the cervix with betadine, [and] insert a small cannula." Gail was not entirely clear as to whether the speculum was inserted by the woman seeking the ME or by other members of the group. More likely than not, this practice shifted between the woman and group members, depending on the woman's own comfort level and familiarity with the process.

Gail continued, "When we got in [the uterus] we would evacuate the uterus by moving the cannula carefully around twice while applying vacuum pressure from a 60 cc syringe attached to tubing. One person would be in charge of the syringe. This job rotated a lot because your arms got tired." It is interesting to note that in Gail's description, her rationale for group members sharing the task of operating the syringe is purely practical – arm fatigue necessitated members taking turns. She gives no ideological rationale here as might be expected given the feminist goal of leveling power differentials and sharing responsibility.

The next step involved inspecting the extracted menses for chorionic villi to determine if the extraction successfully removed the products of conception. Gail explained, "If we didn't see any, we would do it again until we did, or until the woman asked us to stop." Repeating the procedure in the absence of chorionic villi is necessary in order to ensure a complete abortion and to prevent infection. One of the reasons why women might ask the group to stop at this point despite the need to continue may be the pain and discomfort involved.

The group's one major departure from the typical ME procedure described in most published accounts involved insertion of the cannula. The group utilized a tenaculum for holding open the cervix during insertion of the cannula because as Jennifer explained, "Getting in [the uterus through the cervix] was always the tricky part." This practice was not always adhered to, and disagreements over the use of the tenaculum surfaced within the group. These were not mere procedural disagreements, however. Rather, they reflected a deep-seated fear of discovery by unsympathetic outsiders like emergency medical personnel, who might report the group's activities to the police. The use of the tenaculum and its relationship to fears of infiltration are explored in more detail in the following section.

Infiltration

Both Jennifer and Gail felt that other members' apprehension over the use of the tenaculum was not warranted and identified Margaret, the group's co-founder, as particularly vocal in her opposition.

> Margaret was reluctant to use the tenaculum, partly because of not wanting to cause pain and partly because she thought if the woman presented later for medical care someone might suspect our activity through the marks left by the tenaculum. I always disagreed with her on this point. I

> thought using the tenaculum would make for a shorter procedure with less pain because getting through the cervix tended to be very painful and that there was no way anyone who happened to notice the marks would even think, "Hey, I wonder if this woman got her friends together and tried to abort at home?" (Jennifer).

Both Margaret, who opposed using the tenaculum, and Jennifer, who favored it, used the issue of pain to support their argument. The contention over use of the tenaculum indicates the degree to which fear of infiltration permeated group activities, to the point that it affected the techniques and instruments used.

An inherent tension existed between the stated goals of the group and the achievement of those goals. The goals of the group included practicing ME themselves and disseminating the procedure more widely. Yet, to achieve both goals in practice meant possibly exposing themselves to infiltration and arrest, thereby preventing them from further practicing the procedure and teaching it to others.

The fear of infiltration and arrest was not completely unwarranted. Group members were well aware of what has been dubbed the "Great Yogurt Conspiracy." In September 1972, Carol Downer was arrested and charged with practicing medicine without a license for inserting yogurt into another woman's vagina to treat a yeast infection. Arguing that applying a home remedy to cure a yeast infection is not practicing medicine without a license, Downer was eventually found not guilty (Ruzek, 1978). The verdict was hailed as an affirmation of a woman's right to control her own body. Nevertheless, the case served as a powerful warning to self-help groups throughout the U.S. that police and medical examiners were watchful and that the activities of self-help groups were potentially illegal. This may have been especially threatening to groups practicing menstrual extraction, since this procedure was much more invasive than merely inserting yogurt into the vagina. Thus, when members of the Metrotown group expressed concern over infiltration and arrest, they had in their minds an historical precedent on which to base those fears.

One technique used by the group to minimize the possibility of infiltration and arrest involved carefully screening women to ensure they were sympathetic to their cause. Gail explained that the pregnant women referred to them for ME were not complete strangers to members of the referral group, but rather were "mainly acquaintances – [they] knew someone who knew someone." However, even this level of familiarity did not stifle some group members' anxieties concerning possible infiltration.

Follow-up Care

The second challenge stemming from the abortion referral group, the problem of follow-up care for incomplete abortions, is perhaps the most serious. Jennifer explained, "It [ME] is not as effective a procedure as doing a D&C so there are more complications. Women need to understand the risks." One of the most serious risks associated with ME is an incomplete abortion in which some fetal tissue remains in the uterus. Excessive bleeding, hemorrhaging, and infection can result and if left unchecked could be fatal. Typically a repeat procedure will remove the remaining fetal tissue, but in other cases medical care may be required to subdue infection. Jennifer recounted one particularly bad experience:

> We had to repeat the procedure a couple of times. One of the women freaked out. She was a medical student. I kept telling her we had to redo it, we had to repeat it, but she wouldn't listen. It would have been different if she had been an active member of the group because we would have been able to get on her about it.

The problems with follow-up are apparent in Jennifer's story. Knowing the women as only acquaintances, the close affiliation and friendship network on which most self-help groups thrive and depend was absent in the referral group. As Gail explained, ME "works well with a group who know each other well, who have a group orientation." Outside of such a structure the group pressure that normally would have been exerted to facilitate the repeat procedure became much less effective. In other cases, the group was able to "get on" the women and the repeat procedure was successful. In the case of the medical student, she eventually reported to a local emergency room explaining that she thought she might have suffered a miscarriage.

Gail linked the problems with follow-up to the fact that outsiders were not personally committed to the goals of feminist self-help healthcare. "The problem with the referral group was that [the women who were referred to us] were just looking for abortions. They weren't taking responsibility for untoward outcomes" (Gail). The term "untoward outcomes" is, of course, a nicer way of saying "incomplete abortions" or "failures." Gail's careful phrasing here may indicate an attempt by either Gail herself or by the group as a whole to minimize problems or complications related to ME. Though Jennifer notes above that ME does involve risks and that its efficacy is below that of a D&C, Gail clearly believes that the complications that periodically arose were tied to the level of commitment of the woman undergoing the extraction, rather than to problems inherent in the procedure itself or to problems inherent in feminist self-help gynecology.

Utopian Health Care – Dealing with Unrealistic Expectations

Another challenge presented by the referral group concerned the outsiders' unrealistic expectations of menstrual extraction. Jennifer and Gail recounted the care the group took to explain the procedure fully and realistically to the women referred to them. But just as some commentators have stereotyped ME as a back-alley abortion and equated it with dangerous coat hanger techniques, some women seeking ME from the group equated the procedure with a rosy vision of utopian feminist health care.

> We had to be really careful in screening people. [We had to be sure] that they didn't think it was only going to be wonderful. [Some women] just wanted to remove the unpleasantness [of abortion], which is inherent in the process (Jennifer).

Even the most careful screening and education did not prepare some of the women for the procedure if they clung to this utopian vision of feminist abortion practice, a vision that the Metrotown group themselves exemplified in certain ways and fell short of in others.

STRUCTURAL CHANGE OVER TIME

Power Imbalances

One of the ways that the Metrotown group fell short of the ideals of feminist self-help gynecology is in the ways that power imbalances surfaced within the group. Not all information was shared equally among group members. This was obvious from the different responses I received to a question concerning equipment and supplies.

> DC: What materials and supplies did the group use for these activities and where and how did the group obtain these materials?
> Jennifer: Margaret obtained the supplies. I never asked where she got them from. We had a tenaculum, and cannulas, tubing, syringes, and a collecting bottle.

Gail believed the supplies were obtained from the Feminist Women's Health Center, most likely through Margaret's associations there, though she too was not exactly sure. Given that several of the women were nursing students, and others worked in health services, it is entirely possible that supplies could have been obtained through these connections as well. The women's "ignorance" of where supplies were acquired may very well be a function of how they were acquired, particularly if this was done through their health services contacts. Moreover, these exchanges indicate that a certain level of secrecy was maintained within the group, with some members, namely Margaret, exhibiting a good deal more knowledge and power than other members. It was clear throughout the interviews that Margaret was the distinct, if unofficial, leader of the group. She initiated the group's formation, was a major source of knowledge within the group, obtained many of the supplies, and exerted considerable influence over the particulars of the ME procedure including the use of the tenaculum, which was eventually abandoned at her request.

Group Transformation and Demise

The technical difficulties with follow-up care, fear of infiltration and arrest, personal issues, and changes in the larger political climate surrounding abortion rights combined to eventually lead several key members to re-evaluate the referral group altogether. Members became less inclined to provide menstrual extraction services to women outside the immediate group, shifting the group's focus away from its original political goals of learning and teaching the procedure and facilitating its transformation into a feminist support group.

The group remained active for a number of years, and disbanded "little by little." Neither Gail nor Jennifer could be sure when exactly the group dispersed. Jennifer thought the group existed for "two to three years," remembering that "it started in 1992, spring, and disbanded in 1994." Gail estimated that the group lasted for a total of "three or four years," starting in 1991. Jennifer mentioned a number of different reasons for the group's eventual demise. Some members moved away and others simply lost interest.

> Some people had not been terribly interested in direct self-help beyond familiarizing themselves with the procedures and once that was accomplished they wanted to turn the group into a support/discussion group, which it became for about another year.

Both Jennifer and Gail remained active in the group throughout its various transformations – from its initial formation as a feminist self-help gynecology group to the home abortion referral group to the support group. Gail offered another explanation for its changing character and makeup when she pointed out that "the immediate group members stopped getting pregnant. One experience was enough." While core members like Gail and Jennifer continued with the abortion referral group, others less interested in the direct provision of abortion services stayed active only in the support group or dropped out altogether.

Gail also notes the relationship between the group's eventual demise and their fears of infiltration. She recalled that the publication of *A Woman's Book of Choices* in 1992, which detailed the menstrual extraction procedure and advocated it as an alternative to clinical and physician provided abortions, caused some concern for the Metrotown group. Several women active in the group, particularly those who participated in the abortion referral group, felt the book would bring public scrutiny to their activities. As Gail notes, "It freaked out the people who were doing it." While the book did not identify any particular groups currently practicing ME, and certainly did not point the finger at the Metrotown group, the women were frightened of the heightened public awareness of ME that the book inevitably brought. They were content with providing home abortions to women as long as they felt comfortable and safe to do so, but the book simply made them feel increasingly threatened. Gail commented that the public awareness of ME brought about by Chalker and Downer's book also tended to reduce the need for their services, though this explanation seems less plausible.

The final explanation that both Gail and Jennifer offered, however, stemmed from the rationale behind the group's initial formation. As Gail articulated, "the political climate eased up and it looked like our skills would not be required just yet."

The experiences of and transformations within the Metrotown group offer insight into the political nature of self-help activities like menstrual extraction. Members of the group defined their activities as indispensable in the face of escalating anti-abortion legislation. As the political situation changed, however, so too did members' assessment of the necessity of the group. When the political situation seemed less threatening, members characterized the actual provision of menstrual extraction as less important, and eventually characterized the group's very existence as a feminist self-help health group as less important as well.

THE CHALLENGE OF MEDICAL ABORTION

Several changes have occurred in both the medical and political landscape since the demise of the Metrotown group and the resurgence of ME in the late 1980s and early 1990s. In particular, a new, legal abortion method has become available in the U.S. – medical abortion with either mifepristone or methotrexate. The U.S. Food and Drug Administration's (FDA) approval of mifepristone (formerly known as RU 486) in September 2000, was hailed by women's health advocates as a milestone for women's reproductive choice. Like ME, mifepristone is used for early termination abortion. Unlike ME, however, which is generally used only up to eight weeks LMP, mifepristone can be used up to 49 weeks LMP. Mifepristone may be useful to a larger number of women since it can be used later, when an unwanted pregnancy can be more easily identified. Unless it is used on a monthly basis, women wishing to use ME must have fairly regular menstrual periods and be able to recognize the early symptoms of pregnancy. Mifepristone was preceded by the "off-label"[3] use of methotrexate for elective medical abortion as early as 1993 and has also been used for the treatment of ectopic (tubal) pregnancy. Both mifepristone and methotrexate are used in conjunction with a prostaglandin, typically misoprostol, to aid expulsion.

Except in states that give prescription privileges to non-physicians, medical abortion using methotrexate requires the cooperation of a physician. The use of mifepristone for medical abortion requires the cooperation of a physician in *every* state because of stipulations set out by the FDA at the time of the drug's approval. The FDA mandated that mifepristone must not be dispensed through pharmacists, but rather through qualified physicians who have signed a Prescriber's Agreement and established an account directly with Danco, the sole U.S. distributor. This was done largely in the hopes of ensuring that the drug did not fall outside of the control of medical practitioners (FDA, "Memo to Population Council") and into the hands of laypersons.[4] Furthermore, FDA restrictions have severely limited the use of mifepristone for off-label purposes, including purposes other than abortion, and according to protocols not tested in the U.S. clinical trials. Thus, while trials outside the U.S. indicate that mifepristone can be safely administered by women themselves outside of a doctor's office, self-administration has not been approved for use in the U.S. Women must take the drug in the presence of a physician and altering this protocol will place the physician in violation of the Prescriber's Agreement. These restrictions place mifepristone clearly within the realm of medicalized abortion and therefore severely undercut its radical potential.

While both mifepristone and methotrexate offer an alternative to surgical procedures, neither offers an alternative to *medicalized* abortion. While pro-choice feminists had to overcome great political obstacles in order to bring mifepristone into the U.S., they did so by forging alliances with pro-choice physicians, politicians, and family-planning organizations, thus leaving the medical monopoly on abortion unscathed. The radical potential of ME derives from the fact that it is a woman-centered, woman-controlled abortion method that exists outside the medical model. The conditions of mifepristone's approval ensure that it remains firmly entrenched *within* the medical model.

This is not to say that women cannot find ways to "seize the means of reproduction" (Bart, 1981) with medical abortion, as they have done with surgical abortion. In fact, women have already done just that. For example, Gail recounted her own experience with medical abortion using methotrexate and compared this to her previous surgical abortion experiences. Because of connections she had in the medical community, she was able to obtain a prescription for methotrexate and misoprostol. She explained, "I did it at home the day I chose, and had several friends with me. I got to recover in my own bed." While she noted that "it hurt a lot more and a lot longer" than her previous surgical abortions, she felt that "it was exciting to be doing it by myself. It was a lot more autonomous . . . I would never do it any other way. A home abortion allows the woman all the support and freedom she needs."

Yet, an at-home medical abortion like Gail's, with either methotrexate or mifepristone, may be inaccessible to most women. Gail was able to use methotrexate at home only because her close healthcare contacts were willing to go to great lengths to help her obtain the supplies of the drugs she needed. Given the present restrictions on medical abortion, most women will not be able to obtain the methotrexate or mifepristone regimen. Thus, for the time being, medical abortion is likely to remain firmly within the medical arena.

To paraphrase Rothman, medical abortion, like surgical abortion before it is not the fundamental revolt. It is not a woman-centered or woman-controlled approach to reproduction. Menstrual extraction, on the other hand, remains the only non-medicalized, woman-centered abortion alternative. While the majority of women do not participate or know someone who participates in gynecological self-help, the information necessary to do so is readily available in feminist publications. Yet, the question remains – is menstrual extraction a viable alternative to legalized abortion? As critics have maintained, if abortion rights were completely erased or severely restricted within the next several years (which is plausible given abortion-foe George W. Bush's current leadership), it appears that ME itself would only help a small percentage of those in need of abortion services. This is the case not only because of the lack of trained practitioners and the uncertain legal status surrounding ME, but also because of limitations built into the procedure itself – namely, that it is effective only up until about eight weeks LMP. After that point, it is increasingly likely that the extraction may miss the pregnancy or that the low-level suction used would not be enough to remove the pregnancy tissue.

The more important question for feminist social scientists seems to be not whether ME is a viable or practical alternative to legal abortion. Rather, the question remains – what lessons can be gleaned from the most recent resurgence of menstrual extraction? Practical issues aside, menstrual extraction is a powerful symbolic affirmation of a woman's right to control her reproductive destiny. It illustrates feminist resilience in the face of strong political threats to women's hard-earned rights. It serves as a powerful example, indeed, one of only a few examples of feminist alternatives to medicalized abortion.

CONCLUSION

Women's health activists pioneered self-help gynecology and menstrual extraction in the early 1970s. With the advent of legal abortion and the cooptation of many of the movement's initial interests by mainstream medicine, self-help gynecology waned. It resurfaced in the late 1980s and early 1990s as a response to the anti-abortion political climate and the erosion of women's right to safe and legal abortion. The political aims of the group I studied, which appear to reflect those of other feminist self-help groups at the time, were recounted succinctly by Gail: "It's not a matter of *if* abortion will happen, it is a matter of *in what context* it will happen." Many feminist self-help health groups pledged to provide abortions in a caring, humane, safe context in which women themselves could play an active role, should *Roe* be overturned. When *Roe* was not overturned many of these groups disbanded. Nevertheless, the political impact will be felt for generations since the knowledge participants acquired will remain and resurface again should abortion rights be severely threatened in the future. With abortion foe George W. Bush currently in the White House parroting the sentiments of anti-choice groups across the country, severe threats to abortion rights loom large on the horizon. Thus, conditions may be ripe for yet another re-emergence for menstrual extraction. Women will continue to "rise up in fundamental revolt" in pursuit of "the key to the temple of liberty." Menstrual extraction remains one element of that key.

NOTES

1. All names have been changed, including the names of non-participants whom interviewees mentioned during the course of the interviews.
2. It is not entirely clear whether the name Anonymous Queers refers to a distinct organization or whether it is used to describe a more loosely affiliated group. Thanks to Jessica Nathanson for bringing this pamphlet to my attention.
3. "Off-label" use refers to prescribing a drug for a purpose other than that for which it was tested and labeled. For a discussion of the issues surrounding the use of methotrexate for medical abortion and the legality of "off-label" uses of FDA approved drugs, see Lakomy (1996).
4. For a fuller discussion of the political and social ramifications of the FDA approval process for mifepristone, see Copelton (2002).

ACKNOWLEDGMENTS

An earlier version of this paper entitled, "Menstrual Extraction as a Woman-Centered Home Abortion Method. The Experience of One Feminist Self-Help Health Group" was presented at the Annual Meeting of the Midwest Sociological Society, April 19–22, 2000 in Chicago. I would like to thank the following people for commenting on earlier drafts: Brian Fletcher, Mary K. Zimmerman, Jessica Nathanson, and Janet Dean. I would also like to express my gratitude to those anonymous women who agreed to be interviewed for this research. This paper would not have been possible without their help and courage.

REFERENCES

An Abortion How-To (1979). *WomenWise*, *2*(3), 6.

Anonymous Queers (1992). *Do it yourself abortion* [Brochure].

Bart, P. (1981). Seizing the means of reproduction: An illegal feminist abortion collective – how and why it worked. In: H. Roberts (Ed.), *Women, Health, and Reproduction* (pp. 109–128). Boston: Routledge & Kegan Paul.

Bauerlein, M. (1992). Life after *Roe v. Wade*. *Utne Reader* (May/June), 17–20.

Boston Women's Health Book Collective (with B. Reinhard) (1991). Resurgence of self-help programs. *Ms.*, *2*, 94.

Brody, D., Grusky, S., & Logan, P. (1982). Self-help health. *Off Our Backs*, *12*(7), 14.

Chalker, R., & Downer, C. (1992). *A woman's book of choices: Abortion, menstrual extraction, RU-486*. New York: Four Walls, Eight Windows.

Copelton, D. (2002). Assessing of the social impact of mifepristone in the U.S.: A pro-choice perspective. *Kansas Journal of Law and Public Policy*, *11*, 333–362.

Dixon-Mueller, R. (1988). Innovations in reproductive health care: Menstrual regulation policies and programs in Bangladesh. *Studies in Family Planning*, *19*, 129–140.

Do-it-yourself abortion is dangerous to your health (1989). *Newsweek*, *25*.

Dorrough, V. (1992). League of women voters' stand on abortion is defended. *St. Petersburg Times* (August 16, p. 3D). Retrieved March 1, 2000, from Lexis-Nexis database.

Dreifus, C. (1977). *Seizing our bodies: The politics of women's health*. New York: Vintage Books.

Federation of Feminist Women's Health Centers (1981). *A new view of a woman's body*. New York: Touchstone.

Federation of Feminist Women's Health Centers (1994). Helping ourselves: The first self-help clinic. *Organizing Strategies in Women's Health: An Information and Action Handbook* (Jan. 31), 59.

Fenly, L. (1989). Abortion kit earns friends, enemies. *San Diego Union-Tribune, Lifestyle Section*, *1* (August 21). Retrieved March 15, 2000 from Lexis-Nexus database.

Ferree, M. M., & Hess, B. B. (2000). *Controversy and coalition: The new feminist movement across four decades of change*. New York: Routledge.

Food and Drug Administration, Center for Drug Evaluation and Research (2000). *Office memo to population council* [On-line]. Available: http://www.fda.gov/cder/drug/infopage/mifepristone/memo.pdf.

Foreman, J. (1991a). Going underground: Self-help groups teach 'menstrual extraction' abortion method, but feminists are divided over method's safety, legality. *Houston Chronicle*. *Lifestyle Section*, *7* (September 22). Retrieved March 1, 2000, from Lexis-Nexis database.

Foreman, J. (1991b). 'Home abortion' safety issues a pro-choice dilemma. *The Boston Globe* (August 26). Science and Technology Section, 33.

Frankfurt, E. (1972). *Vaginal politics*. New York: Bantam.

Fried, D. L. (1991). Activists promote home abortion technique. *San Diego Union-Tribute* (November 17, B1). Retrieved March 1, 2000, from Lexis-Nexis database.

Fugh-Berman, A. (1982). Self-help: The movement and a book. *Off Our Backs*, *12*(7), 14.

Gartner, A. (1990). A typology of women's self-help groups. In: A. H. Katz & E. I. Bender (Eds), *Helping One Another* (pp. 35–45). Oakland, CA: Third Part Publishing.

Gehorsam, J. (1992a). In the hands of women; as legal hopes dim, home abortions gain advocates. *The Atlanta Journal and Constitution* (January 7, D1). Retrieved March 1, 2000, from Lexis-Nexis database.

Gehorsam, J. (1992b). Legal climate spurs home abortion advocates. *St. Louis Post-Dispatch, Everyday Magazine* (February 6, 1E). Retrieved March 1, 2000, from Lexis-Nexis database.

Hamm, S. (1989). Women's groups endorse legal abortion over self-help aids. *BC Cycle, United Press International* (November 14). Retrieved March 1, 2000, from Lexis-Nexis database.

Harrison, M., & Gilbert, S. (Eds) (1993a). *Abortion decisions of the U.S. Supreme Court: The 1980s*. Beverly Hills, CA: Excellent Books.

Harrison, M., & Gilbert, S. (Eds) (1993b). *Abortion decisions of the U.S. Supreme Court: The 1990s*. Beverly Hills, CA: Excellent Books.

Hendrick, S., & Hayes, A. P. (1994). Remembering EUE. *WomenWise, 17*(2), 8.

Imber, J. B. (1986). *Abortion and the private practice of medicine*. New Haven, CT: Yale University Press.

Japenga, A. (1991). The new abortionists. *In Health, 5*, 50–57.

Joffe, C. (1986). *The regulation of sexuality*. Philadelphia: Temple University Press.

Just call 'Jane' (1990). In: M. G. Fried (Ed.), *From Abortion to Reproductive Freedom: Transforming a Movement* (pp. 93–100). Boston: South End Press.

Kaplan, L. (1995). *The story of Jane*. NY: Pantheon.

Katz, A. H. (1981). Self-help and mutual aid: An emerging social movement? *Annual Review of Sociology, 7*, 129–155.

Katz, A. H. (1993). *Self-help in America: A social movement perspective*. New York: Twayne.

Katz, A. H., & Bender, E. I. (1990). *Helping one another: Self-help groups in a changing world*. Oakland, CA: Third Party Publishing.

Kaufmann, K. (1992). Reproductive options for women. *San Francisco Chronicle, Sunday Review, 5* (November 29). Retrieved March 1, 2000, from Lexis-Nexis database.

Key United States Supreme Court abortion and privacy cases (1990). In: M. G. Fried (Ed.), *From Abortion to Reproductive Freedom: Transforming a Movement* (pp. 45–48). Boston: South End Press.

Kolata, G. (1989). As new tactic, do-it-yourself abortions taught. *New York Times*, (October 23, B12). Retrieved March 1, 2000, from Lexis-Nexis database.

Lakomy, M. (1996). A meaningful choice: Two FDA approved drugs are combined to perform medical abortions. *Women's Rights Law Reporter, 18*, 49–65.

Lanzerotti, R. (1992). Women's health in women's hands: Practices and politics of self-help groups. *Sojourner, 17*(7), 5H.

Luker, K. (1984). *Abortion and the politics of motherhood*. Berkeley, CA: University of California Press.

Maines, R. (1999). *The technology of orgasm*. Baltimore, MD: Johns Hopkins University Press.

Marieskind, H. (1975). The women's health movement. *International Journal of Health Services, 5*(2), 217–223.

Marieskind, H. (1977). The women's health movement: Past roots. In: C. Dreifus (Ed.), *Seizing Our Bodies* (pp. 3–12). New York: Vintage Books.

Marieskind, H. I., & Ehrenreich, B. (1975). Towards socialist medicine: The women's health movement. *Social Policy*, Sept/Oct, 34–42.

Martin, P. (1990). Rethinking feminist organizations. *Gender and Society, 4*(2), 182–206.

McGuire, J. M. (1992). Groups not seen here yet. *St. Louis Post-Dispatch, Everyday Magazine* (February 6, 1E). Retrieved March 1, 2000, from Lexis-Nexis database.

Morgen, S. (1990). Contradictions in feminist practice: Individualism and collectivism in a feminist health center. *Comparative Social Research, 1*, 9–59.

NARAL (National Abortion and Reproductive Rights Action League) (1999). Supreme Court decisions concerning reproductive rights: A chronology, 1965–1998. Retrieved September 21, 1999 from http://www.naral.org/publications/whod.html.

O'Brien, K. (1989). An outlaw operation. *The Record* (September 17, L01). Retrieved March 1, 2000, from Lexis-Nexis database.

Planning for the day that abortions are restricted (1992). *U.S. News and World Report, 64* (May 11). Retrieved March 1, 2000, from Lexis-Nexis database.

Punnett, L. (1990). The politics of menstrual extraction. In: M. G. Fried (Ed.), *From Abortion to Reproductive Freedom: Transforming a Movement* (pp. 45–48). Boston: South End Press.

Rothman, B. K. (2000). *Recreating motherhood.* New Brunswick, NJ: Rugers University Press.

Rothman, L. (1978). Menstrual extraction: Procedures. *Quest: A Feminist Quarterly, 4*(3), 44–48.

Ruzek, S. (1978). *The women's health movement: Feminist alternatives to medical control.* New York: Praeger.

Ruzek, S. (1980). Medical responses to women's health activities: Conflict, accommodation and cooptation. *Research in the Sociology of Health Care, 1*, 335–354.

Ruzek, S. (1981). The women's self-help health movement. In: P. Conrad & R. Kern (Eds), *The Sociology of Health and Illness* (pp. 563–570). New York: St. Martin's.

Salstrom, R. (1992). Menstrual extraction: Is self-help making a comeback? *WomenWise, 15*(1), 6.

Shepos-Salvatore, K. (1992). Menstrual extraction: Women take control. *Off Our Backs, 22*(4), 1.

Simonds, W. (1996). *Abortion at work: Ideology and practice in a feminist clinic.* New Brunswick, NJ: Rutgers.

Taylor, V. (1996). *Rock-a-by baby: Feminism, self-help, and postpartum depression.* NY: Routledge.

Toufexis, A. (1989). Abortions without doctors. *Time, 134*, 66.

Trueheart, C. (1991). Clash looms over at-home abortion. *The Washington Post* (October 22, C7). Retrieved March 1, 2000, from Lexis-Nexis database.

Uzelac, E. (1989). Group: Do-it-yourself abortion is an option. *St. Petersburg Times* (July 30, 3A). Retrieved March 1, 2000, from Lexis-Nexis database.

Women turn to self-help groups for abortions, despite the risks (1992). *New York Times* (September 9, C13). Retrieved March 1, 2000, from Lexis-Nexis database.

Zimmerman, M. K. (1987). The women's health movement: A critique of medical enterprise and the position of women. In: B. B. Hess & M. M. Ferree (Eds), *Analyzing Gender: A Handbook of Social Science* (pp. 442–472). Newbury Park, CA: Sage.

GENITAL SURGERIES AND STIMULATION IN NINETEENTH CENTURY PSYCHIATRY

Carol A. B. Warren

INTRODUCTION

The medical suppression of female sexuality in Victorian society has long been the subject of historical and cultural scholarship, with documentation not only of textual threats by religious and medical "experts," but also of surgical assaults on female reproductive systems (Longo, 1979, 1986; Scull & Favreau, 1986; Sheehan, 1997). Less well known is the apparent obverse: the use of medical techniques to stimulate the female genitalia as a means of treating hysteria and other mental disorders (Maines, 1999; Schleiner, 1995). In this paper, I trace the cultural history (mainly Anglo-American) of the psychiatric enhancement, as well as repression, of female sexual pleasure, through various genital treatments, including the surgical and the electrical.[1] I then make the case that these "opposite" treatments are, in the context of Victorian society, two sides of the same coin of the patriarchal, medical control of female sexuality.[2]

This patriarchal, medical control of female sexuality is part of our western cultural heritage, involving both the woman's physical body and her social place. Psychiatric diagnosis is one of the many ways in which women in Europe and America have, for centuries, been kept "in their place": in the marriage bed, the household, and the private sphere, outside the public world of education, work, and politics. And from ancient times into the present, women's reproductive

Gender Perspectives on Reproduction and Sexuality
Advances in Gender Research, Volume 8, 165–197

ISSN: 1529-2126/doi:10.1016/S1529-2126(04)08006-3

systems have been defined by medical and psychiatric experts as the source of their deficits of social place, emotion, and behavior.

I also discuss the genital treatment of psychiatric disorders among men in the nineteenth century. Nineteenth century clinical psychiatry included cases of males diagnosed in the context of gendered and sexual expectations, and treated genitally. But both quantitatively and qualitatively, the genital-psychiatric literature on males in Victorian times was much less than that on females. Although at times male symptomatology – such as spermatorrhea or impotence – was made the object of psychiatric interpretation and intervention, it was more likely to be defined as a somatic rather than a mental disorder, and treated as such. And while Victorian gynecology was a burgeoning specialty, giving impetus to the surgical and genital treatment of women's mental disorders, the parallel male specialty of andrology never achieved anything like gynecology's professional success.

In addition to gender, class and ethnicity were significant elements of Victorian psychiatric diagnosis and treatment. Hysteria was thought to be a disorder of civilization and of the idle upper classes, as well as one of the female genitalia, although from the time of Galen onward there were published case histories of male and of lower class hysterics.[3] Diagnoses were often fitted to class or status; Beard and Rockwell, for example, proposed three subtypes of neurasthenia related to social place: "spinal neurasthenia (caused by physical labor or women's work), cerebrasthenic neurasthenia (caused by mental activity) and lithemic neurasthenia or autointoxication (caused by overindulgence)" (Cushing, 1995, p. 435). Treatments for these and other disorders were also classed and raced as well as gendered, thought to be more or less suited to a particular class, ethnic group, or nationality. Electrotherapy, for example, was viewed in nineteenth century psychiatry as wasted on the bodies of Irish immigrants, African-Americans, or the poor (Kneeland & Warren, 2002). Some of the genital treatments discussed in this paper were, however, attempted with poor, immigrant or lower class mental patients, for example the use of pelvic surgeries in state asylums.

I use several kinds of text to make my case. To document the use of genital treatments for insanity I use late eighteenth to early twentieth century American and other English language medical case histories.[4] For a contextual understanding of premodern to modern psychiatric medicine I rely on secondary sources in the cultural history of medicine. These secondary sources include an interdisciplinary and a feminist array of scholars from classicists Hanson (1990), King (1993), and Sissa (1990) to canons of history of medicine scholarship such as Laqueur (1990), Micale (1991), Oppenheim (1991), Shorter (1992), and Scull (Scull & Favreau, 1986).

I use "genital" and "sexual" as overlapping but not interchangeable terms. The ancients wrote unabashedly about the genitalia and their sexual response; by the Victorian era, many physicians had separated the genital from the sexual in accounts of psychiatric treatment. Some nineteenth century physicians, however, did allude to the sexual aspects of the genital for patients, while a few, especially in the early twentieth century, referenced patients' sexual responses directly (see, for example, Flint, 1874; Smith, 1903). It would have been as unthinkable for these nineteenth century physicians to write about the possibility of their own sexual arousal as the same confession would be for contemporary gynecologists performing vaginal examinations (Emerson, 1971).

Contemporary scholars are less reticent about the sexuality of psychiatric treatments than the physicians themselves. Ann Douglas Wood (1973) describes Silas Weir Mitchell, the "father" of the rest-cure in the treatment of mental disorders, as skating "on the edge of a theory of primitive healing through mesmeric sexual powers" (1973, p. 38). She adds that

> His admirers delighted to tell how, when a strangely recalcitrant patient refused to rise from bed after Mitchell had decreed that her rest cure was over, Mitchell threatened to move into bed with her if she did not get up, and even started to undress. When he got to his pants, she got up. Although the story may well be apocryphal, its spirit is not (Wood, 1973, p. 39).

Similarly, Taylor (1983) suggests that electrotherapy involved a fusion of the body of the patient with that of the physician through the latter's electric hand; the operator "experienced the same exhilaration and tonic effects from the current passing through their bodies as did the patients" (p. 282).

Direct sexual references in psychiatric texts became more commonplace in the early twentieth century than during previous decades, in the context, perhaps, of Freud's foregrounding of the sexual in his theory of psychoanalysis. Lunbeck (1994), analyzing case histories of female patients from the Boston Psychopathic Hospital during the 1900s, recorded several references to the sexualization of therapy on the part of physicians or patients, with one psychoanalyst referring to a teenage patient as "highly erotic . . . as she lies on the couch, is apt to expose a part of her legs." One patient asked him "how he had the nerve to ask the questions he did. 'Your questions rouse one's passions,' she told him. 'I was wondering if your passions were roused and how you could control them' " (Lunbeck, 1994, p. 224).

It is tempting to read sexuality into accounts of interactions whose meanings might not, at the time, have included sexual ones. Consider the following account of electro-mesmeric treatment in England in 1848. A Miss Aglonby reported that her mesmerist, "Mr Nixon," had sent her into a trance while applying galvanic shocks. During the first treatment, on June 7th, "Mr Nixon retreated a few steps from me . . . I felt drawn irresistibly to him as the needle by the magnet." On June 16th, "My mesmeriser, by taking my aunt by the hand, placed her *en rapport* with me; but here some cross-mesmerism seemed to take place, for I felt confused, and alternately repelled from and attracted to both." The next day, after treatment, she was left "mesmerised and lying on the sofa with the organ of language excited." Nixon returned within thirty minutes, but "some minutes before he arrived, I felt a glow of warmth with a perspiration all over me, and my breathing became quick, panting, and difficult" (*The Zoist*, 1848, pp. 238–240).

My stance is to try to take the genital at its face value, and not assume sexuality unless sexuality is also part of the primary text (although *The Zoist* tempts me to side with Wood & Taylor). And at the point where our story begins – in ancient hysteria and the wandering womb – both sexuality and genitalia were integral to the text.

ANCIENT HYSTERIA AND THE WANDERING WOMB

Whether the sexual implications of psychiatric interventions were or were not commented on by nineteenth century psychiatrists, the history of female insanity and its treatments is closely bound up with the sexual as well as the genital. Although many female (and to a much lesser extent male) diagnoses such as neurasthenia and melancholia were treated genitally, it was mainly hysteria, with its wandering womb, to which nineteenth century sexual psychiatry attended; an association which has a long and ancient lineage in the West. Plato, famous for his designation of hysteria as the wandering womb, described its journeys in a canonical passage from the (satirical) *Timeaus*. This passage has been mined for its reference to the womb, but not so much for the equally mobile penis:

> Wherefore also in men the organ of generation becomes rebellious and masterful, like an animal disobedient to reason, and maddened with the sting of lust, seeks to gain absolute sway, and the same is the case with the so-called womb or matrix of the woman. The animal within them is desirous of procreating children, and when remaining unfruitful long beyond its proper time, gets discontented and angry, and wandering in every direction through the body, closes up the passages of the breath, and, by obstructing respiration, drives them to extremity, causing all varieties of disease, until at length the desire and love of the man and the woman, bringing them together and as it were plucking the fruit from the tree, sow in the womb, as in a field, animals unseen by reason of their smallness and without form; these again are separated and matured within; they are then finally brought out into the light, and thus the generation of animals is completed (Plato, 1953, p. 1210).

Despite the Platonic penis's movement, "a creature instinct with life . . . bent on carrying all before it" (Adair, 1996, p. 156) few (and not canonical) etiologies or treatments were derived from this male "wandering animal."[5] By contrast, physicians derived numerous etiologies, symptomatologies, and sites of treatment from the wandering womb. The Platonic uterus wandered when it was sexually dissatisfied; it got into many parts of the body, including the throat, causing a plethora of symptoms. The Hippocratic uterus – although it was not an " 'animal, desirous of childbearing' . . . peevishly stray[ing] through the body" – still wandered: "a dry uterus goes off in search of moisture" (Hanson, 1990, p. 319).

An alternative etiological theory for hysteria to the wandering womb – but with similar treatment consequences – was that of retention. Retention of bodily fluids when they should be discharged was a symptom, for the ancients, of various forms of physical or mental distress. The retention of menstrual blood was interpreted from the time of the Hippocratics into the Victorian era as a symptom of hysteria and other mental disorders in women, to be treated in the same manner as other retentions: by purging with techniques ranging from bloodletting to massage (see, for example, Pallen, 1879).

The retention of female "semen" formed another etiological link between hysteria and purging. In what Bodemer (1973) refers to as a cervical theory of insanity, first century C. E. physician Galen argued that hysteria was caused by retention of sperm, which could – since both sexes were seen as producing seed – occur in the "abstinent of both sexes"; thus men could suffer from hysteria as well as women (Simon, 1978, p. 265). Galen (who presumably had seen anchored wombs during dissections), thought that the uterus was not really an animal nor did it wander, although it was animal-like because it "sucks the male semen . . . with a force like that of a magnet" (Roccatagliata, 1986, p. 205).

Despite different etiologies for the Platonic and Hippocratic uterii (and the Galenic cervix), their symptoms and treatment regimens were similar. "Symptoms of uterine suffocation are apparently common to both tradition[s]," including gnashing of teeth, rolling of eyes, loss of voice, choking, and throat strangulation – the hysterical "suffocation of the mother" of later Renaissance writers (Hanson, 1990). Even after dissections (of animals and perhaps humans) established that the uterus was anchored in place (Laqueur, 1990), the gynecological writings of Galen and Soranus, as well as the Hippocratics, recommended (among other treatments) aromatherapies "designed to entice a self-directing womb to follow pleasant smells back to its proper position or recoil from fetid ones" (Hanson, 1990, p. 319).

The ancient model of hysteria in women proposed that its symptoms built up to a "hysterical paroxysm," after which the woman would be relieved, a concept which bordered on that of female orgasm. Since female as well as male orgasm was deemed necessary to procreation, anything that might hinder orgasm was the subject of medical intervention (Laqueur, 1990). These medical theories – in one form or another – lasted for more than two thousand years, from Plato and the Hippocratics to the early twentieth century, and perhaps beyond.[6]

The Hippocratic writings recommended becoming a wife and mother as soon as puberty arrived, otherwise madness would ensue. According to the treatise *On the Diseases of Young Women*:

> girls are subject to madness at puberty because their bodies are totally closed and become stifled. The body retains the blood of the first menstrual flow, and this poisonous humor spreads blindly in search of an exit, so that breathing is impaired and there is a consequent impulse toward self-strangulation. When this syndrome occurs, victims should not go off and dedicate their clothing to Artemis, as custom dictates. Rather, the best thing for them is to marry and bear children (Sissa, 1990, p. 359).

From the Hippocratic corpus into the nineteenth century and beyond, women's menstrual cycle and blood, as well as her social role, were implicated in the diagnosis and treatment of insanity. Young women at puberty, older women at menopause, and unmarried women in between, were seen as vulnerable to madness consequent upon the toxicity of retained menstrual blood, or the debilitation of excessive menstruation. Indeed, the only woman not particularly liable to insanity was the young, married, reproductive woman. As Hanson (1990, p. 318) notes, "A constant refrain throughout the gynecology of the [Hippocratic] *Corpus* is the advice that 'She should sleep with, go to her man,' and it is frequently coupled with 'if she becomes pregnant she is healthy.' " This theme remained alive in the medical literature for the next two thousand years.

But what was to be done by the medical profession about women who could not or would not marry – nuns, or widows past the age at which they were likely to remarry? And, worse, what about those women who sought sexual satisfaction outside marriage, perhaps by themselves, with non-husband men or other women, or clitorally rather than vaginally? Throughout the centuries, genital answers (among others) were provided for these genital questions, including clitoridectomies and genital stimulation.

Premodern Clitoridectomies

The clitoris – as an anatomical structure common to all women and as the site of women's sexual pleasure – has had a checkered medical history. Although all women were, in ancient times, presumed to have uteruses, and to use them in marriage and childbirth, there has been no such consensus, in the West, on the clitoris. While some ancient anatomists recognized the clitoris, others confused it with the labia or vulva. But whatever knowledge there was of the clitoris was lost to medical writing during the dark ages, until Fallopia's (Park, 1997) or Columbus's (Laqueur, 1990) "rediscovery" of it during the sixteenth century.

A number of Western and Arab medievial to Renaissance physicians thought that the clitoris was a pathological growth, or that it was found only in "uncivilized" women of other races (Laqueur, 1990; Park, 1997). If the penis-like clitoris was common to all women, then perhaps all women were hermaphrodites (Park, 1997). By the Enlightenment, most physicians believed that the clitoris was indeed common to all women and, unless enlarged, was not pathological. But it could still stir up all kinds of trouble, from tribadism – the assertion of male gender and sexual rights – to being oversexed or hysterical.

According to Hanson, ancient "post Hippocratic gynecologies" favored the clitoridectomy (female genital mutilation, or FGM) as a medical treatment for oversexed women: "An enlarged clitoris is a sign of hypersexuality in a woman, and post-Hippokratic gynecologies recognize clitoridectomy, rather than the traditionally prescribed remedies of pregnancy and motherhood, as an appropriate therapy" (Hanson, 1990, p. 333). According to Shorter (1992, pp. 79–81), clitoridectomies had been performed in Egypt, and were "frequently" mentioned in Roman writings on "nymphomania . . . which usually meant chronic masturbation" (p. 81). Proposals for clitoridectomy continued throughout the Renaissance and Enlightenment in Western societies. One sixteenth century French physician suggested that all Frenchwomen, like Ethiopian women, should have the operation as "a way of disciplining unbridled female sexuality" (Park, 1997, p. 184). But clitoridectomies were not the only answer for women driven to hysteria by their genitalia: genital stimulation was another possibility.

Galen's Widow's Treatment

Genitally stimulative therapies, like clitoridectomies, were recommended in Egyptian, Greek and Roman medical discourse, and practiced throughout the middle ages. Ancient stimulative therapies were directed at the hysterical woman whose (marital) sexuality was inadequate for reproduction. In the Hippocratic corpus, intercourse, as well as "vaginal probes and pessaries 'shaped like a penis,' " straightened out curved and bent reproductive systems in order to make them properly reproductive" (Hanson, 1990, p. 319).

But it was Galen who provided the canonical genital, paroxysmal treatment for a female insanity based in too little, rather than too much, sexuality. He recounts, in one case history, his "widow's treatment" for hysteria-like symptoms; there are many translations and accounts of this case history, of which Helen King's (1993, p. 43) is one of the more recent:

> In a passage from *On the Affected Parts* taken up by the hysteria tradition, Galen describes the case of a woman who had been a widow for a long time and who was told by a midwife that her

> symptoms were due to her womb being 'drawn up.' The woman applied to her external genitalia 'the customary remedies' (details of which are not given here) for this condition and passed a quantity of thick seed; the suggestion appears to be that rubbing in the traditional scented ointments causes orgasm, and thus releases the retained matter. For Galen, both menstrual blood and seed must be evacuated, otherwise they will become toxic and poison the body (King, 1993, p. 43).

Earlier twentieth century translations cover roughly the same genital terrain, but imply that Galen himself administered the rubbing treatment (Simon, 1978), or that a midwife was instructed by Galen to provide it (Roccatagliata, 1986).

Galen's widow's treatment disappeared into the Arab medical literature during the Dark Ages and reappeared in Europe during the Renaissance (Maines, 1999). A number of tenth century writers, including Avicenna, repeated Galen's widow's case history and recommended the treatment. Al-Majusi "repeats the Galenic therapy . . . and states explicitly that this has the same effect as intercourse, in warming and thinning the seed, so that it can drain away and the woman can 'find peace' " (King, 1993, p. 52). By the Renaissance, genital stimulatory treatment for hysteria was taken up as authoritative by physicians still wondering how to treat hysterical women. The treatment, however, was mired in the controversies of a Judeo-Christian era in which it seemed altogether too sexual and not very clerical. Medical writers such as the French physician Ranchin, in 1600, debated the legitimacy of genital stimulation as a treatment for mental symptoms, adding a fake-penis twist to the Galenic original:

> Very serious and extremely important is the difficulty mentioned, namely whether one is allowed to rub women or handle their parts in the hysterical paroxysm. First Galen puts forth the story of some widow restored to health by a midwife inserting her finger in her womb and thus evacuating the semen. From this grew the practice that [most] women use instruments skillfully hollowed out and similar in form to the male penis in order to provoke voluntary pollution and guard against hysterical symptoms. Secondly, Avicenna recommends that midwives insert a finger into the vulva and rub it diligently until the seminal material is expelled (quoted in Schleiner, 1995, p. 120).

Despite theological reservations, Galen's widow's treatment continued to be used throughout the seventeenth and eighteenth and into the nineteenth century. In a 1653 medical compendium, Pieter van Foreest advised for hysterical symptomatology:

> to ask a midwife to assist, so that she can massage the genitalia with one finger inside, using oil of lilies, musk root, crocus, or similar. And in this way the afflicted woman can be aroused to the paroxysm. This kind of stimulation with the finger is recommended by Galen and Avicenna, among others; most especially for widows, those who live chaste lives, and female religious . . . it is less often recommended for very young women, public women, or married women, for whom it is a better remedy to engage in intercourse with their spouses (quoted in Maines, 1999, p. 1).

It would seem possible, even likely, that the rationality and science of the Enlightenment might put an end to uterine theories of madness and its genital treatment, but this was not to be. Despite the rejection (by no means global) of uterine in favor of nerve theories of hysteria in the eighteenth century, and the (by then) indubitable anatomical evidence of the anchoring of the uterus in the body (Laqueur, 1990), the Platonic model of the madwoman's medical problem and its Hippocratic and Galenic solutions continued into the nineteenth and early twentieth centuries, along with models that used the solutions but offered different etiologies.

GYNECOLOGY AND GENITALIA IN NINETEENTH CENTURY PSYCHIATRY

The genital treatment of female – and to a lesser extent male – mental disorder was discussed fairly extensively throughout the nineteenth and into the twentieth century Anglo-American medical literature. Its etiological justification still lay, despite challenges, in the ancient association between the reproductive system and mental symptoms, including the uterus, the ovaries, and the clitoris. With the discovery of the functioning of the ovaries (earlier defined as "female testicles"), these organs joined the uterus as body parts common to all Victorian women – indeed as defining them – but as, like the clitoris, mentally troublesome when "deranged" in some manner.

Some nineteenth century etiologies of mental illness – especially prior to the 1880s – still referenced the womb, menstruation, and associated ancient theories of humors, vapors, and congestions. Dr. Meigs, in the 1950s, proposed that auras and vapors from the "diseased womb" rose to pervade other organs, including the brain (1851, p. 479). Pallen (1879, p. 193; italics in the original) referred to an "*aura*" arising from "functional disturbances" of the uterus and ovaries that caused hysteria. Williams (1863–1864), who linked "defective menstruation" to mania in women, concluded that "congestion" was the causal link (p. 853). Storer proposed an etiology that included the "deficient elimination of carbon from the . . . catamenial fluid" (1866, p. 158).

By the end of the century, the prevailing somatic etiology of mental symptoms was based not on the wandering womb but on nerve or "reflex theory," which could pertain to womb, ovaries, clitoris – or for that matter penis and testicles, stomach or liver. Reflex theory held that the "reflex action of genital pathology" on the brain was one cause of mental illness; psychosis was described as a "genital reflex" (Shorter, 1992, pp. 69–71), and "hysterical psychosis" was ascribed to an "irritable weakness" of the "genital nerves" (Erb, 1883, p. 158). Other theories were based on endocrinology, with "inadequate uterine secretions" in women

(Wood, 1887, p. 67) and a shortage of "testicular juice" in men the sources of mental pathology (Shortt, 1986, p. 157).

Throughout the eighteenth and nineteenth centuries, theorists speculated that psychological or social causes were important in hysteria. Some thought that the attention women got when they went to the physician precipitated hysterical symptoms (Albutt, 1884). Others based their etiologies on social structure, continuing the Enlightenment critique of the impact of civilization on women's uterine and mental health. Sir Benjamin Brodie wrote that

> The liability to hysteria is, in fact, among females, one of the severest penalties of high civilization . . . among the higher classes of society, at least four-fifths of the female patients, who are commonly supposed to labour under diseases of the joints, labour under hysteria, and nothing else (1837, p. 37).

Some Victorian physicians interpreted hysteria culturally, attributing it to the lack of meaningful activities for Victorian girls and women. Zenner (1883) concluded that hysteria in women was caused not by genital symptoms but by the "idle lives of . . . fashionable ladies" who needed "useful employment or earnest study" (p. 525; see also Storer, 1866, p. 158).

Whatever the etiology of Victorian female insanity, technological and medical inventions expanded the options for genital treatment. From the 1860s onward, the growth of the specialties of gynecology and surgery and the development of anaesthesia fostered uterine and other reproductive system surgeries. These movements, together with the invention and use of static, voltaic, galvanic or franklinic electrical (Kneeland & Warren, 2002) and vibratory (Maines, 1999) instruments and machines, formed the scientific context for the Victorians' technological re-deployment of both genital surgery and Galen's widow's treatment. But neither science nor technology displaced the notion of reproductive insanity or the Platonic recommendation of marriage as its cure.

Reproductive Insanity and the Marriage Cure

Nineteenth century physicians, patients and relatives did not hesitate to attribute women's mental illness to their reproductive systems, and not only alienists but the new gynecological specialists had their say. "Like frogs 'just before the period of copulation' mused the gynecologist E. J. Tilt in 1853, women 'subjected to increased ovarian action' revealed nerves 'endowed with the greatest degree of irritability' " (Oppenheim, 1991, p. 188; see also Storer, 1866). Family members of patients at Thomas Kirkbride's Pennsylvania asylum asked if gynecological examinations could be performed in order to determine whether "derangements of the womb" were responsible for their condition (Tomes, 1984, p. 93). One patient's husband told Kirkbride that her menopause was "one great cause of the derangement of her nervous system" (Tomes, 1984, p. 93).

The Platonic notion of women's hysteria as curable through marriage and intercourse continued into nineteenth century medical writings on what to do with these genitally and socially irritated women. Samuel Ashwell, in London (1848, pp. 171–172) proposed that the best "cure" for hysteria was "women married happily and at a sufficiently early age becoming mothers"; he derided those among his colleagues who, like Dewees (1828), challenged the ancient association between female hysteria and the uterus, and thus the medical authority of Galen and the ancients.[7] In the 1875 fifth edition of an American advice book for the "Maiden, Wife and Mother," George Napheys noted that hysteria and mania were "almost exclusively confined to single persons" (1875, p. 386), and that "Marriage exerts a decidedly curative influence" in "chronic nervous ailments" because "Success . . . is always a tonic . . . to women, marriage is a success. It is their aim in social life; and this accomplished, health and strength follow" (pp. 386–387).

Ancient uterine themes also appeared in these nineteenth century treatises. Napheys referred to menopause as a time when she was "finishing her pilgrimage of sexual life" and "shades of moral insanity" appeared; she must curb any sexual desires she has, since this is "contrary to nature" (1875, pp. 392–402). In *Our Family Physician*, published in 1889, Dr. H. R. Stuart (1889) insisted that hysteria was an affliction of the mind, not, as in "ancient times," of the womb. Nevertheless, he claimed that the symptoms of hysteria were almost exclusively the provenance of the widowed and unmarried, while the hysterical paroxysm was associated with the menses (pp. 90–91).

Like Galen before them, nineteenth century physicians faced the problem of treating hysterical women who were not married (perhaps undersexed), and married women who nevertheless seemed hysterical (perhaps oversexed, or "nyphomaniacal"). The Victorians' problems with the oversexed woman are well known; less well known is the fact that they also had problems with the asexual (and therefore non-reproductive) woman. A healthy (if infrequent) sexuality within marriage was encouraged by physicians in order for "the race" – even, indeed especially, the upper and middle classes – to reproduce (Oppenheim, 1991, p. 205).

One set of possibilities, given the obduracy of uterine theories of mental illness causation, was to intervene in the reproductive systems of women in order to treat mental symptomatology with the two sets of local treatments proposed by the ancients: surgical removal or modification of the various sexual parts, or their stimulation. Such local treatment solutions were, however, highly contested terrain. Although the theological arguments of the middle ages against genital treatment were not as persuasive after the Enlightenment, questions of "female delicacy" remained firmly entrenched. The debates revolved around three issues: the legitimacy of male physicians approaching the female genitalia with eyes, fingers or speculum; the question of surgery (clitoridectomy, oopharotomy or the removal of healthy ovaries), pelvic surgery, male castration, and male and female "circumcision") as a treatment for mental illness; and the use of Galen's widow's treatment.

The Speculum, Penetration, and the Gynecological Examination

The invention of the speculum early in the century (Barker-Benfield, 2000), and the development of anaesthesia for surgery, fostered the rapid development of the specialty of gynecology. At the beginning of the nineteenth century, digital examination of the internal female genitalia was not a fit subject for many physicians (as in previous eras, such examinations were often left to midwives, mothers, or other female assistants). After the invention of the speculum, however, digital and mechanical examinations became increasingly commonplace and accepted (Mitchison, 1991). The propriety of examining the uterus with fingers or speculum, and the appropriateness of removing healthy reproductive tissue, were among the themes debated in the medical literature of the Victorian era, exhibiting a "wide range of opinions and practice" (Mitchison, 1991, p. 242). Some physicians believed that penetration defined female sexuality, and, thus, that the use of a speculum violated virginity and marital chastity.

By the late nineteenth century, in the giddy wake of speculum and gynecology, the uterus had taken pride of place in the physician's lexicon. Dr. Philip Zenner lamented that gynecological examinations and treatment had become "only too fashionable" in America (1883, p. 523). From the other side of the Atlantic, Dr. Clifford Albutt, Fellow of the Royal College of Physicians, wrote of the uterus:

> A neuralgic woman seems to be particularly unfortunate . . . she is either told that she is hysterical or that it is all uterus . . . in the second case she is entangled in the net of the gynaecologist, who finds her uterus, like her nose, is a little on one side, or again, like that organ, is running a little, or it is as flabby as her biceps, so that the unhappy viscus is impaled upon a stem, or perched upon a prop, or painted with carbolic acid every week in the year except during the long vacation when the gynaecologist is grouse-shooting, or salmon-catching, or leading the fashion in the Upper Engadine (1884, p. 17).

GENITAL SURGERIES IN NINETEENTH CENTURY PSYCHIATRY

The focus of twentieth century analyses of the local, genital treatment of female mental illness – "pelvic madness" (Shorter, 1992, pp. 69–70) or "oophoro-mania" as well as hysteria – has been on sexual surgery: the removal of all or part of the healthy clitoris (clitoridectomy, associated in particular with Isaac Baker Brown; see Scull & Favreau, 1986; Sheehan, 1997), or the excision of healthy ovaries (oopharotomies; see Longo, 1979; Shorter, 1992). Less attention has been paid to three other nineteenth century forms of sexual surgery for the treatment of insanity: pelvic surgery (encompassing a range of procedures from dilation and curettage to the repair of torn cervixes), male castration, and both male and female "circumcision." Although these various genital operations were controversial even at the time, quite a number of them were performed, especially after the development of anaesthesia in the 1860s (Longo, 1979). Even George Beard (1880) whose electrotherapeutic work has been more often associated with stimulative than operative treatment (Kneeland & Warren, 2002), referred to genital "galvano-cautery" as a "very old" but "good" treatment for neurasthenia, noting that it "is not specially painful, even to the most delicate woman" (p. 173).

Clitoridectomy, Oopharotomy, and Pelvic Surgeries

Nineteenth century clitoridectomies were directed not only at insane, unmarried or sexually "deviant" women, but also at married women whose behavior indicated inappropriate sexuality both in and out of the marital bed. Diagnoses ranging from nymphomania to hysteria were, for nineteenth century physicians, indicators for the removal of the clitoris. The most famous – soon infamous – Victorian physician who performed clitoridectomies for "nervous disorder" was Isaac Baker Brown, an 1854 President of the Medical Society of London (Scull & Favreau, 1986, p. 7). One of Baker Brown's assistants, in 1876, described the procedure:

> Two instruments were used: the pair of hooked forceps which Mr. Brown always uses in clitoridectomy, and a cautery iron. . . . The clitoris was seized by the forceps in the usual manner. The thin edge of the red hot iron was then passed around its base until the original was severed from its attachments, being partly cut or sawn, and partly torn away. After the clitoris was removed, the nymphae on each side were severed in a similar way by a sawing motion of the hot iron. After the clitoris and nymphae were got rid of, the operation was brought to a close by taking the back of the iron and sawing the surfaces of the labia and the other parts of the vulva which had escaped the cautery, and the instrument was rubbed down backwards and forwards till the parts were more effectually destroyed than when Mr. Brown uses the scissors with in effect the same result (quoted in Scull & Favreau, 1986, p. 9).

Scull and Favreau (1986) claim that some of Brown's cases were women who "sought to take advantage of the new Divorce Act of 1847, usually diagnosed as suffering from incipient mania" (p. 8). They quote Case 48:

> Mrs S. M. had developed a 'great distaste for her husband . . . and [for] cohabitation with him. I pursued the usual surgical treatment, which was followed by uninterrupted success; and after

two months' treatment, she returned to her husband, resumed cohabitation . . . and became a happy and healthy wife and mother' (quoted in Scull & Favreau, 1986, p. 8).

Although Dr. Isaac Baker Brown was eventually censured for his surgeries by the medical profession, it was less because of his performance of these surgeries than the fact that he made mention of masturbation in women at all – and because he advertised his operations, something seen at the time as quite inappropriate (Scull & Favreau, 1986). But his operation survived his disgrace. In 1894 McGinness described the removal of an "over-developed clitoris" that "interfered with marital intercourse" (p. 2), while Robert Taylor, a Professor at Columbia University, recommended in 1905 "full excision of the clitoris" for "some" cases of "nymphomania" (p. 425). Clitoridectomies for insanity continued into the 1920s (see Diefendorf, 1923; Paramore, 1921) and perhaps beyond (Sheehan, 1997).

The nineteenth century discovery of the functioning of the ovaries gave physicians a new definition of woman's "nature": where she had been defined by her uterus, now she was to be defined by her ovaries (only deviant women were defined by their clitorises). "Ovarian excitement" could lead to "madness" of a sexual nature (Lightfoot, 1857, p. 79). One of Dr. Lightfoot's patients was

> A young lady, carefully brought up. . . . She has already mingled with society, and that society is of the best . . . [but] From a modest, delicate, tender maid, she becomes a wanton, and makes alarming proposals to every man she meets: there is the madness of lasciviousness in her looks. . . . What has caused this?. . . . A disturbed, perverted . . . condition of those organs whose presence made her a woman (Lightfoot, 1857, p. 79).

Just as an abscessed or cancerous ovary could be treated with ovariotomy, a physically healthy but mysteriously deranging one could be treated with oopharectomy.

Ovariotomies (the removal of diseased ovaries) had been performed since the early part of the nineteenth century, but it was not until the 1860s (too late for Dr. Lightfoot's young lady) that oopharotomies for insanity became commonplace. The operation was named for Robert Battey, an American surgeon who performed many oopharotomies between 1872 and 1890, for ovarian insanity, oophoromania or oophoralgia (Longo, 1979, p. 250). In 1891, at a meeting of the International Medical Congress in England (where the surgery was also popular), Battey reported on 193 cases of oophorectomy by 47 surgeons (with a mortality rate of 18%). One physician claimed that 150,000 women had undergone Battey's operation by 1906 (Longo, 1979, p. 253).

Like Isaac Baker Brown and his clitoridectomies, however, Battey and his operation were not without critics. As Longo (1979, p. 244) notes, the "procedure was dubbed 'castration' . . . 'spaying' . . . 'desexing' and 'unsexing' and decried as a pernicious and dreadful operation. . . . Moreover, surgeons who carried out such procedures were labeled 'gynecological perverts.' " But unlike Baker Brown,

Battey was not drummed out of medicine. Indeed, many physicians remained convinced that oopharotomy was a valuable treatment, and not only because it was believed to cure the mad woman herself. In the words of William Goodell, professor of gynecology at the University of Pennsylvania, "I am not sure that, in the progressive future, it will not be deemed a matter of social policy . . . to stamp out insanity by castrating all the insane men and spaying all the insane women" (1881, p. 639).

In addition to clitoridectomy and oopharectomy, various forms of "pelvic surgery" were used in American and English psychiatry during the later part of the nineteenth century. Dr. Rohe (1893, pp. 325–326), an expert in "lactational insanity," reported on several cases under his care, including one woman diagnosed with melancholia who had her "lacerated cervix" "stitched up with silk-worm gut. The improvement [in her mental state] was noticeable from the day of the operation." And Dr. Hersman, writing in the *Journal of the American Medical Association* (1899, pp. 709–711), described a case of "endometritis" which had caused insanity through "local irritation" of the sympathetic nervous system, cured through curettage. He also claimed that uterine disease was the cause of nymphomania. Rohe summed up the prevailing opinion when he quoted a Dr. Gooch as saying, "we have no power by medical agents in relieving a disordered mind, *excepting indirectly through the disorder of the body with which it is connected*" (1893, p. 326; italics in the original).

Pelvic surgery was attempted as a treatment for insanity during the late nineteenth century in asylums in America and England. In the Maryland Hospital for the insane, 35 gynecological examinations revealed 26 pelvic disturbances; 18 pelvic operations resulted in the improvement or cure of 13. Similar results were claimed at the Norristown Asylum ("The Relation of Pelvic Disease to Psychical Disturbance in Women," 1893, p. 650). In the London Asylum in 1885, genital surgeries included ovariotiomy, dilation and curettage, perineal repair, cervical amputation, uterine suspension, and hysterectomy (Shortt, 1986, p. 157). According to Shortt (1986, p. 143), A. T. Hobbs performed these and other pelvic surgeries on 19 women patients in 1885, and 209 more during the next five years, claiming a two-thirds recovery rate and concluding that

> Through modern gynecology . . . alienists could leave behind the traditional stigma of therapeutic impotence to participate instead in the most spectacular innovation of Victorian medicine (Shortt, 1986, p. 156).

Other physicians were less sanguine, Sir Thomas Spencer Wells commenting in 1886 that "gynecologists will never empty the lunatic asylum" (Longo, 1979, p. 263).

Male Castration and Circumcision

There are occasional references to testicular surgeries for insane males parallel to oopharectomies for insane women, although I have seen references to the removal of penises only for cancerous conditions. Both Longo (1979, p. 254) and Shorter (1992, p. 92) mention the castration (removal of the testicles) of nineteenth century men diagnosed with insanity, epilepsy, masturbatory insanity, homosexuality, or the male equivalent of nymphomania – satyriasis.

Marshall (1865) reported the use of castration as a treatment for a 36 year old inmate of Cleveland City Infirmary, a "Bohemian" physician whose mental disorder was traced to habitual masturbation. Unlike the *un*feminine female victims of oopharotomy, this patient was *hyper*masculine: sexually predatory, "vicious and dangerous," as well as "muscular and athletic" (p. 363). In January of 1864 his testes were removed while he was anaesthetized with chloroform, after which he was "tractable and manageable," a "changed man . . . quiet, kind and docile" (p. 363). He subsequently left the Infirmary and continued his career as a physician (p. 364). Dr. Marshall concluded that castration was a "good idea" when insanity was caused by "masturbation or excess venery" (p. 364).

In his discussion of this case, Marshall noted that "As far as my knowledge extends this is the first instance where castration has been resorted to for insanity" (1865, p. 344), but apparently it was not. A few years earlier, an exchange of letters read to the Boston Society for Medical Improvement referred to a proposal for the psychiatric castration of a hypermasculine, masturbatory mental patient (Bigelow, 1856, 1860). One of the letters, by Dr. Bell, claimed that "At the Ohio Hospital, some years ago, [castration] was tried on quite an extensive scale," but "No improvement followed" (Bigelow, 1859–1860, p. 166). Unlike Dr. Marshall, Dr. Bell (despite citing two cases of "successful" castration of insane "onanist" males, one a self-castration), did not recommend the surgery (1859–1860, p. 166).

Some male genital treatments for insanity stopped short of castration, just as some female ovarian treatments, such as ovarian compression, stopped short of oopharectomy. Three months before castrating his Bohemian patient, Dr. Marshall had severed his *vas deferens*, a procedure which "arrested his loathsome habit," but only "for a few weeks" (1865, p. 363). Mitchison (1991, p. 282) records one physician as suggesting the compression of testicles in male hysterics, comparable to Charcot's and others' compression of ovaries in the treatment of female hysteria.

The foreskin of the male was sometimes implicated in nineteenth century insanity, analogized by some physicians to the female "foreskin," or clitoral hood. Both male and female insanity was treated with "circumcision" by nineteenth century physicians. In the case of males, phimosis – the adhesion of the foreskin to the penis – was seen as a physical cause of masturbation, which then precipitated masturbatory insanity. H. Sutherland (1875, pp. 845–846), for example, described one of his patients as a 26 year old man "addicted to masturbation" whom he diagnosed with "congenital phimosis." "Partial surgery" was the recommended treatment, after which the man stopped masturbating (according to Sutherland), and his "mental symptoms decidedly improved."

Female Circumcision

Although "female circumcision" has been used in the literature to refer to clitoridectomy/FGM, it is likely that in a few instances the term referred to a procedure more akin to male circumcision. The adhesion of the clitoral hood to the clitoris was seen as precipitating mental symptomatology in women just as the foreskin drove men to insanity – an example of the survival of the one-sex body in the era of two-sexes (Laqueur, 1990).

A Dr. R. T. Morris of New York was quoted by another nineteenth century physician as saying that the clitoris was a "little electric button, which when pressed by adhesions rings up the whole nervous system," resulting in masturbation, which in turn led to "reflex neurotic disturbances." (The Far Reaching Influence of Abnormalities of the Clitoris, 1893, p. 645). One of Dr. Morris's patients had been diagnosed with nymphomania for eight years because of this condition. He proposed, as a treatment, "the freeing of the gland from those adhesions," adding that Dr. Isaac Baker Brown's "mistake . . . consisted in cutting that organ away entirely, when all that was required, in many cases at least, was to liberate it from its imprisonment within the prepuce" (The Far Reaching Influence of Abnormalities of the Clitoris, 1893, p. 645).

Similarly, E. H. Pratt, in the *Chicago Journal of Orificial Surgery* (1898), used the term "female circumcision" to refer to the "freeing of the clitoral hood from its attachments" (p. 386). Dr. Pratt made an analogy between the hood of the clitoris and the foreskin of the penis, claiming that a variety of medical and psychiatric troubles were associated with not circumcising:

> Chorea, so frequent in young girls; chlorosis, which comes a little later on, and hysteria, which is also a common affliction, in addition to the same diseases from which boys whose foreskins have been neglected are liable to suffer, have their origin almost invariably in faulty conditions of the hood of the clitoris (p. 386).

Dawson (1915), more than twenty years later, also advocated the freeing of the clitoris from the clitoral hood, arguing that "Chorea, chlorosis, hysteria, and various nerve disturbances, nearly always have their origin in a faulty condition of the hood of the clitoris" (p. 520). The causal connection was, as for Morris, reflex nerve theory: "Irritation in the sexual organs . . . may reach the mental or moral faculties" (p. 521). He reported on six cases of circumcision on females of various ages and with various conditions: a three to four week old baby with colic, a two year old with boils and malnutrition, a seven year old "masturbator," a ten year old with hip-joint disease, a sixteen year old with "nocturnal enuresus," and a forty-six year old widow who had self-diagnosed as a nymphomaniac. All these conditions were reported by Dawson as cured by the circumcision, which he described as follows:

> [it] is performed by cutting a V-shaped piece from the hood over the center of the clitoris. If very redundant, it will require a large piece; if tight, only a slit will be necessary. Grasp the hood in the center with Pratt's plug forceps or a pointed hemostat; *lift it up from the clitoris* and, with scissors, cut each side of the forceps, the cuts meeting above the point of the forceps, taking out a V from the hood. . . . When strong adhesions have been broken up . . . put a drop of flexible collodion *on the clitoris*, holding the hood up until it dries (1915, p. 523, italics added to phrases indicating that the clitoris remained after the "circumcision").

Both Morris (1893) and Dawson (1915) were more concerned with the social control than the liberation of female sexuality through female circumcision. Pratt, however, was more positive toward the clitorises he proposed to free:

> the clitoris and its hood constitute the most sensitive electrical button, which can be pressed to arouse this entire sympathetic nervous system to increased sensitivity. . . . The pencil of nerves which supplies the sexual organs, although scattered in the periphery, unite in a common center, wending their way to the solar plexus as rays of light climb to the sun (p. 391).

Pratt hoped, by freeing the hood of the clitoris from the glans, to provide women with as "healthy" a sexual life as that of the circumcised male, an aim somewhat different from Morris's:

> The state of sexuality dominates the bodily vigor, but the condition of the sexual organs, as a whole, bears no more important relation to the general health of the body than does the condition of the clitoris and its hood to the health and tonicity of the sexual system itself. By all means, then, let the girls have as fair a start in life as the boys (Pratt, 1898, pp. 391–392).

Similarly, Galen's widow's treatment was directed at those whose lack of sexual satisfaction had provoked hysterical symptoms.

GENITAL STIMULATION AND ELECTRICITY IN NINETEENTH CENTURY PSYCHIATRY

During the nineteenth century, gender, sexuality and electricity were intertwined in the diagnosis and treatment of insanity. The ancient diagnosis of hysteria, with its gendered and sexualized implications, was joined by the new diagnosis of neurasthenia, popularized in America by George Beard (Beard & Rockwell, 1881). Although applied, at first, to over- or underworked male upper to middle class American men, the neurasthenic diagnosis was soon extended to other classes and nations, and to women (Micale, 1991). By the turn of the century, neurasthenia had become yet another diagnosis associated with women's "more vulnerable" nervous and reproductive systems (Libbrecht & Quackenbush, 1995). The gendering and sexualization of treatments, as well as diagnoses, was amplified by Victorian gynecology. And, although competitive with gynecology (Longo, 1986), the growing specialty of electrotherapeutics was also harnessed to the genital treatment of a variety of mental disorders, mainly with female neurasthenics and hysterics (Kneeland & Warren, 2002).

Despite the reservations of the Church during the Renaissance, Galen's widow's treatment had survived the centuries into the eighteenth and nineteenth centuries. Although quite controversial, genital stimulation was used during the nineteenth century – even during the "repressive" Victorian era – as a medical treatment for mental disorder, mainly for female hysteria and other neurosis, but also, occasionally, for male madness. Some of these stimulative treatments were non-electrical, similar to the aromatherapies, ointments, and pessaries attempted during the eras from the Hippocratics to the Enlightenment. In 1848, Ashwell proposed treating hysteria in a variety of ways, including water in the face (hydrotherapy), smelling salts (aromatherapy), leeches to the perineum, rectum or cervix, scarification of the cervix, as well as electricity. Some forty years later, Tipton recorded his treatment of "nymphomania" with heated ointments applied once or twice a day on the "pubes and organs" (1882, p. 151). Smelling salts were used not only in the 1850s (Meigs, 1851), but in England (at least) well into the 1950s,[8] for the problem of "vapors" arising from the womb (and other bodily organs) and causing the woman to become hysterical or faint.

Despite the phallocentrism of the nineteenth century – the definition of penetration, only, as constituting sex – physicians such as George Savage (1878) wrote of the use of pessaries (vaginal inserts) in the treatment of insanity caused by ovarian and uterine "irritations." He described one of his patients, a 45 year old woman going through the "change of life," as "neglecting her home duties, or doing them badly.... She wanted to leave home." He cured her prolapsed and heavy uterus, and thus her insanity, by using "a pessary with a bag at the end." Another patient, who was driven mad by clitoral masturbation, was cured by the use of a vaginal pessary. Savage, who referred to the "unpardonable sin" as yet another genital cause of insanity, noted "the importance of investigating the condition of the genitalia in certain cases of insanity" (p. 272).

The Electrification of Galen's Widow's Treatment

In addition to these ancient stimulative treatments, nineteenth century alienists and gynecologists brought electrical machinery to bear in the local treatment of genital-psychiatric distress.[9] Many of the physicians who used Galen's widow's treatment for hysteria relied upon electrical or electromagnetic devices, including probes and pessaries delivering faradic or galvanic electricity and vibrators powered by electricity, while electricity was also used for galvano-cautery of the clitoris (Beard, 1980; McGinnis, 1894). These treatments were indubitably genital, but their sexuality was a more open question.

Victorian physicians who wrote about the electric stimulative treatment of female insanity either did not mention its possible sexual implications, alluded to them indirectly, or – more rarely – spoke of them openly. In 1900, Hedley described the genital electrical treatment of hysteria without reference to the hysterical paroxysm, female orgasm, or even stimulation – as had the ancients – referencing the genitalia but not sexuality:

> If hysterical, five wire currents, one electrode above pubes, the other intra-uterine or intra-vaginal; or the intra-uterine bi-polar electrode may be used (p. 195).

In many nineteenth century clinical accounts of electrical treatment the menses, rather than sexual response, formed the link between genital disturbance and insanity. Tipton's treatment for chlorosis involved bringing on the monthly menses; he recommended that the physician "insert the uterine electrode . . . wet in warm water, per vagina, until it meets the uterus" (1882, p. 148). For hysteria, the positive electrical pole was applied over the uterus and ovaries, and the negative pole between the thighs or attached to the vaginal electrode and "introduced per vagina" (Tipton, 1882, pp. 233–234).[10] George Beard and A. D. Rockwell treated female patients diagnosed with hysteria, neurasthenia, sexual neurasthenia and other ailments with a variety of general and local electrical applications, including internal and external genital stimulation. Among their many case histories was

> A most violent and persistent case of hysteria, in the person of a married lady, aged 40. . . . The menstrual period was delayed nearly two weeks, and to this circumstance it was possible, in part, to attribute the attack. The patient was submitted to thorough general faradization, and immediately after a galvanic current from eight cells was as nearly as possible localized in the uterus. These efforts were followed by decided alleviation of the symptoms, and a tolerably quiet night was the result. The menses, however, did not appear, and on the following night we gave again the same treatment, slightly increasing the tension of the galvanic current. Before morning, menstruation became manifest, and there was no further evidence of nervous disturbance (Beard & Rockwell, 1881, p. 422).

A few physicians made what a twenty-first century reader might consider indirect allusions to sexuality. Tripier, recorded by Maines (1999) as one of the physicians who employed Galen's widow's treatment, referred to a uterine faradic attachment as "The uterine exciter" (1894, p. 140). Wood (1887, pp. 377, 617), recommending the faradization of the "pubes," "pelvis," and "uterus" to "restore secretions," noted that it "stimulates the muscles to involuntary contractions." In a similar vein, Erb (1883) commented that the electrical current is useful because of its "vigorous stimulating actions upon uterine contractions" (p. 352).

Other practitioners referred to the hysterical paroxysm or to sexual response directly in their case histories. Ashwell, lecturing at Guy's Hospital in London (1848), recommended treating women patients' "hysterical paroxysm" with electricity, as well as the other treatments noted above. He added that "the paroxysm and its immediate results have been materially relieved, and in some cases entirely cured, under the influence of the electric treatment" (1848, pp. 177–178). Neiswanger, an electrotherapist, noted that "vibration over the hypogastric plexus . . . influences the bladder, rectum, and sexual organs; causes sexual emotions" (1908, p. 244). He added that "a good vibrator should constitute a part of the armamentarium of every progressive physician" (p. 238; and see Maines, 1999).

But whether evasive or overt about the sexual meanings of electrical genital treatment, nineteenth century physicians continued to write the ancient linkages between women's reproductive system – its organs and functions – and the diagnosis and treatment of insanity. In a treatise on neurasthenia and its treatment, the influential electrotherapist George Beard referred to "irritations of the reproductive apparatus" as one cause of female mental disorder, noting that

> In females, excessive child-bearing, the injuries that follow parturition, and uterine and ovarian congestions resulting from various causes, are often the starting-points of every conceivable phase of functional nervous disorders, from mild and transient neurasthenia through all the gradations to severe melancholia (1880, p. 180).[11]

Beard proposed that, despite the "war" between proponents of local and general treatment, both should be considered in any given case (1880, p. 179); according to the electrotherapy of the day, "The future will show that very much can be done for congestion, atrophy, and engorgement of the womb by carefully localized electrization" (Beard & Rockwell, 1881, p. 541). As late as 1923, the author of a textbook on clinical psychiatry recommended that psychiatric diagnosticians should pay attention to the female "sexual organs," for which "*mechanical therapy*" including electricity, massage, and hydrotherapy, "can be relied upon to produce excellent results" (Diefendorf, 1923, pp. 472–473).

Electrical Stimulative Treatment of Male Insanity

Women were the main, but not the only recipients of genital stimulation as a treatment for insanity. Based on a genital etiology for male mental disorder, the Victorian medical literature occasionally referenced male hysteria (Micale, 1991), and the electrical stimulation of male penises or testes as a treatment.[12] Meigs, in a case history of male hysteria that he treated electrically, claimed that hysterical men had "frequent erections" as well as "globus" and suffered the "morbid aphrodisiac element of unrequited love" (1851, pp. 480–481). Jewell and Bannister's (1874) study of 38 cases of hysteria must have included at least half men, since they found electrical treatment effective with "nineteen cases of pollution and impotence" (p. 325). Erb (1883, p. 353) claimed that for men with "sexual disorders," a "majority of cases . . . require direct electrical treatment of the genitals" with the galvanic current. He also recommended the application of electricity for "hysterical psychosis," but did not specify the site of application (1883, p. 158). Mills (1898, p. 205) mentions the application of the rheophore to the spinal column or the urethra with an electric bougie for conditions such as "spermatophobia" as well as spermatorrhea and impotence.

Masturbation was often proposed as the cause of male sexual dysfunctions and consequent mental disorders. Electrotherapist George Beard (1880, p. 180) claimed that male "self-abuse, especially when begun in early years, before or just after puberty," caused neurasthenia and other disorders. Beard and Rockwell reported the local treatment of a 17 year old boy with spermatorrhea associated with "hypochondriacal depression"; the youth "attributed his symptoms to the vice of masturbation, which he had practiced for years." Treatment involved a catheter electrode in the boy's penis, together with local and general faradization and central galvanization (1881, p. 563). Ives (1879, p. 61) recommended galvanization of the "parts" for "real or imagined diseases of the organ of procreation, such as impotence or spermatorrhea."

Male patients' mental problems were sometimes associated with spermatorrhea or impotence just as women's were with menstruation; psychiatric diagnoses were mediated through genital organs and bodily fluids. Tipton (1882) equated male spermatorrhea with female nymphomania and recommended similar electrical treatment. He suggested putting a pint to a quart of water in a mug, and putting the penis and testicles in it with the positive electrode, while moving the negative electrode, with a long cord "over the lumbar vertebrae . . . If a female a sponge roll may be placed between the labia . . . Otherwise treat the same as males" (pp. 150–151). A similar equation of female and male parts was made by de Watteville (1885), who reported that he had "frequently had the opportunity in the out-patients' room to observe the beneficial effect of the current on the penis and sense of weariness or discomfort depending upon various ovarian or uterine derangements" (p. 196).

Medical accounts of local, genital treatment of men's behavioral or mental disorders are even more textually distant on the issue of sexuality than those concerned with women's. But there are hints. Ives (1879, pp. 81–82) recommended the "use of the wire brush to the parts" in cases of impotence (caused by hypochondriasis, the nineteenth century male equivalent of hysteria). Mr John Birch, London Surgeon, recounted a 1799 case history of a 28 year old gentleman afflicted with impotence. This young man was referred to Birch by another physician, who had treated him unsuccessfully with "medicines." Birch then tried local electricity:

> I therefore passed gentle shocks through both the testes, supposing their deficiency of secretion was the cause of the complaint. These were continued daily, and before the end of one week it was evident their secretion was restored. The patient, however, was so impressed with the *timor animi*, that he chose to continue the remedy a month before he satisfied himself of a perfect cure (Birch, 1799, p. 547).

Despite my anti-anachronistic intentions, I could not help but read this 1799 report on the patient's three months of continuing genital stimulation as tongue-in-cheek.

Controversies Over Genital Stimulation

The use of genital stimulation for the treatment of mental disorders was quite controversial during the nineteenth century, especially where women patients were concerned – and critics, unlike many practitioners, were not reluctant to attribute sexual meanings to genital treatments. In the early part of the century, the sexually stimulative potential of Galen's widow's treatment was recognized and sometimes deplored; in 1802, a French author described, in Latin (the preferred language for delicate subjects), the "shameful practice" of "tickling a woman's clitoris to stop her hysterical fits" (Shorter, 1992, p. 92). In the later part of the century, much of the debate involved the issue of the internal and penetrative, vs. the external and non-penetrative, sexual possibilities of the treatment.

Some of the practitioners of electrical genital stimulation as a treatment for hysteria seemed worried about sexual imputations that might be made by others. In 1800, John Birch published an essay on the use of electricity in the cure of female genital "obstructions," assuring the reader that there was no "*indelicacy*" to the "mode of treatment" (p. viii). He described the electrical procedure using a Leyden jar and two glass rods he called "Directors" which were placed

> below the peak of her stays . . . the wheel is turned and the shock passes immediately through that part of the Pelvis which is included between the Directors. . . . The nerves and vessels . . . [of] the uterus must be affected by the passage of the electric fluid (pp. ix–xi).

Apparently, however, Birch disapproved of the Galenic use of the treatment; he notes that "when obstruction is . . . attended with symptoms which require relief, the application of *shocks* are [sic] often very improper" (p. xiii), adding defensively: "I hope that no imputation of harboring a secret can be imputed to me; for that is a crime" (p. xv). Eighty years later, Zenner lamented "the frequent inutility or needlessness of local treatment," citing his belief that hysteria was not always caused by uterine disturbance (1883, p. 524). He also warned his readers of the possible involvement of locally-treating physicians in patients' sexual fantasies:

> Peretti, physician to an asylum for the insane, gives details of a number of cases in which gynecological examination or treatment were directly productive of injury. In some, local treatment, in others, a mere examination, were the direct exciting causes of an outbreak of insanity, or greatly aggravated the condition of those in whom the disease already existed. In proof of the direct relationship between the gynecological measures and the mental condition, he mentions that the patients usually had delusions or hallucinations of a sexual type, in which the examining physician was a central figure (Zenner, 1883, p. 525).

Early twentieth century physicians continued to criticize genital treatments for female insanity – implying that it was still being used. Reynolds warned that "with intractable neurotics, local treatment, whether operative or minor, only fixes the attention of the patient and increases the evil" (1910, p. 113). Paramore cited the case of a 29-year-old woman treated vaginally with a pessary with neurasthenia; she was operated upon and subsequently became worse, diagnosed with melancholia (1921, p. 116). In 1923, Diefendorf suggested that the surgical removal of healthy ovaries should be "discarded today," although pressure "upon the hysterogenic zones" and "simple suggestion" might be useful.

Other nineteenth and early twentieth century writers distinguished between internal (penetrative) and external stimulation of the female genitalia, apparently on the grounds that only penetration was "really" sexual, and approving of external but not internal stimulation of the woman's genitalia (Maines, 1999). In discussing Galen's widow's treatment for hysteria, Lee Benjamin warned that "Manipulating" the female reproductive organs "directly through the vagina, as recommended by Reeves Jackson and others, is not sufficient to counterbalance the serious objections to the procedure on the score of delicacy and the risk of inducing involuntary erotic manifestations on the part of the patient" (1891, pp. 332–333). Dr. Charles Neiswanger proposed that

> The employment of vibratory stimulation *within* the rectum, urethra, or female pelvis cannot be too strongly condemned, although in many instances it may be used upon the *outside* for the relief of pelvic disturbances (1908, p. 241).

Eberhard (1913, p. 148), however, approved of intra-vaginal electrification, noting that "A physician who condemned the vaginal applicator severely at first . . . now considers this one of the most valuable applicators on the list." He prescribed for uterine diseases, amongst which he included hysteria, vibratory

> intra-vaginal treatment with the special vaginal applicator, or with author's uterine applicator, and short or medium rotary stroke, lasting one and one-half to three minutes, [as] may be required (1913, pp. 108, 147–148).

These intra-vaginal considerations were particularly salient for Victorian physicians when young girls, presumably virgins, were involved. Rockwell, echoing the sentiments of both the age and ages, noted in 1891 that internal local treatment was not "wise" and was sometimes impossible for young girls (p. 106). His recommendation for the local galvanic treatment of menstrual disorders associated with hysteria is so convoluted as to be not entirely clear: one form of the treatment "tends to induce a condition of nervous irritation that is exceedingly unpleasant," while another produces "strong subjective sensations" (p. 208). The recommendation seemed to be, in the end, to apply electrical treatment "over some portion . . . in front . . . of the abdomen" (p. 208).

Although these were indeed serious matters for many physicians, others were not above making a joke of the relationship between female genitalia and insanity. An "Observer" (1878), in a letter to the editors of the *British Medical Journal*, reported an "Effectual Treatment of the Hysterical Paroxysm" that he had observed when he was called into a home. On a bed lay

> the prostrate form of a buxom lass in the paroxysm of hysteria . . . in rushed the family doctor. . . . Having laid hold of a tuft of hair which graced her pubes, he gave it a vigorous tug. The effect was electrical. . . . I never saw this remedy in the books, but it acted like magic (p. 470).

The "Observer" wondered if he might have been a witness to a "criminal assault."

DISCUSSION

Both the genital surgical treatment of female (and to a lesser extent male) insanity, and the stimulatory genital treatment of insanity during the nineteenth century are instructive in the context of scholarly debates over Victorian sexuality, insanity, and anatomy. The electrical genital treatment of hysteria and allied disorders continued and expanded a long tradition of Platonic, Hippocratic, and Galenic explanations and treatments for hysterical symptoms into a post-Enlightenment, Cartesian era supposed by some scholars to have moved from uterine to nervous-system explanations of mental illness. Even Charcot, Freud's mentor, official proponent of a nerve theory of male as well as female hysteria, recommended ovarian compression in some cases, and is reported as insisting of female hysteria that "c'est toujours une chose genitale" (Maines, 1999, p. 43).

The contemporary canon of the cultural history of the body, Thomas Laqueur (1990), has proposed a movement, during the nineteenth century, from an anatomical theory of the one-sex to the two-sex body, with its consequent definition of women as qualitatively, not just quantitatively different from men (a shift with political and social, as well as anatomical implications). The continuation of what are essentially humoral approaches to treating hysteria indicates that this shift was not (as Laqueur himself points out) global or total, and may have affected anatomical and cellular studies, perhaps, more than a clinical medicine still partially grounded in the authority of the ancients.

The Victorians, from our twentieth century standpoint, have been portrayed as sexually repressive, not only guarding female virginity and female and male heterosexuality and marriage, but also warning against male and female masturbation, with its connotations of material wastefulness and social isolation. Galen's widow's treatment was both genital and orgasmic, reflecting the ancient association between conception and female (as well as male) orgasm (King, 1993; Laqueur, 1990). The stimulative local treatments of the Victorian era were sometimes textually genital, but rarely textually sexual; it was mainly the critics of stimulatory treatment (internal or external) who referenced its pleasurable possibilities for the patient.

But what was and is constant is the interposition of medical authority, and mostly male medical authority at that, between a woman's body and her social experience of it, and a woman's social role and her body. From the Hippocratics to the Victorian era and into the twentieth century, Western culture has established the expert as a source of knowledge and authority, and the medical expert as the site of knowledge and authority over the body – especially the female body, and its sexualities.[13] And where the body (its humors, hormones, organs, or genes) is framed as the source of sane or insane behavior or feelings, then it is medical authority that functions as the arbiter of the borderline between the sane and the insane – between those who do, and those who do not, fit their gendered (and class, race, age) place within the social order. Dr. Laycock, in 1850, described the symptoms of cerebral hysteria or moral insanity in women – which he treated with electro-galvanization of the pelvis and abdomen – as deficits of social place:

> The gentle, truthful and self-denying woman has unaccountably become cunning, quarrelsome, selfish . . . there is no regard for appearances, or for the feelings or interests of others. . . . In short, there is such a complete perversion of the character, that . . . it can only be considered as a state of disease (p. 57).

Men have, indeed, had their genitalia subjected to medical social control over the millennia, and certainly during the nineteenth century. There were parallels between male and female insanity in Victorian times, with the psychiatric linking of bodily fluids, reproductive systems, and mental pathologies into diagnoses. But the genital treatment of women's madness was both quantitatively and qualititatively different from men's. There are many more female surgical operations to be found in the case histories of the genital treatment of insanity than men's – and the discipline of gynecology flourished past the *fin de siecle*, while that of andrology (although it still exists, and indeed appeared on almost 30,000 websites as of 2001) is little spoken of. Both men's and women's mental disorders were embodied, linked with the humoral, the genital and the sexual, and both were social, linked with the social roles available at the time – but women's sexual and social limitations were (and are) far greater than men's in Western culture (Barker-Benfield, 2000).

It is women who have at all times from the Platonic to the present been caught within the net of sexological and medical expertise, judged in one era or one situation as too asexual and others as too sexual; as too reproductive, or not reproductive enough. And these definitions have been interwoven into the fabric of psychiatric symptomatology, diagnosis, and treatment. Clitoridectomy as a "treatment" for women who were psychiatrically diagnosed because they masturbated, committed adultery, were interested in clitorial stimulation with other women or men or even with their husbands, or who behaved in ways unbefitting their gender, was part of Western medicine from the Hippocratic corpus into the early twentieth century. Both genital stimulation and "female circumcision" as "treatments" for women who were psychiatrically diagnosed because they did not reproduce, did not experience sexual pleasure or orgasm, or who behaved in ways unbefitting their gender, were also a part of the same medical tradition. One was not liberatory in opposition to the repressive; rather, both were aspects of the Western cultural dominance of the expert, and of medical social control. We know that the end of female genital mutilation for the treatment of insanity in the West came somewhere between the 1920s and the 1940s, but what of "female circumcision" and Galen's widow's treatment, the two pathways to an (albeit medically normalized) orgasm?

The last references to the involvement of female genitalia in psychiatric diagnosis and treatment that I have been able to find were in the 1950s. In 1959, Dr. W. G. Rathmann published an article entitled "Female Circumcision: Indications and a New Technique." Like Pratt more than sixty years earlier, Rathmann writes from the point of view of women's right to sexual satisfaction, and his main concern is with "redundancy or phimosis of the female prepuce" interfering with clitoral sensation. (His use of the term for the male foreskin in describing the clitoral hood indicates the tenacity, still, of the one-sex body). Rathmann recounts a case history of "psychosomatic illness" caused by the inability to have an orgasm – which, in turn, was caused by "rather severe redundancy and phimosis" (1959, p. 116):

> After being circumcised, she remarried the last man she had divorced and has had no further sexual problems. She stated that she 'wasted four perfectly good husbands.' While having the five marriages and divorces, she had a great number of psychosomatic symptoms and illnesses (1959, p. 116).

Galen's widow's treatment also survived into the mid-twentieth century in a textbook on electroshock therapy at a Pennsylvania asylum (Steinfeld, 1951). Steinfeld and his colleagues treated 47% of their postpartum psychiatric patients and 27% of all their female patients monthly during their periods with electroshock. They also treated some of these female patients with male hormones, reasoning that this would "break down inhibitions" and "increase clitoral excitability." The resulting "direct genital gratification," as in the case of Galen's widow, would then provide "alleviation . . . of some of the symptoms" of mental disorder through masturbation (1951, pp. 207–208). They reported that "nine patients were treated with this aim in mind. All of them responded with a heightened sexual excitability and some improvement in their capacity for adjustment" (1951, p. 209).

The female genitalia appeared in these researchers' accounts in the context of psychotherapy and somatic treatment as well as hormones. They described one case of a female "psychoneurotic" aged 22 treated with 24 sub-coma insulin shocks and 14 superimposed electroshocks to facilitate transference:

> The therapist . . . spent considerable time with the patient . . . [who] began to form a strong positive transference, the very intensity and *genital character* of which was later to clash with her weakened, aggressive ego (Steinfeld, 1951, p. 138; italics added).

Sexually stimulative psychiatric treatment, having lasted almost two thousand years, seems not, however, to have survived into the third millennium. But even without genitalia, the involvement of gender and gynecology in women's psychiatric diagnoses continued through the twentieth and into the twenty-first century, with (as just one example), older women treated by gynecologists with psychopharmacology for the "symptoms" of menopause. Although now without the local treatment of genitalia, Anglo-American psychiatry continues to involve gynecology in the diagnosis and treatment of women as mentally ill, implicating their hormonal fluids and the configurations of their social roles in their psychologies and pathologies. Nevertheless and despite the Renaissance, the Enlightenment, and the rise of modernity:

> Deaf to pleas from anatomy and experience, the [hysteria] texts continue to tell one another the traditional stories. The language may shift – the womb travels, vapors rise, sympathy transmits symptoms through the body – but the message remains the same: women are sick, and men write their bodies (King, 1993, p. 64).

NOTES

1. In researching and writing this essay, I have been helped enormously by a number of people and institutions. I want to thank Susan Case in particular for her assistance, first at the Logan Clendening Library of the History of Medicine at the University of Kansas Medical Center, and later of the Anschutz Library of the K. U. Lawrence campus. Without her help, this project would have been impossible. I would also like to thank the staffs of the Bakken Institute (a museum and library of electricity) in Minnesota, and the K. U. Spencer Rare Books Library for their assistance. Rachel Maines, Darlaine Gardetto, Jennie Kronenfeld, Marcia Texler Segal, and Vicky Demos provided valuable insights and suggestions during the writing of this manuscript. University of Kansas undergraduate student Sara Sipe was most helpful in locating some of the primary sources used in this study, as was Vickie Kennedy, KU Sociology graduate student, who acquainted me with contemporary andrology on the internet. Special thanks to Lynn Porter of the wordprocessing office of the University of Kansas College of Liberal Arts and Sciences, who endured, with great patience, competence, and good humor, many drafts of this paper.

2. For a popular media portrayal of a nineteenth century genital treatment, among other treatments, see the movie and the book *The Road to Wellville* (Boyle, 1994).

3. Some physicians, especially during the Renaissance, used the diagnosis of hypochondria to classify the hysteria-like symptoms of men, tracing its physical origins to the spleen. Today, of course, the term hypochondria is used with a quite different meaning.

4. I use mostly secondary rather than primary sources when discussing genital surgeries for the treatment of female insanity, because this ground has been well covered in published sources, especially Longo (1979, 1981), Scull and Favreau (1986), Sheehan (1997), Shorter (1992), and Shortt (1986).

5. This is not to say that no etiologies or treatments for mental illness were derived from the Platonic penis (see below); only that there was no canonical parallel to Galen's widow's treatment.

6. In the late 1950s, when I was growing up in Europe, I was told by my mother that I should not run around too much in case my male genitalia, inside, dropped out and made me into a male. As recently as the 1990s I heard about a young woman who thought her headaches were caused by her uterus rising from its place.

7. Prior to the Enlightenment, medical knowledge – for example in medical texts – was based on the authority of prior experts such as Galen or Avicenna. With the development of empiricism, observation, and experimentation, a clinical medicine developed that was based on these forms of evidence rather than on authority. But even as late as the 1800s, Dewees and other physicians had to remind the reader that just because Galen had proposed an etiology and a treatment thousands of years earlier, clinical medicine might propose a different etiology and treatment.

8. As a child in England during the early 1950s, I was given smelling salts to carry, and my mother also carried them.

9. Medical treatment is either general or local. Some nineteenth century electrical treatments, such as static electrical baths, were general treatments, directed at the body in general, and working through the blood, nerves, or cells. Other electrical treatments were local, directed at the site of the proposed lesion held responsible for the mental symptoms, for example electric shock to the brain or electrification of the genitalia.

10. Like his successors, the electroshock practitioners of the twentieth century, Tipton also applied the electric current with "mild force" to the head (1882, p. 227).

11. Nineteenth century physicians commonly believed in the progression of mental illnesses over time from the less to the more serious diagnoses.

12. Perhaps not surprisingly – given the homoerotic implications of male physicians genitally treating male patients – I have found no instances of *non*-electrical (or at least non-technological, using the hands only) stimulation of male genitalia in the treatment of insanity.

13. There were other medical arenas where new developments were seen as threatening to women's "delicacy." Mary Poovey (1989) contrasts the adoption of chloroform in surgery with its resistance in childbirth during the nineteenth century. Chloroform was suspected of causing women under its influence to have sexual dreams or make orgasmic movements, something too shocking for either the women or their physicians to contemplate.

REFERENCES

Adair, M. J. (1996). Plato's view of the 'Wandering Uterus'. *Classical Journal*, *91*, 153–163.

Albutt, C. T. (1884). *Visceral neuroses*. London: Churchill.

Ashwell, S. (1848). *A practical treatise on the diseases peculiar to women*. Philadelphia: Lea and Blanchard.

Barker-Benfield, G. J. (2000). *The horrors of the half-known life* (2nd ed.). London: Routledge.

Beard, G. M. (1880). *A practical treatise on nervous exhaustion (Neurasthenia)*. New York: William Wood.

Beard, G. M., & Rockwell, A. D. (1881). *On the medical and surgical uses of electricity* (8th ed.). New York: William Wood.

Benjamin, L. (1891). Swedish movements and massage. In: H. A. Hare (Ed.), *A System of Practical Therapeutics* (Vol. 1, pp. 247–338). Philadelphia: Lea Brothers.

Bigelow, H. J. (1859–1860). Castration as a means of cure for satyriasis. *Boston Medical and Surgical Journal*, *61*, 165–166.

Birch, J. (1799). A letter to the author. In: G. Adams (Ed.), *An Essay on Electricity*. London: R. Hindmarsh.

Birch, J. (1800). *Consideration of the efficacy of electricity in removing female obstructions* (2nd ed.). London: T. Cadell.

Bodemer, C. W. (1973). Historical interpretation of the human uterus and cervix uteri. In: R. J. Blandau & K. Moghiri (Eds), *The Biology of the Cervix* (pp. 1–11). Chicago: University of Chicago Press.

Boyle, T. C. (1994). *The road to Wellville*. New York: Signet.

Brodie, Sir B. C. (1837). *Lectures illustrative of certain local nervous affections*. London: Longman, Rees, Orme, Brown, Green and Longman.

Cushing, P. (1995). *Constructing the self, constructing America: A cultural history of psychotherapy*. Reading, MA: Addison-Wesley.

Dawson, B. E. (1915). Circumcision in the female: Its necessity and how to perform it. *American Journal of Clinical Medicine*, *22*(June), 520–523.

Dewees, W. P. (1828). *Treatise on the diseases of females*. Philadelphia: Carey, Lea and Carey.

Diefendorf, A. R. (1923). *Clinical psychology: A text book*. London: Macmillan.

Eberhard, N. M. (1913). *A brief guide to vibratory technique* (3rd ed). Chicago: New Medicine Publishing Co.

Emerson, J. (1971). Behavior in private places: Sustaining definitions of reality in gynecological examinations. In: H. P. Dreitzel (Ed.), *Recent Sociology*, (Vol. 2, pp. 73–97). London: Collier-Macmillan.

Erb, W. (1883). *Handbook of electro-therapeutics*. New York: William Wood and Co.

Far Reaching Influence of Abnormalities of the Clitoris, The (1893). *Journal of the American Medical Association*, *10* (June 10), 645.

Flint, A. (1874). *The physiology of man, Vol. V: Special senses*. Generation. New York: D. Appleton and Co.

Goodell, W. (1881). Clinical notes on the extirpation of the ovaries for insanity. *Transactions of the Medical Society of the State of Pennsylvania*, *13*, 638–643.

Hanson, A. E. (1990). The medical writers' woman. In: D. M. Halperin, J. F. Winkler & F. I. Zeitlin (Eds), *Before Sexuality: The Construction of Erotic Experience in the Ancient Greek World* (pp. 309–337). Princeton, NJ: Princeton University Press.

Hedley, W. S. (1900). *Therapeutic electricity and practical muscle testing*. Philadelphia: P. Blakiston Son and Co.

Hersmann, C. C. (1899). Relation of uterine disease to some of the insanities. *Journal of the American Medical Association*, *32*(Sept. 16), 709–711.

Ives, J. (1879). *Electricity as a medicine and its mode of application*. New York: John T. Ives Jr.

Jewell, J. S., & Bannister, H. M. (1874). Therapeutics of the nervous system and mind. *Chicago Journal of Nervous and Mental Disease*, *1*, 100–107.

King, H. (1993). Once upon a text: Hysteria from Hippocrates. In: S. L. Gilman et al. (Eds), *Hysteria Beyond Freud* (pp. 3–90). London: University of California Press.

Kneeland, T., & Warren, C. A. B. (2002). *Pushbutton psychiatry: A history of electroshock in America*. Westport, CT: Praeger.

Laqueur, T. (1990). *Making sex: Body and gender from the Greeks to Freud*. Cambridge, MA: Harvard University Press.

Laycock, Dr. (1850). On the treatment of cerebral hysteria, and of moral insanity in women, by electro-galvanism. *Medical Times* (New Series 1, July 6 to Dec. 28), 57–58.

Libbrecht, K., & Quackenbush, J. (1995). On the early history of male hysteria and psychic trauma. *Journal of the History of the Behavioral Sciences*, *31*, 370–384.

Lightfoot, T. (1857). On the mental, nervous and convulsive disorders traceable to physiological or pathological conditions of the sexual organs in women, and more especially to the ovaria. *Lancet*, *1*(July 24), 79–80.

Longo, L. D. (1979). The rise and fall of battey's operation: A fashion in surgery. *Bulletin of the History of Medicine*, *2*(Summer), 244–267.

Longo, L. D. (1986). Electrotherapy in gynecology: The American experience. *Bulletin of the History of Medicine* (Fall), 343–366.

Lunbeck, E. (1994). *The psychiatric persuasion: Knowledge, gender and power in modern America*. Princeton, NJ: Princeton University Press.

Maines, R. P. (1999). *The technology of orgasm: 'Hysteria,' the vibrator, and women's sexual satisfaction*. Baltimore, MD: Johns Hopkins University Press.

Marshall, J. H. (1865). Insanity cured by castration. *Medical and Surgical Reporter*, *13*, 363–364.

McGinness, E. (1894). The uses of electricity in obstetrics: Galacotorrhoea; sore nippleism. In: H. R. Bigelow (Ed.), *An International System of Electro-Therapeutics* (pp. 1–10). Philadelphia: F. A. Davis Co.

Meigs, C. D. (1851). *Woman: Her diseases and remedies* (2nd ed.). Philadelphia: Lea and Blanchard.

Micale, M. (1991). Hysteria male/hysteria female: Reflections on comparative gender construction in nineteenth-century France and Britain. In: M. Benjamin (Ed.), *Science and Sensibility: Gender and Scientific Inquiry, 1780–1945* (pp. 200–201). Oxford: Basil Blackwell.

Mills, C. K. (1898). *The nervous system and its diseases*. Philadelphia, PA: Lippincott.

Mitchison, W. (1991). *The nature of their bodies: Women and their doctors in victorian Canada*. Toronto: University of Toronto Press.

Napheys, G. H. (1875). *The physical life of woman: Advice to the maiden, wife and mother* (5th ed.). Philadelphia: Fergus, Watts & Co.

Neiswanger, C. S. (1908). *Electrotherapeutic practice: A Ready reference guide for physicians in the use of electricity* (15th ed.). Chicago: Ritchie & Co.

Observer, A. (1878). Effectual treatment of the hysterical paroxysm. *British Medical Journal*, *1*(March 30), 470.

Oppenheim, J. (1991). *'Shattered nerves': Doctors, patients and depression in victorian England*. New York: Oxford University Press.

Pallen, M. A. (1879). The insanities of females. *American Gynaecological and Obstetrical Journal*, *1*, 190–202.

Paramore, R. H. (1921). The neurasthenic element in mid-wifery and gynecology. *British Medical Journal*, *11*, 768–769.

Park, K. (1997). The rediscovery of the clitoris: French medicine and the tribade, 1570–1620. In: D. Hillman & C. Mazzio (Eds), *The Body in Parts* (pp. 171–193). London: Routledge.

Plato, *The Dialogues* (1953) (4th ed.), Trans. B. Jowett. Oxford: Jowett Copyright Trustees.

Poovey, M. (1989). *Uneven developments*. London: Virago Press.

Pratt, E. H. (1898, March 6). Circumcision of girls. In: *The Journal of Orificial Surgery* (pp. 385–392). Chicago.

Rathmann, W. G. (1959). Female circumcision: Indications and a new technique. *GP* XX, September, 115–120.

Relation of Pelvic Disease to Psychical Disturbance in Women, The (1893). *Journal of the American Medical Association*, *20*, 650.

Reynolds, E. (1910). Gynecological operatons on neurasthenics: Advantages, disadvantages, selected cases. *Boston Medical and Surgical Journal*, *CCXII*, 113–117.

Roccatagliata, G. (1986). *A history of ancient psychiatry*. New York: Greenwood Press.

Rockwell, A. D. (1891). Electro-therapeutics. In: H. A. Hare (Ed.), *A System of Practical Therapeutics* (Vol. 1, pp. 133–226). Philadelphia: Lea Brothers.

Rohe, G. H. (1893). Lactational insanity. *Journal of the American Medical Association*, *10*(Sept. 2), 325–326.

Savage, G. H. (1878). Uterine displacement corrected – insanity cured. *Brain: A Journal of Neurology*, *1*(April–January), 270–272.

Schleiner, W. (1995). *Medical ethics in the renaissance*. Washington, DC: Georgetown University Press.

Scull, A., & Favreau, D. (1986). 'A chance to cut is a chance to cure': Sexual surgery for psychosis in three nineteenth century societies. In: *Research in Law, Deviance and Social Control* (Vol. 8, pp. 3–39). London: JAI Press.

Sheehan, E. A. (1997). Victorian clitoridectomy: Isaac Baker Brown and his harmless operative procedure. In: R. N. Lancaster & M. di Leonardo (Eds), *The Gender Sexuality Reader* (pp. 325–334). New York: Routledge.

Shorter, E. (1992). *From paralysis to fatigue: A history of psychosomatic illness in the modern era*. New York: Free Press.

Shortt, S. E. D. (1986). *Victorian lunacy: Richard M. Bucke and the practice of late nineteenth century psychiatry*. Cambridge: Cambridge University Press.

Simon, B. (1978). *Mind and madness in ancient Greece: The classical roots of modern psychiatry*. Ithaca, NY: Cornell University Press.

Sissa, G. (1990). Motherhood without maidenhead: The female body in Ancient Greece. In: D. M. Halper, J. J. Winkler & F. I. Zeitlin (Eds), *Before Sexuality: the Construction of Erotic Experience in the Ancient Greek World* (pp. 339–364). Princeton: Princeton University Press.

Smith, E. H. (1903). Masturbation in the female. *Pacific Medical Journal* (n.v. Feb.), 76–83.

Steinfeld, J. I. (1951). *Therapeutic studies on psychotics*. Des Plaines, IL: Forest Press.

Storer, H. R. (1866). The causation, course, and treatment of insanity in women: A gynaecist's idea thereof. *The Transactions of the American Medical Association*, *XVI*, 121–254.

Stuart, H. R. (1889). *Our famiy physician*. New York: Smith and Hillman.

Sutherland, H. (1875). Notes on a case of insanity indirectly caused by phimosis. *British Medical Journal*, *1*(June 26), 845–846.

Taylor, E. (1983). The electrified hand: Therapeutic implications. *Medical Instrumentation*, *17*(July–August), 281–282.

Taylor, R. W. (1905). *A practical treatise on sexual disorders of the male and female* (3rd ed.). New York: Lea Bros.

Tipton, A. W. (1882). *Electrical medication*. Chicago: Chas. C. Johnson.

Tomes, N. (1984). *A generous confidence: Thomas Story Kirkbride and the art of asylum-keeping, 1840–1883*. Cambridge: Cambridge University Press.

Tripier, A. (1894). Engorgement and displacements of the uterus. In: H. R. Bigelow (Ed.), *An International System of Electro-Therapeutics* (pp. 135–147). Philadelphia: F. A. Davis Co.

de Watteville, A. (1885). *A practical introduction to medical electricity*. New York: J. H. Vail.

Williams, S. W. D. (1863–1864). Cases illustrating the action of amenorrhoea as a cause of insanity. *The Journal of Mental Science*, *9*, 344–353.

Wood, A. D. (1973). 'The fashionable diseases': Women's complaints and their treatment in nineteenth century America. *Journal of Interdisciplinary History*, *4*(Summer), 25–52.

Wood, H. C. (1887). *A treatise on therapeutics* (6th ed.). Philadelphia: J. B. Lippincott.

Zenner, P. (1883). The value of gynecological treatment in hysteria and allied affections. *The Journal of the American Medical Association* (n.v.), 523–525. Chicago.

Zoist, the Journal of Cerebral Physiology and Mesmerism and their Application to Human Welfare (1848–1849). London: Hyppolyte Balliere.

A DEMOGRAPHIC PARADOX: CAUSES AND CONSEQUENCES OF FEMALE GENITAL CUTTING IN NORTHEASTERN AFRICA

Kathryn M. Yount and Deborah L. Balk

ABSTRACT

Ritual female genital practices, widespread throughout Africa, are essential to gender identification and often are a pre-requisite for marriage. More severe forms of the practice, which are common in parts of Northeastern Africa, are also believed to enhance a woman's childbearing capacity. Here, we critically review the gender- and class-based theories that explain the origins and persistence of female genital practices and the factors that precipitate social change. We also critically review evidence of the association of certain forms of the practice with various health, demographic, and social consequences. Our review exposes several methodological limitations of existing research that preclude population-based inferences about the medical and social implications of these practices and suggest that existing policies targeting such practices draw more on concerns over human rights than on scientific evidence about their sequelae. This review nevertheless exposes a potential contradiction between local justifications for and consequences of certain forms of the practice. Namely, despite an intended function of female genital practices to enhance a woman's marital capital, certain forms may

Gender Perspectives on Reproduction and Sexuality
Advances in Gender Research, Volume 8, 199–249

ISSN: 1529-2126/doi:10.1016/S1529-2126(04)08007-5

ironically lead to marital instability and dissolution through their negative effects on the health and reproductive capacity of women. We conclude with recommendations for research to examine the salience and implications of this potential paradox for women in Northeastern Africa.

INTRODUCTION

Ritual female genital practices have existed for millennia (see Gordon, 1991; Kassamali, 1998; Kennedy, 1970; Leonard, 2000; Mackie, 1996) and persist in some form in Western, Central, North Eastern, and Eastern Africa as well as Indonesia, Malaysia, the Arab Peninsula, and immigrant communities worldwide (Isa, Shuib & Othman, 1999; Leonard, 2000; Shell-Duncan & Herlund, 2000). Of the approximately 25 African countries with data, estimated prevalences vary from 18% in Tanzania (Bureau of Statistics and Macro International, 1997) to 98% in Somalia and Djibouti (in Shell-Duncan & Herlund, 2000). Among those African countries with representative data, the highest prevalence (97%) occurs among ever-married Egyptian women of reproductive age (Carr, 1997; El-Zanaty et al., 1996). Although estimates are tentative and vary by and within countries, approximately 130 million women have experienced some form of genital cutting, and 2 million women are at risk of genital cutting annually, most of whom live in 28 African countries (World Health Organization, 1996).[1]

The perspectives from which to understand these practices come from a diverse group of social scientists, clinicians, and activists. Anthropologists and sociologists argue that most women and men in populations that adhere to these practices believe that they exist and should continue for various long-standing reasons. Most prominently, these practices are thought to ensure a daughter's prospects for marriage and motherhood (e.g. Boddy, 1982; Cloudsley, 1983; Gordon, 1991). Others suggest that this custom is an integral part of gender identification (e.g. Talle, 1993; van der Kwaak, 1992) and the political economy (e.g. Gruenbaum, 1988, 2001; Toubia, 1985). As a consequence, women may be important perpetuators of this practice not only as mothers and grandmothers who favor continuation (e.g. Candib, 1999; Hayes, 1975; Mackie, 1996, 2000), but also as midwives whose livelihoods depend in part on these and associated practices (e.g. Gruenbaum, 1982). Clinical studies attribute an array of demographic and health consequences to various forms of the practice, ranging from minor infection to infertility and death (e.g. Aziz, 1980; Cook, 1979; Dirie & Lindmark, 1991; El Dareer, 1982; Inhorn & Buss, 1993; Jones et al., 1999; Knight et al., 1999; Mawad & Hassanein, 1994; Momoh et al., 2001; Morison et al., 2001; Shandall, 1967; Verzin, 1975). For these reasons and interests in safeguarding human rights, a large, activist's literature calls for "eradication" of these practices (e.g. Allam et al., 2001; Barstow, 1999; Eke & Nkanginieme, 1999; Hosken, 1982; Koso-Thomas, 1987; Lax, 2000; McLean & Graham, 1983; Slack, 1988; Toubia, 1993, 1994).[2]

In a context of diverse perspectives and uneven quality of data, this paper has two aims. First, we seek to understand the causes and consequences of female genital practices. To do so, we adopt an approach that is based both in positivism and cultural relativism (Gordon, 1991; Lyons, 1981). In particular, we acknowledge our external cultural and Western feminist predisposition (sometimes shared with cultural "insiders") to view these practices as contrary to women's and children's well-being or a violation of basic human rights. At the same time, we recognize that discovering the logic behind behaviors that are foreign to the analyst requires an understanding of the socio-cultural context and relations of power within which these behaviors occur, and that policies "targeting" female genital practices are likely to be ineffectual when formed in a cultural vacuum (e.g. Gordon, 1991; Lyons, 1981; van der Kwaak, 1992).[3] Therefore, we acknowledge that many women, especially those who favor and participate in some form of female genital cutting, identify it as an acceptable and even welcomed ritual that is central to a woman's social identity and economic security in the contexts where these practices persist (Boddy, 1991; Gordon, 1991; Gulick, 1976; Hicks, 1993; Talle, 1993).

A second aim of this monograph is to encourage greater attention to female genital practices in the socio-demographic literature about Africa. Historical inattention to these practices among demographers is ironic because much of this literature has been influenced by demographers who are likely to call attention to socio-cultural factors. (Recent exceptions include Balk (2000), Caldwell, Orubuloye and Caldwell (1997, 2000), El-Gibaly et al. (1999, 2002), Jones et al. (1999), Larsen (1994, 1995, 2000), and Yount (2002).) For example, Lesthaeghe's edited volume on reproduction and social organization (1989), with a notable exception (see Larsen, 1989), does not consider the role of female genital practices in the production or survival of children. Except until recently (Caldwell, Orubuloye & Caldwell, 1997, 2000), the Caldwells' extensive research on Africa includes little about female genital cutting. In 1983, they acknowledge this deficit with the following explanation: "We, and other researchers, have ignored the possibility of primary sterility arising from infection at the time of clitoridectomy. One reason is that the incidence of cliterodectomy does not appear to be associated with that of primary sterility. Another reason is that girls appear to be too old at the time of the operation for infection to have resulted in sterility by the time of marriage. Yet the practice of clitoridectomy, and the type practiced, is culture-specific, so perhaps we may be premature in ignoring it" (Caldwell & Caldwell, 1983, p. 20).

To achieve these aims, we critique the existing literature that seeks to understand the origins and persistence of female genital practices and the factors that precipitate social change. We also critique the clinical and epidemiological literature that addresses the potential effects of various forms of the practice. In reviewing these bodies of literature, we often refer to the experiences of women in Northeastern Africa (Egypt, Eritrea, Ethiopia, Djibouti, Somalia, and Sudan) because some of the highest prevalences and most varied forms of female genital cutting exist in this region. Our critique motivates a discussion of the following demographic paradox: the very practices that are often central to the formation of women's marital capital in many African societies may be a cause of marital instability and dissolution in these same settings, in part due to the effects of certain forms of the practice on the health, reproductive capacity, and psychological and sexual well-being of African women. At the same time, declines in the practice of female genital cutting that have been observed in several African settings (Caldwell et al., 2000; El-Gibaly et al., 1999, 2002; Yount, 2002) may not be sustainable if female genital practices remain a normative prerequisite for marriage. The reviews and analysis in this paper establish a framework for methodologically sound research, without which we can neither answer outstanding medical, social or political questions about these practices nor frame appropriate policy questions.

DESCRIPTION OF THE PRACTICE AND NOMENCLATURE

Several systems of classification have been proposed to categorize the major forms of female genital cutting (Hosken, 1982; Toubia, 1998; World Health Organization [WHO], 1997). According to these systems, there are generally five recognized forms of the practice and other forms that are found in settings like Sudan and Egypt (Table 1). Table 1 provides descriptions of these major forms and estimates of the prevalence of each form in Northeast African countries with representative data from the Demographic and Health Surveys (DHS).

The first type, often called *symbolic* circumcision, involves nicking the clitoris with a sharp instrument to cause bleeding but no long-term damage. *Symbolic* circumcision reportedly occurs in settings like Indonesia and Malaysia (Hosken, 1982; Isa et al., 1999) and may be increasing in prevalence in settings where more extensive procedures have been practiced (Ibrahim, personal communication, January, 2002). A second form, known in Arabic as *sunna* circumcision,[4] involves removal of the prepuce, or the layer of skin covering the clitoris. An estimated 13% of Sudanese women have experienced *sunna* circumcision (DHS, 1991);

Table 1. Types of Ritual Female Genital Practices.

WHO System of Classification	Detailed Descriptions of Types of Female Genital Cutting	DHS Estimated Prevalence (%)		
		Sudan[a]	Egypt[b]	Eritrea[c]
	Symbolic circumcision: nicking of the clitoris in order to cause minor bleeding. Usually doesn't cause long term damage and leaves the sexual function of the genitalia intact. Low chance of complications.	0.0	0.0 (0.0)	0.0
Type I: Excision of the prepuce, with or without excision of part or all of the clitoris	Sunna circumcision: figuratively means tradition or duty in Arabic. Removal of prepuce of the clitoris. Sometimes also includes removal of the tip of the clitoris, but usually the gland and body of the clitoris are left intact. Permanent alteration to genitalia may include a reduction of sexual response. Chance of complications.	13.2	0.0 (0.0)	0.0
Type II: Excision of the clitoris with partial or total excision of the labia minora.	Excision: removal of the clitoris, generally along with the parts of the labia minora. Permanent alteration to genitalia including probable complete loss of clitoral orgasm. Increased chance of complications.	0.0	64.0 (98.6)	65.9

Table 1. *(Continued)*

WHO System of Classification	Detailed Descriptions of Types of Female Genital Cutting	DHS Estimated Prevalence (%)		
		Sudan[a]	Egypt[b]	Eritrea[c]
Type III: Excision of part or all of the external genitalia and stitching/narrowing of the vaginal opening (infibulation)	Intermediate or Matwasat circumcision: includes excision, removal of the anterior parts or all of the labia minora, and some or all of the labia majora. The two sides are stitched together (i.e. infibulated) leaving a moderately sized opening. Varies considerably. Permanent alteration to genitalia. Clitoral orgasm highly unlikely. Complications likely.	2.4	9.4 (0.7)	34.0
	Infibulation, Pharaonic or Sudanese circumcision[d]: removal of clitoris, labia minora; and most or all of the labia majora is scraped or cut away. The wound is stitched closed leaving a tiny opening, roughly the size of a match stick to allow for the passage of urine and menstrual blood. The girl's legs are often tied together (i.e. ankles, knees, thighs) and she may be immobilized for up to 40 days. High risk of infection and complications, with long term implications, are common. Clitoral orgasm highly unlikely. (Often requires de-infibulation for intercourse.)	73.4	0.0 (0.0)	0.0

Table 1. *(Continued)*

WHO System of Classification	Detailed Descriptions of Types of Female Genital Cutting	DHS Estimated Prevalence (%)		
		Sudan[a]	Egypt[b]	Eritrea[c]
Type IV: Unclassified: includes pricking, piercing, incising the clitoris and/or labia; stretching the clitoris and/or labia; cauterization by burning of the clitoris and surrounding tissue; scraping tissue surrounding the vaginal orifice (angurya cuts) or cutting of the vagina (gishiri cuts); introduction of corrosive substances or herbs into the vagina to cause bleeding or for the purposes of tightening or narrowing it; and any other procedure that falls under the WHO definition of female genital mutilation.	Cutting of labia minora only: This practice is common in Egypt.		7.8	
	Clitoridectomy: removal of the clitoris. Permanent alteration to genitalia including probable complete loss of clitoral orgasm. Increased chance of complications.		18.7	

Sources: Procedure descriptions are compiled from Hosken (1982), Kheir et al. (1991), and WHO (1997); Data from the 1989/1990 Sudan Demographic and Health Survey, National Population Coucil-Egypt and Macro International Inc. 1995, Egyptian Fertility Care Society 1996, National Statistics Office-Eritrea and Macro International Inc. 1995.

[a] These figures are DHS estimates of prevalence for 1989–1990. Eighty-nine percent report having had some form of circumcision. The remaining 11% of women indicated that they had no form of circumcision.

[b] These figures are DHS estimates of prevalence for 1995. Figures outside parentheses are taken from a clinic-based study, and those in parentheses are taken from a nationally representative sample of ever-married women aged 15–49 years. Figures from the clinic-based study are not nationally representative. This study was undertaken by the Egyptian Fertility Care Society and included 1,339 women. "Any excision of labia majora" is classified here as Matwasat circumcision. In the population-based survey, most (98.6%) circumcised women (97% of ever-married women) report that their vaginal area was not sewn, suggesting that they had excision or clitoridectomy only. Only 0.7% of circumcised women report that their vaginal area was sewn closed, suggesting that <1% of women are infibulated. Vaginal area sewn closed is classified here as matwasat circumcision. 0.6% of circumcisions were of unknown type.

[c] These figures are DHS estimates of prevalence in 1995. 94.5% report having had some form of circumcision. The DHS classification of "Infibulation" is noted here as matwasat circumcision.

[d] In the literature, the terms infibulation, pharaonic, and Sudanese circumcision are used interchangeably, although in the Sudan infibulation occurs both in pharaonic and matwasat procedures.

however, the term *sunna* may refer to a variety of genital practices, which makes cross-cultural comparisons using this terminology difficult (Gruenbaum, 2001).

A third form, known as *clitoridectomy*, involves removal of the prepuce and the clitoris only, leaving most or all of the labia minora and majora intact (Inhorn & Buss, 1993). An estimated 61.5% of women in Eritrea and 19% of women in Egypt have experienced clitoridectomy (El-Zanaty et al., 1996; National Statistics Office [NSO], 1997). A fourth form, known as *excision*, entails clitoridectomy along with removal of parts or all of the labia minora. According to the DHS, this type is not found in Sudan but is believed to occur among women in Eritrea (4%), Egypt (64%), and certain groups in West Africa (El-Zanaty et al., 1996; Hosken, 1978; NSO, 1997).[5]

A fifth form of cutting is known as *infibulation*, which also has been called *pharaonic* circumcision. The most extreme form of infibulation involves a complete excision, the scraping or cutting away of most of the labia majora, and the stitching of the labia majora, leaving a small hole for the passage of urine and menstrual fluid (see El Dareer, 1982; Hicks, 1993; Kennedy, 1970; Slack, 1988; Verzin, 1975).[6,7] Infibulation is the most common form of female genital cutting in Somalia and Djibouti (Toubia, 1993), and an estimated 73% of ever-married women of reproductive age in Sudan (DHS, 1991), 34% in Eritrea (NSO, 1997), and 1–9% in Egypt (El-Zanaty et al., 1996) have experienced this form of practice.

Other forms are common in certain settings. *Matwasat* (meaning intermediate circumcision) is believed to have emerged in Sudan as an alternative to the more extreme form of infibulation when the latter was outlawed in 1946 (El Dareer, 1982).[8] The severity of *matwasat* circumcision may vary but it is generally considered more moderate than infibulation. Two percent of Sudanese women identified themselves as having had a *matwasat* circumcision (Kheir, Kumar & Cross, 1991). A final major form of the practice that is common in parts of Egypt involves removal of the labia minora only (El-Zanaty et al., 1996; Yount, 2002): approximately 8% of Egyptian women of reproductive age in a clinic-based study experienced this form of cutting (El-Zanaty et al., 1996).

In 1997, the World Health Organization (WHO), The United Nations Children's Fund (UNICEF), and the United Nations Fund for Population Activities (UNFPA) proposed a new system to classify forms of female genital cutting for standard use across different cultures (WHO, 1997). These forms are described in the left-most column of Table 1. Despite promotion of this system, at least four factors challenge its application in cross-cultural research on the practice.

First, researchers collecting data on female genital cutting in face-to-face interviews may encounter biases in women's reporting of the exact form of female genital cutting that they have undergone. This reporting bias may be due in part to the legal status of female genital practices at the time of data collection (see Yount, 2002). More likely, reporting bias may be due to variation in date of (first) genital cutting and age at interview. While circumcision is usually performed before puberty in most settings in Northeastern Africa, there is substantial variation (e.g. Hicks, 1993). Estimates of the age of first circumcision range from 4 to 11 in Sudan with means ranging from 6 to 8 years (El Dareer, 1982; Hicks, 1993; Ministry of Planning, 1979). By contrast, the median age at circumcision is four years for women aged 15–49 years in Eritrea (National Statistics Office, 1997) and about 10 years among ever-married mothers and their daughters in Egypt (El-Zanaty et al., 1996; Yount, 2002). Given these differences, it is plausible that accurate recall about the exact nature of the procedure that is (first) undertaken may vary by age at first circumcision and age at which women are interviewed about their circumcision status.

Second, existing systems of classification fail to identify critical point(s) of variation in forms of female genital cutting that are practiced in specific cultural contexts. For example, the system proposed by WHO, UNICEF, and UNFPA would not capture distinctions between the different kinds of infibulation that exist in Sudan, nor the practice of removing only the labia minora in Egypt, nor the emergence of symbolic forms of the practice. These distinctions may have important implications for other aspects of Sudanese and Egyptian women's lives.

Third, existing systems of classification do not capture variation across settings in the number of times that women experience some form of genital cutting over their lifecourse. While less extensive forms of genital cutting are believed to occur once in a woman's lifetime, this assumption may be incorrect, and evidence suggests that even some women who have been excised may require de-infibulation at marriage or childbirth because their remaining labia have fused together (e.g. Agugua & Egwuatu, 1982; Hosken, 1982; also see examples cited in Widstrand, 1964). It is suggested that women who are initially infibulated commonly require de-infibulation for sexual intercourse or childbirth, and re-infibulation may occur after childbirth, among women whose husbands are absent from the household, and among divorced and widowed women who wish to remarry (e.g. Boddy, 1982; Cloudsley, 1983; El Dareer, 1982; Hayes, 1975).[9] Therefore, the extent of cutting at any point in time may reflect an accumulation of various procedures that are performed at numerous points in a woman's life, and this cumulative experience may be important to document if repeated cutting is independently associated with specific health effects.

Finally, despite some effort to standardize terminology, persistent use of popular nomenclature to refer to the range of ritual female genital practices reinforces ambiguities in meaning and measurement. English terms that refer to the collectivity of practices include female circumcision, female genital mutilation (FGM), and female genital operations, surgeries, and procedures (see Abd el Salam, 1999; Obermeyer & Reynolds, 1999a, b; WHO, 1997). More precise English terms include clitoridectomy, excision, and infibulation (see Abd el Salam, 1999; Assaad, 1999; Obermeyer & Reynolds, 1999a, b). The classical Arabic word for the general practice is *khifad*, which means "reduction," and colloquial Arabic words for the practice are *tahur* or *tahara*, which mean "cleanliness" or "purity." As others have pointed out (Abd el Salam, 1999), choice of terminology is subjective and symbolic and represents individual- and community-level biases about these practices. In addition, sole use of any of these terms is in some way problematic because the term may not accurately describe all forms of the practice, may not acknowledge the ritualistic meanings of the practice, or may be value laden.

Because of the limitations of any single word or phrase to describe the full range of ritual female genital practices, we have not adopted a single term to refer to the entire set. Rather, we use a combination of the above terms, as appropriate. For the sake of simplicity, however, we rely most heavily on the phrases "(ritual) female genital cutting" and "(ritual) female genital practices." Despite our objection that the first phrase fails to capture important differences in forms of the practice, the term "cutting" is less value laden and a more accurate description of the most basic act involved in performing any form of the procedure. The term "practices" also is less value-laden and emphasizes the ritualistic significance of female genital cutting in practicing populations.

CAUSES AND PERSISTENCE OF FEMALE GENITAL PRACTICES

In examining the causes, persistence, and consequences of female genital practices, we review literature mainly from the social and medical sciences. Social scientists tend to review critically the sociocultural underpinnings of these practices while speculating about their medical sequelae, whereas medical and public health professionals tend to oversimplify the social and cultural roots of these practices while providing illuminating studies of their health effects. Medical anthropologists are notable insofar as they often consider the origins and consequences of these practices (e.g. Gordon, 1991; Gruenbaum, 1991, 2001; Hicks, 1993; Inhorn & Buss, 1993). Otherwise, because of "natural" divisions in the literature, the sections of this paper that focus on the causes of and social change in female genital practices draw largely on the accounts of social scientists, and sections that address the health-related and demographic consequences of various forms of the practice draw heavily on the writings of medical and public health professionals. We also touch upon but do not review systematically the activist literature that addresses these practices, since this literature focuses heavily on eradication rather than on the processes of social change. Because our review uncovered considerable repetition in reviews and ritual descriptions across discplines, we rely most heavily on those references that present original data or points of view. We begin by placing the study of female genital practices in historic context.

Evolution of Research

Female genital practices have long been considered integral to the events of a woman's life course in Northeastern Africa (e.g. Barclay, 1964; Ibrahim, 1979; Kennedy, 1970; de Villeneuve, 1937). The exact origins of these practices are uncertain, but painted records of them date back as far as 2340–2180 B.C. in Egypt (Ghalioungui, 1962 in Kennedy, 1970). The earliest written account of these practices is found in the writings of historian Pietro Bembo (who was sent to Ethiopia as secretary to Pope Leo X), which were published posthumously in 1551 or 1552 (Cloudsley, 1983; Widstrand, 1964).

Considerable attention has been given to understanding the causes and context of female genital practices only in this century, and especially in the last 20–30 years. The rigor and style of these writings has varied depending upon the mode of expression and means of investigation of the period. Travelers, explorers, and traders to the region provided most of the early descriptions of practices like excision and infibulation (see Widstrand, 1964). Then, with the notable exception of de Villeneuve (1937), the work of male social scientists (e.g. Barclay, 1964; Hansen, 1972/1973; Kennedy, 1970; Widstrand, 1964) and male and female medical practitioners (e.g. Sequeira, 1931; Shamma, 1949; Shandall, 1967; Worsley, 1938) dominated. In 1975, Hayes wrote, "to the best of my knowledge, no other female social scientist has conducted an investigation of infibulation in Sudan, and the strict seclusion of Sudanese females from unrelated males, especially European or any other non-Sudanese males, has almost completely prevented male social scientists from interviewing female informants on the subject" (p. 618). Hayes further notes that until that time, there had been at most half a dozen other social scientific investigations of these practices. Barclay's (1964) was perhaps the only work in Sudan by an anthropologist, but he relied on male informants and secondary sources and treated the matter descriptively and largely in the context of analyzing the secularization of village life (Hayes, 1975). Writing at about the same time, Hansen (1972/1973) implicitly criticizes female scholars of the past 25 years for ignoring the subject.

Since the mid-seventies, and probably the rise of feminist scholarship and female social scientists, both female and male social scientists have examined the practice more analytically (e.g. Abdalla, 1982; Boddy, 1982; Ericksen, 1989; Gordon, 1991; Gruenbaum, 1991, 1996, 2000, 2001; Hayes, 1975; Hicks, 1993; Lowenstein, 1978; van der Kwaak, 1992). Around the same time, a number of Sudanese and Egyptian feminist physicians began to bring international attention to the subject (e.g. El Dareer, 1982; El Saadawi, 1982; Toubia, 1985), and an activist literature emerged among "insiders" and "outsiders" to practicing populations (e.g. Abu Daia, 2000; Hosken, 1978, 1981, 1982; Koso-Thomas, 1987; Maendeleo Ya Wanawake Organization, 1991; McLean & Graham, 1983; Toubia, 1993).

Except until recently, little extensive fieldwork has been conducted on the subject of female genital practices (Gordon, 1991). Rather, these practices are often considered in more general works on "at risk" populations, on the position of women in society, and on women's rights (Berhane et al., 2001; Mensch et al., 1999; Santow, 1995). This historical neglect of female genital practices has limited our understanding of their causes and persistence, and the recent politicization of the practice has encouraged a proliferation of both editorials that lack supporting data and research that lacks generalizability (e.g. Obermeyer, 2003; Obermeyer & Reynolds, 1999a, b; Yount & Balk, 2002). Acknowledging these caveats, the literature suggests several reasons for the existence and perpetuation of female genital practices.

Patriarchal Control and Gender Identificiation

The literature that addresses the reasons for female genital practices gives greatest attention to two, closely related themes of gender – patriarchal control and the social construction of feminine identity: "the operation renders her [a girl] marriageable; undergoing it is a necessary condition of becoming a woman..." (Boddy, 1982, p. 683).

From the perspective of practicing societies, one immediate function of female genital cutting is the "protection" of females. Narrowly, the practice (and infibulation in particular) is believed to protect girls and women from sexual assault (e.g. Cloudsley, 1983; Hayes, 1975; Talle, 1993). In discussions of the trading of female slaves, for example, infibulated female slaves commanded a higher price than uninfibulated slaves.[10] Others even suggest that infibulation is an evolutionary response to pastoral life, because it renders women "odorless," and therefore less vulnerable to wild animals (Grassivaro-Gallo & Viviani, 1992). More broadly, the practice is believed to protect women from "social condemnation" (Hayes, 1975; Yount, 2002): "...a woman who is known not to have been circumcised is considered to be a prostitute, in behavior if not in profession . . . a woman or girl must be protected from the suspicion of sexual misconduct as much as from . . . sexual assault or voluntary intercourse" (Hayes, 1975, p. 627).

Because the social standing of male elders and their families rests in part on the chastity of unmarried daughters, protecting the virginity of daughters through female genital cutting also serves to maintain honor in the patrilineage (e.g. Gruenbaum, 1982; Hicks, 1993; Talle, 1993; Yount, 2002). The practice is thought to diminish female wantonness, which if not controlled would bring shame to a girl's father and her family (Constantinides, 1985; Hayes, 1975). As it ensures an unmarried daughter's virginity, infibulation also may ensure a wife's fidelity (e.g. Barclay, 1964).

The underlying purpose of protecting a girl's virginity and of preserving her family's honor is to ensure a proper marriage. Not surprisingly, therefore, the perceived enhanced marriageability of circumcised daughters is a leading explanation for the practice (e.g. Ammar, 1954; Ericksen, 1989; Hicks, 1993; Kennedy, 1970; van der Kwaak, 1992; Widstrand, 1964). "Among the populace [in Northern Sudan], no one would marry an uncircumcised woman" (Lightfoot-Klein, 1989a). Even as public health measures have been implemented to change people's attitudes toward and awareness of the consequences of the practice in Sudan, "the definition of marriageability continues to include virginity, which is largely constructed through infibulation" (Gruenbaum, 1991, p. 642). Virginity and marriage are so closely linked in the Sudan and other countries where infibulation is common that divorced and widowed women who want to remarry may be re-infibulated to appear virginal (e.g. MacDonald as cited in Barclay, 1964; Boddy, 1982; Cloudsley, 1983; El Dareer, 1982; Hayes, 1975; Lightfoot-Klein, 1989b; Talle, 1993).

In addition to its links with virginity and marriage, the practice persists also because it is believed to be cleansing (Yount, 2002), aesthetically appealing (Yount, 2002), and central to the construction of gender identity (e.g. Ammar, 1954; Boddy, 1982; Constantinides, 1985; Kennedy, 1970; Talle, 1993; van der Kwaak, 1992). Much of this literature stresses the identification in practicing societies of a pre-infibulated vagina or a pre-circumcised clitoris with a penis, and vice versa (e.g. Boddy, 1982; Ericksen, 1995; Talle, 1993), and beliefs exist in settings like Minia, Egypt that cutting a girls' clitoris will prevent it from growing (Yount, 2002; see also Eke & Nkanginieme, 1999). Although the practice of female genital cutting is undertaken well before either puberty or marriage, it certifies a girl as "non-male" and therefore normal, whole, pure, and on the right path to womanhood (Yount, 2002). Boddy (1982, p. 683) argues further that infibulation is used symbolically and physically to enclose – and therefore make more important, sacred, and scarce – the womb, which represents a woman's reproductive center, and fertility her "one great gift."

Studies outside of infibulating areas may place less emphasis on the symbolic association of genital cutting and fertility, yet there is ample suggestion throughout the region of its relationship to gender roles: "By insisting on circumcision for their daughters, women assert their social indispensability . . . not as the sexual partners of their husbands . . . nor . . . as their servants, sexual or otherwise, but as mothers of men" (Boddy, 1982, p. 687). In this sense, female genital cutting is associated in many practicing societies with positive images of women's social identity and womanhood, which complement and reinforce ideologies of male dominance (Fig. 1).

From the perspective of a critical outsider (including cultural insiders who view the practice critically), female genital practices exist in patriarchal societies where women have historically been the property of men, where women often are economically dependent on their natal and marital families, and where women's sexual purity and fidelity are central to marriage and to the honor of the patrilineage. In such settings, female genital cutting represents one of many "codes of modesty" that ensure the social and sexual control of women. Other mechanisms include segregation of the sexes or the seclusion of females, the veiling of women in public, child betrothal, and tests of virginity on the wedding night. Patriarchal control is preserved by making female genital cutting a marker of virginity, virginity a prerequisite for marriage and essential to the honor of the patrilineage, and marriage one of the few means by which women acquire social acceptance and economic security (Fig. 1).

Women's Roles in Maintaining the Practice

Despite the presumed origins of female genital practices in patriarchal institutions, women often are centrally involved in their continuation. While there is variation in the ceremonial aspects of the practice among different groups, mothers, grandmothers, and female circumcisers each play an integral part: the practice is often described as "being performed on small girls, by women, in the company of women, and in the absence of men" (Gulick, 1976, p. 182; also see Boddy, 1982; Chalmers & Omer-Hashi, 2000; Mackie, 1996, 2000; Ntiri, 1993).[11] Proposed reasons for women's involvement in female genital practices are many. First, women who are dependent on their marital families for economic security and who derive their status primarily from their roles as successful wives, mothers, and grandmothers have direct incentives to maintain the honor of the lineage (e.g. Hayes, 1975). Second, in settings like Sudan and Somalia, older women play an integral role as partner in the patrilineage (Hayes, 1975; van der Kwaak, 1992; See discussions on works by Boddy & Talle, below.). In particular, husbands and wives who are

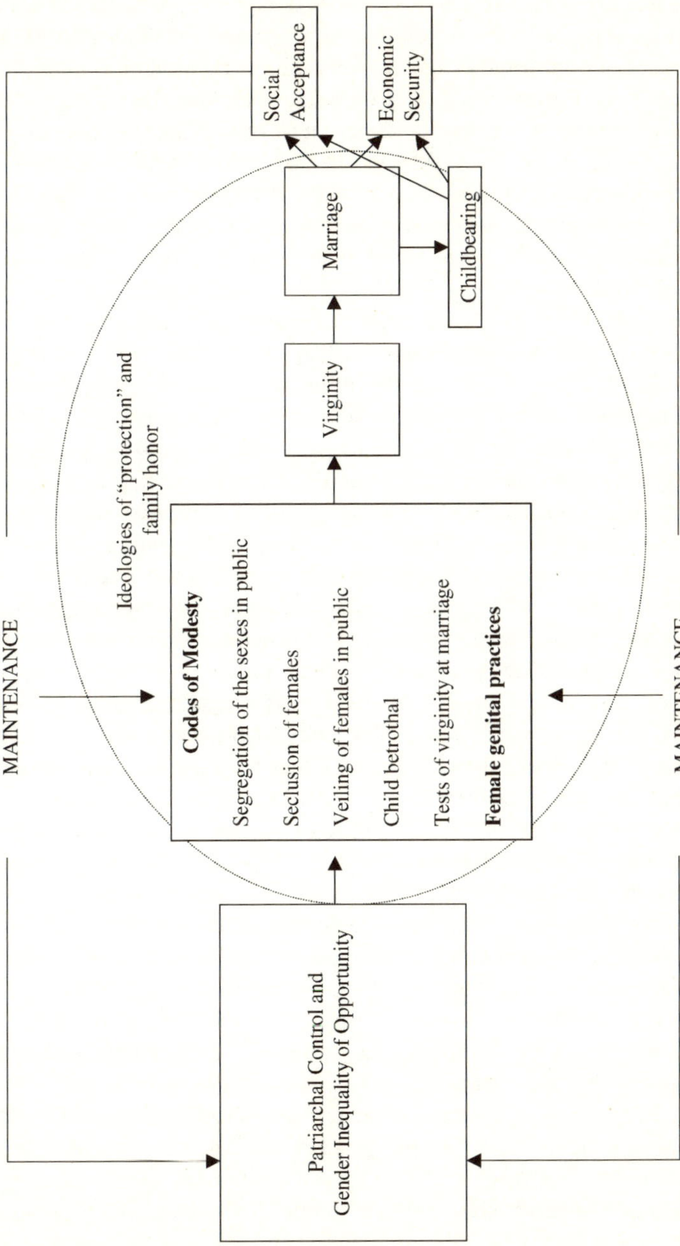

Fig. 1. Causes of Female Genital Practices.

co-founders of a lineage section enjoy considerable power, which they in turn may apply to ensure that their female relatives are circumcised. Third, in the absence of other sources of opportunity outside of marriage and motherhood, mothers and grandmothers may be unwilling to jeopardize their daughters' marriageability and subsequent financial security by rejecting or modifying an expected tradition (Chalmers & Omer-Hashi, 2000; Mackie, 1996, 2000; Ntiri, 1993; Yount, 2002).

Fourth, female genital cutting may in some settings serve as a bargaining tool in marriage. From this perspective, even though the practice may weaken their own sexual desires, women may accept it because they believe that it enhances the sexual pleasure of men (e.g. Barclay, 1964; Boddy, 1982; Cloudsley, 1983; Gruenbaum, 1991), in whose domain sexuality appropriately falls (e.g. El Saadawi, 1982; Ericksen, 1995; Hansen, 1972/1973; Talle, 1993; van der Kwaak, 1992).[12,13] For this reason, women in infibulating societies may even seek re-infibulation because they wish to please their husbands sexually (Cloudsley, 1983; El Dareer, 1982; Gruenbaum, 1982). By providing sexual satisfaction in marriage, a woman may seek to encourage her husband's reciprocity in the form of gift giving and to avoid the possibility that her husband will exercise his legally guaranteed rights to unilateral divorce or polygynous marriage (Gruenbaum, 1982).[14]

Ironically, studies conducted among men suggest that the association between female genital cutting and men's sexual pleasure may be a rationalization for the practice among women that is inconsistent with men's experiences, particularly in infibulating societies. In fact, Sudanese men who oppose the practice report insufficient sexual satisfaction as a leading reason (Kheir et al., 1991; Koso-Thomas, 1987).[15] In another study of Sudanese men ($n = 59$), 63% reported sexual and physical complications that they attributed to severe forms of female genital cutting (Almroth et al., 2001), and no man mentioned sexual satisfaction as a reason for preferring a wife to be genitally cut; rather, those men who wished their wives to be genitally cut gave social acceptance or tradition as the main motivation (Almroth et al., 2001). Other studies have found that men in African settings like Sierra Leone often do not want their wives to be infibulated or re-sutured after childbirth because of the pain that infibulated women experience during sexual intercourse (Lightfoot-Klein, 1989a; Passmore, 1981).

In addition to inconsistencies between women's beliefs about men's sexual desires and men's reported experiences, women's own beliefs about the role of female genital cutting in marital sexuality varies in Northeastern Africa. In settings like Minia, Egypt, where less severe forms of female genital cutting are common, some women state that the practice enhances the sexual pleasure of the husband and wife (Yount, 2002). Therefore, female genital cutting in this setting is seen as a means both to preserve family honor by protecting the chastity of unmarried daughters and to enhance women's and men's sexual pleasure in marriage. Regardless of the particular belief about the role of female genital cutting in marital sexuality, their link nevertheless remains a strong justification among some women to continue the practice.

Roles of Religion and Class

Although more attention has been given to explaining the roots of female genital practices in patriarchal control and gender ideologies, others have proposed that religion and social class are important factors as well. Regarding the role of religion, Hicks (1993) argues that although the form of female genital cutting varies widely in Africa, the practice of infibulation exists largely within closed Islamic societies and has spread with the Islamitization of Northeastern Africa. Therefore, the role of infibulation in gender identification and the maintenance of women's position relative to men must be understood within the context of closed Islamic societies (Hicks, 1993). Other research from the Sudan also suggests that religion is the most commonly mentioned reason among men and the second most commonly mentioned reason among women to favor the practice (El Dareer, 1982), and adoption or continuation of female genital cutting reportedly serves as an important marker of local religious identity (Johnson, 2000).

The association that Hicks (1993) makes between Islam and the practice of infibulation is problematic for several reasons, however. First, female genital cutting as a general practice predated the advent of both Christianity and Islam to Northeastern Africa (Assaad, 1980; Gruenbaum, 2001; Mackie, 1996, 2000). Second, milder forms of the practice have persisted, and symbolic forms of the practice may be emerging, in largely Islamic settings like Egypt (El-Zanaty et al., 1996; Ibrahim, personal communication, January 2002; Yount, 2002, 2004). Third, the adoption and spread of certain forms of female genital cutting have occurred among Christians in settings like Chad (Leonard, 1996, 2000). For these reasons, other researchers have resisted association of specific forms of the practice with certain religious denominations (e.g. Obermeyer & Reynolds, 1999b).

Regarding the role of class in the adoption and maintenance of female genital practices, modernization theory posits that female genital cutting was a practice of patrilineal societies in which male family members inherited land and women acquired access to these resources through marriage, for which female genital cutting was a prerequisite (Hayes, 1975; Kennedy, 1970). Mackie (1996, 2000) argues that female genital cutting originated under conditions of resource inequality whereby high-ranking men attracted multiple potential wives, whose families became motivated by competition to enforce codes of modesty (including female genital cutting) upon their unmarried daughters (Mackie, 1996, 2000). Therefore, both theories stress that female genital cutting emerged as the means by which women acquired access to resources by marrying men who controlled these resources.

Findings from Sudan demonstrate a positive relationship between class and the persistence of female genital practices. Balk (2001) finds clear evidence of strong middle-class adherence to the practice, and socioeconomic status always raises the odds of being circumcised and infibulated. El Dareer (1982) notes that among the Beni Helba (of western Sudan), women from families of high social status were infibulated while all other women had *sunna* circumcisions, and Tubiana (1984) finds that among the Beri of Sudan and eastern Chad, female circumcision is practiced only among the daughters of royal clans. Regarding other markers of socio-economic status, El Dareer (1982) finds that re-infibulation is associated with urban residence and higher levels of education and notes that midwives reportly charge more for re-infibulation, which suggests that women who seek post-partum re-stitching are those who can afford it.[16]

Concerning the recent adoption and spread of female genital cutting among groups that did not traditionally circumcise in Sudan, Gruenbaum (1988, 1991, p. 640) finds that circumcision serves as a marker of ethnic identity and associated class privilege: "Rare indeed was the Kenyana woman who had thought of giving up pharaonic circumcision, . . . a mark of her ethnic superiority." Grassivaro-Gallo (1986b) similarly finds in Somalia, that "the practice of infibulation has become more widespread and has been accepted as a sign of nobility and ethnic identity at a time when the practice appears destined to disappear" (p. 155, cited in Grassivaro-Gallo & Viviani, 1992). In attempts to assimilate or gain acceptance, groups that formerly did not practice female genital cutting or practiced milder forms also began circumcising and infibulating, respectively (El Dareer, 1982; Gruenbaum, 1988). Finally, Lightfoot-Klein (1989b) reports that "recircumcisions" were unknown 50 years ago, and guesses that their introduction was through wealthy (westernized) Sudanese women's desire for a "vaginal tuck" (p. 381).

Evidence from elsewhere in Northeastern Africa, however, suggests that a positive association between female genital practices and social class is not universal. The Cairo Family Planning Association, for example, has stated that female circumcision is not practiced by many middle- and upper-class Egyptians (see Inhorn & Buss, 1993), and data from Minia, Egypt show no association between family wealth and the decision to circumcise uncircumcised daughters (Yount, 2002). These differences suggest that the contribution of class to the adoption or continuation of female genital practices may vary across cultural contexts.

CONSEQUENCES OF FEMALE GENITAL PRACTICES

Understanding the forms of female genital cutting provide some clues about their potential consequences. Several studies have reviewed and described the major health consequences in detail (e.g. Abdalla, 1982; Cook, 1979; El Dareer, 1982; El Saadawi, 1982; Gordon, 1991; Hosken, 1982; Koso-Thomas, 1987; Obermeyer, 2003; Obermeyer & Reynolds, 1999a, b; Yount & Balk, 2002), and three general themes emerge from this literature. First, the more severe the procedure, the more severe the short- and long-term complications are likely to be (Verzin, 1975). In a comparison of urinary complications among *sunna* circumcised and excised women in Nigeria, severe early or delayed complications are relatively rare among *sunna* circumcised women (Agugua & Egwuatu, 1982). Infibulated women in Sudan also have a higher incidence of sterility (in the five years preceding a 1978/1979 survey) than do uncircumcised or less severely circumcised women (Larsen, 1989). Lastly, the risk of a complicated delivery has been shown to increase with the severity of prior genital cutting in clinics in rural Burkina Faso and urban and rural Mali (5% among uncut women, 18% among women with Type I circumcision, 30% among women with Type 2 circumcision, and 36% among women with Type 3 circumcision) (Jones et al., 1999; Moore, 2000).

A second theme emerging from this literature is that repeated performance of some form of cutting, especially the practice of de-infibulation and re-infibulation, may increase independently the risk of medical complications (e.g. El Dareer, 1982; Laycock, 1950; Mustafa, 1966). A few studies have shown that de-infibulation, in particular, may lead to sepsis and other complications (El Dareer, 1982; Laycock, 1950). A third theme from the literature is that most forms of genital cutting may be associated with difficult-to-measure emotional, psychological, and sexual complications, although these complications are less well-documented (Chalmers & Hashi, 2000; El-Defrawi et al., 2001).

One caveat in distilling these themes is that, despite a recent proliferation of studies on the health consequences of female genital cutting, generalizable evidence regarding the prevalence of various complications in practicing populations remains sparse (see Obermeyer, 2003; Obermeyer & Reynolds, 1999a, b; Yount & Balk, 2002). To assess the quality of recent studies about the health consequences of female genital cutting, we conducted a search of articles published from 1990 to the present using Medline and SocioAbs databases. The following terms served as keywords in both searches: circumcision, female circumcision, genital cutting, genital mutilation, infibulation, clitoridectomy, and excision. In addition, Medline permitted selection of articles that were classified under a sub-heading entitled "adverse effects" of the main heading "female circumcision." Additional sources were identified from the reference lists of all articles that were located during the initial search.

Of the 28 studies conducted after 1990 that we identified, Table 2 provides a summary of the basic characteristics of their designs.[17]

Table 2. Design Characteristics of Studies of the Health Consequences of Female Genital Cutting (1990 to Present).

	Studies ($n = 28$)	
	n	%
Source of sample[a]		
Hospital/Clinic	21	70
School	1	3
Population	8	27
Sampling strategy[a]		
Census	1	3
Probability	3	10
Non-probability	15	50
Systematic/complete period	5	17
Unclear	6	20
Sample size[a]		
1	5	17
2–9	3	10
10–49	2	7
50–99	5	14
100–499	9	31
500–999	1	3
1000+	4	14
Unknown	1	3
Response rate (%)[b]		
<50	0	0
50–69	0	0
70–89	2	22
90+	5	56
Unreported	2	22
Geographic distribution		
Egypt[c]	3	11
Ethiopia	1	4
Eritrea	1	4
Gambia (Farafenni)	1	4
Eastern Nigeria	1	4
Somalia[d]	4	14
Sudan[e]	2	7

Table 2. (*Continued*)

	Studies ($n = 28$)	
	n	%
Burkina Faso & Mali	1	4
Ismailia	1	4
Immigrant populations[f]	13	46
Sources of data		
Case report (clinical exam)	7	25
Interviews/self-report	8	29
Medical records	5	18
Medical records and self-report	1	4
Clinical exam and self-report	2	7
Focus group interviews	1	4
Interviews/medical records	1	4
Clinical exam, self-report, lab analysis	2	7
Interview, observations, clinical exam	1	4
Classification of female genital cutting		
All circumcised (type unspecified)	4	14
All circumcised (type specified/no-little variation)	11	39
All circumcised (type specified/variation)	2	7
Not all circumcised (type unspecified)	4	14
Not all circumcised (type specified)[g]	4	14
Circumcision status unclear	2	7
Study of men[h]	1	4

Note: Studies included are Dirie and Lindmark (1991, 1992), Ozumba (1992), Baker et al. (1993), Calder et al. (1993), Ericksen (1995), Inhorn and Buss (1993), Ntiri (1993), Mawad and Hassanein (1994), McCleary (1994), Erian and Goh (1995), Hanley and Ojeda (1995), McCaffrey et al. (1995), Walker and Morgan (1995), Sayed et al. (1996), Davis et al. (1999), Jones et al. (1999), Knight et al. (1999), Chalmers and Hashi (2000), Kroll and Miller (2000), Missailidis and Gebre-Medhin (2000), Almroth et al. (2001), Brisson et al. (2001), El-Defrawi et al. (2001), Epstein et al. (2001), Momoh et al. (2001), Morison et al. (2001), Rouzi, Aljhadali et al. (2001).

[a] Two studies included multiple methods, so those studies are counted twice in the denominator ($n = 30$).

[b] Percentages are based on studies using censuses, probability samples, and systematic sampling for a specified period ($n = 9$).

[c] Including a village near Assiut, a hospital in Alexandria, Cairo, and the Nile Delta.

[d] Including Mogadishu, Juba (Southern Somalia), and one unknown location within Somalia.

[e] Including Khartoum and a village in the Gezira scheme along the Blue Nile.

[f] Immigrant populations include but are not limited to those from Somalia, Sudan, Central Africa, Ethiopia, Eritrea, and Djibouti who migrated to the United States, Canada, England, Saudi Arabia, and Australia.

[g] No empirical distinction is made between types and subsequent complication.

[h] Men's attitudes about female genital cutting were not clearly distinguished by type of cutting.

Several features of the sampling strategies used in these studies are noteworthy. First, most (70%) of the studies are clinic-based, which suggests that their results cannot be generalized to an identifiable community-based population. Second, relatively few (13%) of the samples included in these studies were drawn either by taking a census or by using probability-based sampling strategies. Therefore, findings even from those studies that are "community-based" are not necessarily generalizable to the communities from which study participants were drawn. Third, among the nine studies that relied on censuses or probability samples, response rates were unreported for two. Fourth, about half of the studies were based on sample sizes of less than 100 participants, which limits the scope of health consequences that can be explored. Fifth, about half of the studies (46%) were conducted among immigrant populations originating from countries in Northeastern Africa (e.g. Sudan, Somalia, Ethiopia, Eritrea, Central Africa, and Djibouti) and migrating to more industrialized settings (e.g. United States, Canada, England, Australia, and Saudi Arabia). Although understanding the behavior of immigrant populations is valuable in its own right, their practices and experiences may not be representative of groups in either their sending or receiving countries.

Also noteworthy are characteristics pertaining to the method and quality of data collection in these 28 studies. First, sources of data and means of data collection include self-reports, medical records, and clinical and laboratory exams, and findings from studies of reproductive and gynecologtical morbidity from the region (e.g. Khattab, 1992) suggest that estimated prevalences of complications that are derived from different sources of data may not be comparable. Second, researchers do not always make optimal use of the methods of data collection that they select. For example, case reports have the potential to provide valuable information about the physical and psychological effects of female genital cutting for individual women; however, some case reports do not clearly specify the type of circumcision that the woman experienced. Third, studies differ in the extent to which sufficient variation in types of genital cutting is obtained to permit analysis of the association of type with specific complications.

Morbidity, Pain, and Psychological Ill-Health

With these caveats in mind, Table 3 provides a list of the major complications that have been found to be associated with female genital cutting, along with their estimated prevalences. Table 3 includes findings from the reviews of Obermeyer and Reynolds (1999a,b) and additional studies that we located during our review.

Table 3. Complications of Female Genital Cutting: Summary of Major Findings.

Main Complication	Detailed Complication	Range in Frequency (%)	Study[a]
Bleeding problems	Hemorrhage/shock	0–52	1, 7, 17, 18
	Bleeding/serious bleeding	6–81	6, 8, 9, 11, 13, 15
	Septicemia	1–8	7, 15
Infections	Infection (not specified)	2–37	6, 13, 15
	Wound infection/fever	0–81	1, 2, 7, 9
	Vulvar abscess/swelling	0–5	1, 2, 17
	Abscess at site of excised clitoris	9	10
	Vaginal infection	8	12
	Pelvic infections	22	13
	Bacterial vaginosis	OR = 1.66	16
	Any genital infection	OR = 1.72[b]	18
Urinary problems	Urine retention	0–84	1, 2, 6, 7, 9, 13, 15
	Pain at micturition	20	7
	Urinary infection	4–66	1, 2, 9, 12, 15
	Poor urinary flow	58	15
	Incontinence	1–11	9, 15, 18
Scars and cysts	Keloid scars	0–62	1, 2, 15, 18
	Inclusion/Bartholin's cysts	0–2	1, 2
	Clitoridal cysts	12	7
	Dermoid cysts	12–55	10, 15
	Perineal cysts	24	13
	Perineal scars	54	13
	Gynetresia (stenosis of the vagina)	[c]	20
Reproductive problems	Tubal-factor infertility	OR = 0.9	5
	Dyspareunia	0–76.5	2, 12, 15
	Menstrual problems	16–80.5	9, 12, 13, 15, 19
	Difficulty conceiving	9	15
Labor and delivery problems	Prolonged labor (stage II)	14	4
	Postpartum hemorrhage	5	4
	Caesarean section	0–4	3, 4
	Chronic pelvic infection	4–13	1, 2
Sexual complications	Overall	22–78	6, 13
	Vaginal dryness during intercourse	48.5	19
	Lack of sexual desire	45	19
	Less frequency of sexual desire per week	28	19
	Less initiative during sex	11	19
	Being less pleased by sex	49	19

Table 3. (*Continued*)

Main Complication	Detailed Complication	Range in Frequency (%)	Study[a]
	Less orgasmic/less frequency/difficulty reaching	25–60.5	19
Other	Pain	3–84	6, 9, 11, 13, 15
	Psychological complications	8	6
	Slow healing	52	9
	Fainting	45	9
	Foul-smelling discharge from circumcision	35	9
	Narrowed introitus	79	12
	Vaginal stenosis	13–20	10, 18
	Edema/swelling	50	13
	Perineal tears	0.6–62	13, 17
	Male difficulties to penetrate	92	14
	Male wounds, bleeding, inflammation on penis	27	14
	Herpes simplex virus II	OR = 4.71	16
	Dysuria	73	9
	Postcoital/postnatal circumcision trauma/injury	2	17
	Vesicovaginal fistula	1	18
	Rectovaginal fistula	0–1	18
	Apareunia	18	12
	Vaginal obstruction	6–8	18
	Vaginal synechia	2–6	18
	Haematocolpos (requiring vaginal widening)	7	15

Note: The information summarized here includes and adds to that which is provided in Obermeyer and Reynolds (1999a).

[a](1) Shandall (1967), hospital study ($n = 4{,}283$) in Sudan; (2) El Dareer (1989), survey ($n = 3{,}104$) in Sudan; (3) Beradi et al. (1985), hospital study ($n = 852$) in France; (4) De Silva (1989), hospital study ($n = 2{,}157$) in Saudi Arabia; (5) Inhorn and Buss (1993), hospital study ($n = 130$) in Egypt; (6) Gadallah et al. (1996), survey ($n = 782$) in Egypt; (7) Dirie and Lindmark (1992), survey ($n = 290$) in Somalia; (8) Leonard (1996), survey ($n = 91$) in Chad; (9) Calder et al. (1993), survey ($n = 105$) in Somalia; (10) Dirie and Lindmark (1991), hospital study ($n = 118$) in Somalia; (11) Sayed et al. (1996), survey ($n = 1732$) in Egypt; (12) Knight et al. (1999), hospital study ($n = 51$) in Australia; (13) Chalmers & Hashi (2000), interviews ($n = 432$) in Canada; (14) Almroth et al. (2001), interviews ($n = 59$) in Sudan; (15) Momoh et al. (2001), hospital study ($n = 108$) in London, England; (16) Morison et al. (2001), survey & clinical exam ($n = 1{,}138$) in Gambia; (17) Mawad and Hassanein (1994), hospital study ($n = 13{,}768$) in Sudan; (18) Jones et al. (1999), clinic study ($n = 7, 259$) in Burkina Faso and Mali; (19) El-Defrawi (2001), hospital study ($n = 250$) in Ismailia; (20) Ozumba (1992), review of medical records of confirmed gynetresia ($n = 78$).

[b]In Burkino Faso only (comparing cut to uncut women).

[c]Prevalence unavailable because this study was based on a sample of medical records with the reported complication.

The complete list of health consequences presumed to be associated with some form of female genital cutting is long: among the 20 studies included in Table 3, the number of complications exceeds 58. Most often cited complications (e.g. cited in five or more sources) include bleeding, retention of urine, urinary tract infection, menstrual problems, and pain. Health consequences that are cited by at least two sources include: hemorrhage and serious bleeding, urinary tract infections and reproductive tract infections (RTI), pelvic inflammatory disease (PID), vaginal stenosis, urinary retention and dysuria, urinary incontinence, infection and septicemia, dyspareunia, dysmenorrhea and other menstrual problems, obstruction of the urethra, injury to the rectum, scarring and keloid scarring (e.g. fibrous tissue formed at the site of scar), perineal tearing, cysts, vaginal stenosis, vulvar abscesses and/or swelling, fistulas (e.g. an abnormal passage between two hollow organs), difficult and painful childbirth, birth defects, painful intercourse or sexual complications, and psychological complications (e.g. Agugua & Egwuatu, 1982; Aziz, 1980; Calder et al., 1993; Chalmers & Omer-Hashi, 2000; De Silva, 1989; de Villeneuve, 1937; Dirie & Lindmark, 1991, 1992; El Dareer, 1982; Hosken, 1982; Jones et al., 1999; Knight et al., 1999; Leonard, 1996; Maendeleo Ya Wanawake Organization, 1991; Mawad & Hassanein, 1994; Momoh et al., 2001; Mustafa, 1966; Sayed et al., 1996; Shandall, 1967; Shaw, 1985; Silberstein, 1977; Verzin, 1975; see Toubia, 1985, 1994 for reviews of this literature).[18]

When interpreting findings in Table 3, it is important to note that certain commonly mentioned complications (e.g. bleeding and pain) occur in settings where less and more severe forms of cutting are practiced (e.g. Egypt and Sudan), whereas other commonly mentioned complications (e.g. retention of urine) occur *largely* in settings where more severe forms of cutting are practiced (e.g. Somalia and Sudan). Therefore, even though Table 3 does not provide information on the individual-level risk of specific complications by severity of cutting, general relationships may be inferred from the geographic distribution of studies (with known prevalences of certain forms of genital cutting) in which specific complications are reported.

Also notable is the wide range of estimated prevalences for most complications listed in Table 3. The extent of this variation may be a function of differences across studies in the relative frequencies of observed types of cutting, source of data used to estimate the prevalence of complications, sample selectivity, or any combination of the above differences. Therefore, while the information in Table 3 provides some insight into the range and magnitude of complications associated with some form of female genital cutting, it also exposes limits in our ability to make precise (or even accurate) inferences about observed associations.

Less well represented in Table 3 but thought to be commonly associated with circumcision-related morbidity are on-going psychological, physical, and emotional hardships resulting from the practice. For example, many circumcised women complain of painful urination and intercourse (e.g. Agugua & Egwuatu, 1982; Calder et al., 1993; El Dareer, 1982; Ozumba, 1992), whereas other studies cite sexual complications of the practice more generally (Chalmers & Omer-Hashi, 2000; El Defrawi, 2001; Passmore, 1981). Other researchers document psychological consequences including chronic anxiety and depression (e.g. Baasher, 1979; de Villeneuve, 1937; Toubia, 1994). Although much is not known about the relationship of circumcision to STDs and AIDS, its potential importance also should not be overlooked (e.g. Brady, 1999; Hardy, 1987; van Roosmalen et al., 1992; see Gausset, 2001 for an alternative point of view). Notably absent from studies of female genital cutting are qualitative assessments of the extent to which its more visible consequences affect the quality of life of circumcised women.

Fertility and Sterility

Also poorly represented in Table 3 are estimates of any fertility-related effects of female genital cutting. Nevertheless, research on African fertility suggests that levels of infertility (e.g. childlessness) and subfecundity are high in regions where certain forms of female genital cutting are practiced (e.g. Bongaarts, Frank & Lesthaeghe, 1984; Frank, 1983; Mammo & Morgan, 1986). But, high proportions of childlessness are commonly attributed to the widespread incidence of sexually transmitted infections (STIs) (e.g. Frank, 1983; Mammo & Morgan, 1986; McFall & McFall, 1984) rather than female genital cutting. For example, no mention of female genital cutting is found in Frank's (1983) paper, however, some form is practiced in over half of the 21 countries in her analysis.[19] Further, although Mammo and Morgan (1986) argue that sexually transmitted infections probably play a large role in explaining infertility in rural Ethiopia, they acknowledge that the evidence supporting a theory of infections as the sole cause is unconvincing. Nevertheless, they do not fully consider the evidence regarding female genital practices, despite the fact that most rural Ethiopian groups perform some type of the procedure.[20]

Anecdotal accounts and case study evidence suggest that the greater the severity of genital cutting should imply greater difficulty in getting pregnant, staying pregnant, and bearing healthy babies (e.g. Dewhurst & Michelson, 1964). These effects have been difficult to demonstrate, however, due in large part to the lack of appropriately designed studies, the use of self-selected samples (particularly in clinical studies), exclusive use of infertile couples, and resistance or inability on the part of women to associate problems of fertility with their circumcision status and history (e.g. Dirie & Lindmark, 1992; El Dareer, 1982; Inhorn &

Buss, 1993; Meuwissen, 1966). We review those studies that consider whether the following occur at higher rates in circumcising, and especially in infibulating, groups: (1) pregnancy loss and stillbirths; (2) secondary sterility (e.g. infertility after a known pregnancy); (3) primary sterility (e.g. unable to conceive despite exposure over a prolonged period); and (4) infections (e.g. PIDs and RTIs) that cause infertility.[21]

One recent study identified difficulty conceiving as a possible complication of female genital cutting (Momoh et al., 2001). Belsey (1979) proposes generally that rituals involving the female genital organs may produce infection or injury that interferes with conception or increases the risk of pregnancy wastage. Stillbirths may result from a number of causes, but evidence from the medical literature suggests that infibulation increases the probability of a stillbirth, largely because labor is obstructed by an extreme narrowing of the vagina and accumulated fibrous and scarred vulvar tissue that fails to dilate during contractions (e.g. Gordon, 1991). A clinic-based study of women aged 15–55 in rural Burkina Faso and rural and urban Mali shows a significant positive association between the severity of genital cutting and the probability that a woman experiences obstetric complications; the outcomes of these deliveries, however, were not examined (Jones et al., 1999). Using case-study evidence from Sudan, Laycock (1950, pp. 448–449) speculates "the mutilation of the vulva produced by infibulation, and more particularly by subsequent septic infection, should produce a condition of the soft tissues incompatible with parturition." In a controlled study of Sudanese expatriate women in Saudi Arabia,[22] De Silva (1989) finds that circumcised women are three times more likely than uncircumcised women to experience prolonged (stage II) labor; however, they appear not to be more likely to have a pregnancy end in a stillbirth or early neonatal death (also see Daw, 1970).[23,24] Infants born to circumcised women, however, are more likely to experience severe asphyxia, which may lead to brain damage, other morbidities, and death (De Silva, 1989). In another study of twelve Somali refugee women in the United States, of whom 11 were circumcised, 4 out of 48 pregnancies resulted in stillbirths, a much higher rate than that found in non-infibulating populations (Arbesman et al., 1993).[25]

The issue of primary and secondary sterility has been addressed in a few studies,[26] mostly through consideration of infertility-causing infections. Lenzi (1970), for example, discusses four Somalian case studies due to chronic inflammation of the fallopian tubes secondary to an ascendant infection contracted at the time of infibulation. In a clinical study of PID, Rushwan (1980) suggests that female circumcision is likely its leading cause in Sudan. (He has no direct assessment of the effects of circumcision, except to note that of the 147 patients in which organisms were isolated and tested for gonorrhea, all but one were circumcised, with infibulation being overwhelmingly prevalent.)[27] In a study of 398 women in infertile marriages in central Ghana, Meuwissen (1966) finds that vaginal changes (mostly the hardening and narrowing of the vaginal passage) resulting from ritual circumcisions and native treatments occur in 10% of women. Although this finding suggests that circumcision may contribute to infertility, the study design precludes a firm conclusion.[28] De Silva (1989) also finds a much higher incidence of urinary and genital tract infections among circumcised Sudanese women in Saudi Arabia. In a study of over 4,000 obstetric and gynecological patients attending the outpatient clinic at the Khartoum General Hospital between 1962 and 1966, Shandall (1967) finds among 436 cases of non-tuberculous chronic pelvic infection that the incidence among those who are infibulated is over three times that among those who are *sunna* circumcised. However, Shandall (1967) also finds that uncircumcised women were about 1.5 times *more* likely to have chronic pelvic infection than *sunna* circumcised women and attributes this finding to the larger share of low-income, southern and western Sudanese women in the uncircumcised group.

The association of female genital cutting to infertility is strongly supported in a case-control study of tubal-factor infertility (TFI) among 190 Egyptian women in Cairo and Alexandria (Inhorn & Buss, 1993).[29] Here, women with TFI are more likely to have had an excision (rather than a strict cliterodectomy) and to have had their circumcision performed by a traditional provider than are their fertile controls. Controlling for other factors, "women who had had either an excision or a cliterodectomy by a traditional provider are at 2.0 times greater risk of TFI than are women who had had neither, and women who had had both excision and a traditional practitioner are at a four times greater risk of TFI than are women who had had neither" (Inhorn & Buss, 1993, p. 232).

Surprisingly few socio-demographic studies have considered the possible effects of female genital practices on infertility (or subfecundity), either directly or indirectly through their effect on the transmission of STIs, and notably few of these studies use population-based, representative samples of women. Among those that do, findings are mixed. In a cross-national analysis, Larsen (1994) finds that primary sterility (measured by the proportion childless among women who married before reaching age 20) is relatively high (5%) as measured in 1978–1979 and relatively low (2%) as measured in 1989–1990.[30] She also finds that sterility is quite high in the upper age groups (in both periods) relative to other African countries. In another study in Sudan, Larsen (1989) finds that those who were infibulated have a higher (adjusted) incidence of sterility (in the five years preceding the 1978–1979 World Fertility Survey) than all other women but that they do not have a higher prevalence of sterility overall; she adds that although there may be real downward pressure on fertility by circumcision, it is difficult to identify in a population with so little variation in the practice. Larsen's lack of a significant finding also may be due to her classification of circumcision types: she groups the relatively few cases of circumcised women who were not infibulated in one category, thus combining women with *matwasat* circumcisions and those with milder *sunna* forms.

In a study using nationally representative samples of women aged 15–49 in the Central African Republic (CAR), Côte d'Ivoire, and Tanzania, Larsen and Yan (2000) find that circumcised women had *lower* childlessness, *lower* infertility by age, and *higher* total fertility rates than uncircumcised women in Tanzania and Côte d'Ivoire, whereas the reverse pattern prevailed in the CAR. In all countries, circumcised and uncircumcised women grouped by age at circumcision had similar adjusted odds of infertility and having a child. Although the authors conclude that "the practice of circumcision does not have a statistically discernable effect on women's ability to reproduce" (Larsen & Yan, 2000, p. 313), they acknowledge that more severe forms of cutting may affect women's fertility. Data from Tanzania were sufficiently detailed to test this hypothesis, but the prevalence of infibulation was too low to estimate its effects.

Therefore, the extent to which more severe forms of female genital cutting affect fertility and sterility in nationally representative samples remains an outstanding question for future research. Given the social importance of fertility for many women in Africa and the belief in some settings that female genital practices enhance fertility, documentation of the effects of these practices on fertility is likely to provide meaningful information to women in practicing settings.

Participation in Social Life Prior to Marriage

Even more sparse and variable in quality is evidence of the social effects of female genital practices either before or after marriage. Complications and ill-health associated with certain forms of female genital cutting, however, may have a number of social consequences for unmarried adolescent girls. Although some researchers suggest that adolescents in parts of Egypt welcome the event as an important marker of maturation (Lane & Meleis, 1991; Leonard, 2000), others speculate that the health-related complications of the practice may interfere with a girl's ability to participate fully in social life (Rushwan, 2000). Complications with urination, for example, may cause particular problems for schoolgirls, whose teachers may accuse them of avoiding lessons because they spend so much time in the bathroom (McCaffrey, 1995). Beyond speculation, however, little is known about the effects of various forms of female genital cutting on the ability of girls to participate fully in school-related and other social activities that would enhance their future prospects for social and economic security.

Quality of Marriage and Marital Stability

Researchers from many disciplines have hypothesized that the effects of female genital cutting are likely to become most apparent at first marriage. While the main justification for female genital cutting in practicing societies is to enhance the marital capital of unmarried daughters, female genital cutting may reduce marital stability in two ways that relate to its effects on women's physical and psychological well-being. First, psychological and physical difficulties arising from a woman's initial or subsequent circumcision may affect the quality of sexual relations. Second, infertility and ill-health effects that are associated with more severe forms of genital cutting may prevent women from fulfilling certain prescribed roles in marriage. Each of these pathways is reviewed in turn.

Regarding the first pathway, women who have had any form of genital cutting may experience pain or anxiety during sexual intercourse that leads to frigidity and unsatisfying sexual relations, and women who have had more severe forms may experience coital difficulty, foul odors resulting from chronic retention of urine and menstrual fluids, and/or the development of fistulae that preclude or seriously hinder their ability to have sex.[31] In either case, persistent difficulties may reduce the overall quality of marital relations and may lead the husband to seek divorce or a second marriage (e.g. El Dareer, 1982; Fourcroy, 1998; Hezekiah & Wafula, 1989; Jordan, 1994; Morris, 1999; Rushwan, 2000; Toubia, 1985; Warsame, 1989 in Toubia, 1994). Among 300 Sudanese men married to infibulated and *sunna* circumcised or uncircumcised women, 20% stated that they married their second, non-infibulated wife because they disliked having to break the scars of their infibulated wives to have sex (Shandall, 1967, pp. 195–196). A more recent study of Sudanese men showed that most men would have preferred to marry an uncut woman (55% of young men and 13% of grandfathers), citing more sexual satisfaction as the main reason for this preference (Almroth et al., 2001).

Regarding the second pathway, female genital cutting may also affect the ability of a woman to fulfill her prescribed roles in marriage. In particular, if marital unions are established in large part to produce children for the lineage, as they often are in Northeastern Africa, then a failure to produce children may logically dissolve the marriage (e.g. Brady, 1998; Inhorn & Buss, 1993; Morris, 1999; Rushwan, 2000). Indeed, when women are unable to produce children, the likelihood that they will be divorced or that the husband will take another wife has been shown to increase (e.g. Ammar, 1954; Larsen, 1995; Meuwissen,

1966; Sami, 1986; van der Kwaak, 1992).[32] In Somalia, "one of the commonest and most important contributory factors in the break-down of a marriage is infertility. In most cases the marriage histories of barren women reveal a series of short unions. Men, certainly, readily divorce a woman who after a few years of marriage has borne no children, unless other attributes compensate for her sterility" (Lewis, 1994, p. 63). Among northern Somali pastoralists, between 24 and 32% of marriages end in divorce (Lewis, 1994). In Sudan, infibulated women have over twice the adjusted odds of being currently divorced compared to uninfibulated women, and such effects may occur through the effect of cutting on fertility as well as by reducing marital quality in other ways (Balk, 2000).

Polygynous remarriage or informal separation may be other consequences of infertility. In East Africa, "women in polygynous unions as well as women with a high frequency of remarriage have a higher incidence of childlessness than those in monogamous unions who are married only once" (Henin, 1981, p. 696). While being in a polygynous union may or may not reduce the relative welfare of women, divorce due to infertility carries especially harsh consequences for women and their natal families (see Inhorn & Buss, 1993 for evidence in Egypt).[33]

A DEMOGRAPHIC PARADOX

The above review suggests that female genital cutting, particularly in Northeastern Africa, is a valued institution that co-exists with the institutions of marriage and reproduction, and which together form the basis of women's social identity and economic security. So closely associated are these institutions that women in practicing populations often insist on circumcising their daughters, because not to do so would likely reduce or eliminate a daughter's ability to marry, become a mother, and acquire financial protection from a husband and his family. All forms of female genital cutting are thus closely associated with attributes that contribute to the formation of a woman's marital capital. As a marker of marriageability, female genital practices ultimately serve to maintain a system of patriarchal control and honor. While certain forms of female genital cutting may further serve as markers of ethnic and class division, the meaning and significance of these practices for certain social classes and ethnic groups likely vary.

Although important for these reasons, female genital cutting comes at a high cost for those women who experience any ill-effects of the practice. Although population-based estimates of the adverse physical and psychological consequences resulting from some form of this practice are lacking, small-scale studies, clinic-based studies, and case reports show strong associations between certain immediate consequences (e.g. bleeding, pain) and all forms of the practice.

Selected studies also show associations between certain long-term or delayed consequences (e.g. chronic retention of urine, urinary tract infections, selected gynecological and obstetric complications) and more severe forms of cutting. Psychological and physical difficulties arising from initial or subsequent female circumcisions may also affect the quality of marital sexual relations, and infertility and ill-health effects that are associated with more severe types may prevent women from fulfilling social expectations that they reproduce. Ironically, any of these intermediate effects may challenge the stability of the marital unions for which female genital cutting is a prerequisite.

Herein lies the "demographic paradox" in the justifications for and consequences of female genital cutting. Infibulation, in particular, may inhibit a woman's lifetime marriage potential and may decrease her fertility despite the fact that Northeastern African societies practicing infibulation have identified one or both of these outcomes as its primary function(s) (Balk, 2000). In the face of this paradox, one might ask whether the circumcision-related risks that all women face (e.g. initial marriageability) would outweigh those risks that only some women experience (e.g. childlessness or marital disruption). If yes, then the perceived greater good of maintaining the current social structure would justify the diminished welfare that a sub-group of women and their families experience. Further supporting this paradox is the likelihood that women who suffer the more severe ill-effects of genital cutting are also the least likely to continue the practice, either because they have the fewest children to circumcise or because they are the most likely to be divorced and thus to lose access to their children. From this perspective, the families of women who benefit from these practices may be the most likely to perpetuate them – and these families are likely to be a majority in the settings where some form of female genital cutting is common.

CONSEQUENCES OF SOCIAL CHANGE

Explaining Recent Declines in the Prevalence of Female Genital Practices

Related to an understanding of the consequences of female genital practices is an appreciation for the consequences of changes in these practices. The most recent findings from Northeastern Africa suggest that the prevalence of female genital cutting has declined in settings where the prevalence has historically been among the highest (El-Gibaly et al., 1999, 2002; Yount, 2002). In part because of different suppositions about the origins of the practice, modernization theory, convention theory, and feminist theory offer different explanations for change in its prevalence. Because modernization theory identifies female genital cutting as a prerequisite for women to gain access to landed inheritance in patrilineal societies, the theory predicts that attitudes about marriage and women's position will change and the relevance of female genital cutting will diminish as rising levels of urbanization, education, wage labor, communication, and economic development decrease the value of landed inheritance (Hayes, 1975; Kennedy, 1970).

Evidence about the role of modernization in the changing prevalence of female genital cutting is mixed, however. Although urban residence is negatively associated with female genital cutting and its perceived necessity in Egypt and Southwestern Nigeria (El-Gibaly et al., 1999; El-Zanaty et al., 1996; Olenick, 1998; Orubuloye, Caldwell & Caldwell, 2000), Hicks (1993) has attributed the absence of change in some urban areas to continued socio-economic ties with rural settings. Certain aspects of modernization have also been associated with the adoption of less severe forms, expansion (Balk, 2001; El Dareer, 1982; Leonard, 1996, 2000; Mackie, 1996; Obermeyer & Reynolds, 1999b; Pia Gallo & Franco Vivani, 1992 in Shell-Duncan & Herlund, 2000), and medicalization of the practice (Carr, 1997; El-Gibaly et al., 1999; Mackie, 1996; Shell-Duncan, 2001; Yount, 2002).

By contrast, convention theory predicts that female genital cutting will disappear rapidly if the "belief trap" that marriage necessitates the practice can be broken. Mackie (1996) proposes that three ingredients are necessary for this rapid decline: (1) introduction of a "superior alien convention," or the common practice elsewhere of NOT performing female genital cutting; (2) promulgation of information about the harmful effects of female genital cutting and the advantages of intact genitalia; and (3) formation of pledge associations committed to eradication of the practice.

Interventions in Egypt and Senegal that have met these conditions are reported to have had some positive effect (CEDPA-Egypt, 1999; TOSTAN, 1999). The sustainability of these effects is debated, however (Caldwell, Orubuloye & Caldwell, 1997; Gray, 1998; Kassamali, 1998; Mackie, 1996, 2000; Spadacini & Nichols, 1998), and analyses that have attributed recent declines in female genital cutting in Egypt to activities surrounding the 1994 International Conference on Population and Development, for example, are limited by the challenge of linking individual outcomes to distal events (El-Gibaly et al., 1999). Also missing from Mackie's (1996) thesis is sufficient acknowledgement of politically powerful anti-eradication groups that are counteracting eradication efforts (e.g. Abu-Sahlieh, 1994; Hicks, 1993; Kassamali, 1998). Finally, because promotion of a "superior alien convention" does not alter gender-biased opportunity structures that oblige women to acquire economic security through marriage, Mackie (1996, 2000) may underestimate women's reliance on customary sources of security, for which female genital cutting is a prerequisite.

Feminist theory offers a third explanation for change in the prevalence of female genital cutting. Some feminists posit that female genital cutting represents patriarchal control over women's bodies and sexuality and a "social and moral order... in which... women are expected... to be silent, subservient,... pure" (Leonard, 2000, p. 162). Members of the Egyptian Task Force have similarly stated that, "FGM [female genital mutilation] is one of the most severe... means of 'educating' women about their subordinate status..." (Abd el Salam, 1999, p. 123). Other feminists recognize that female genital cutting, particularly in Northeastern Africa, is a means by which women define their collective *social* identity, by which women acquire protection and economic security through marriage, and by which women acquire some authority in the private sphere of the family (Hicks, 1993). Despite their differences, both strains of feminist theory predict that sustained change in the prevalence of female genital cutting will occur with fundamental changes in the opportunities that are open to women (Althaus, 1997; El Dawla, 1999; Gruenbaum, 2001; Kassamali, 1998).

Evidence of the effects of mothers' and fathers' educational attainment provides clues about the micro-dynamics of gender-biased opportunity structures. National and community-based studies in Egypt show that better-educated women less often approve of female genital cutting and less often decide to circumcise their daughters (El-Zanaty et al., 1996; Sayed et al., 1996; Yount, 2002) and that higher levels of education may have the greatest effects (Allam et al., 1999; El-Gibaly et al., 1999; Yount, 2002). Fathers' education is weakly associated with daughters' circumcision status and positively associated with consulting a doctor among Egyptian adolescents nationally and among daughters in Upper Egypt (El-Gibaly et al., 1999; Sayed et al., 1996; Yount, 2002). Similarly, most uncircumcised girls in urban Southwest Nigeria had parents, and particularly mothers, with at least some secondary education (Orubuloye et al., 2000; Williams & Sobieszczyk, 1997). Critiques of this perspective point to the fact that even educated and economically independent women are frequently genitally cut (Carr, 1997; Obermeyer & Reynolds, 1999b). Others acknowledge, however, that "women usually undergo genital cutting at too young of an age for [their own] education to have any influence on the likelihood of their being cut" (Carr, 1997, p. 17). Therefore, such critiques incorrectly attribute woman's *own* circumcision status to their *own* educational attainment, when a girl's family jointly determines these two decisions.

More puzzling for feminists is the apparent paradox that women support and perpetuate the practice (Candib, 1999; Leonard, 2000), which has led some to define female genital cutting as a form of violence performed by women on women (El Dawla, 1999; Kassamali, 1998; Mackie, 1996, 2000; Toubia, 1998). To explain this paradox, Hicks (1993) and Gruenbaum (1996) contend that analyses of female genital cutting must consider the history and context of populations in which female genital cutting is practiced. In many such settings, while men largely derive their social status through activities in the public sphere, women largely derive their social status and economic security through their roles as wives, mothers, mothers-in-law, and grandmothers (Gruenbaum, 1988; Hicks, 1993). Sanctioned public scrutiny of women's adherence to social expectations, and the priority of a community over an individual's interests, creates powerful incentives for women to conform. In this way, "belief systems about maleness and femaleness get encoded in social structure . . . the result is a complex system of constraints and opportunities that . . . [shape] the experiences that men and women can have, what they can know, and who they can become" (McAdam, 1992, p. 1213 in Hicks, 1993).

For these reasons, several researchers (Gruenbaum, 1988, 1991, 2001; Robertson, 1996; Toubia, 1985; van der Kwaak, 1992) argue that it is necessary to expand the choice-set for women. By creating viable and attractive social and economic opportunities for women that are not constructed through rigid sex-specialization, women will not be solely dependent on their roles as virgins, brides, wives, and mothers; thus, no longer rendering female genital cutting a *sine qua non*. Recent evidence from Minia, Egypt suggests that age-specific probabilities of genital cutting are indeed lower among daughters than mothers and among younger than older daughters, and that mother's (particularly higher) education is negatively associated with her intent and decision to circumcise a daughter (Yount, 2002).

Implications of Social Change

As our critiques of the above theories have pointed out, the process of social change with regards to female genital practices is neither deterministic nor linear. In those contexts where the prevalence of female genital cutting has declined, however, a question that emerges is the extent to which uncircumcised and circumcised daughters will have the same prospects for marriage. A few analyses provide empirical evidence of the real or perceived difficulty in finding husbands for uncircumcised women who belong to circumcising social groups (e.g. Dirie & Lindmark, 1991; Gruenbaum, 1991; Huddleston, 1949; Lowenstein, 1978; Sequeira, 1931). If the ideological link between genital cutting and marriage persists among some sub-groups within the populations, then one might expect to observe at least four different responses to initial change. First, the circumcision status of girls may become a more central component of marital negotiations, and the age at girls' circumcision may simply rise without a change in their overall risk of circumcision. Second, circumcised and uncircumcised women may begin to marry in different marriage markets, one in which the ideological link between circumcision and marriage has remained intact and one in which this ideological link has dissolved, respectively. Third, uncircumcised women may experience a higher rate of non-marriage than circumcised women. Finally, in settings where brideprice is a part of marital negotiations, circumcised brides may command a higher bride price than uncircumcised brides (e.g. Constantinides, 1985; Grassivaro-Gallo, 1986a; van der Kwaak, 1992; Widstrand, 1964).

A fifth possibility is that declines in female genital cutting will have no effect on girls' marital capital because the link between female circumcision is weaker among men than among women. A recent study conducted among older and younger Sudanese men suggests that only 17% believed that no villager would marry an uncircumcised woman or would divorce her for not having been genitally cut (Almroth et al., 2001). The same study showed that 86% of young men reported that they would have accepted a non-genitally cut woman to be the wife of his son or grandson, compared to 57% of older men. The extent to which attitudes that men express in a context of widespread infibulation would survive in a context of precipitous declines in female genital cutting (or a changes to less severe forms of the practice) is uncertain, however, and a study of circumcision among adolescents in Egypt showed that girls aged 10–19 were already half as likely as same-age boys to view female genital cutting as necessary for marriage (El-Gibaly et al., 1999, 2002). To our knowledge, the consequences for marriage of declines in the prevalence of female genital cutting have not been systematically studied.

RECOMMENDATIONS FOR FUTURE RESEARCH

Notably, some scholars have been skeptical of the disproportionate attention that female genital cutting has received in political and scientific circles at the possible expense of concerns that are more salient to local women (e.g. Walley, 1997). Without question, researchers and practitioners need to view female genital cutting with sensitivity to the full range of social and economic constraints that circumcised and uncircumcised women face. At the same time, researchers and practitioners cannot ignore the realities that female genital cutting occupies a central place in both the lives of women and the scientific community and that the perceived importance of the practice among both groups is unlikely to disappear in the near future. Persistent local and international interest in female genital practices therefore imposes an even stronger responsibility on researchers who are engaged in efforts to understand the practice to pursue their research with methodological rigor and attention to cultural contexts.

In this light, an agenda for future research on the subject of female genital practices should highlight the need for more nuanced understandings of the causes and consequences of various forms of the practice, multi-method research designs, innovative approaches to data collection, inclusion of a broader range of study participants, inclusion of representative samples when population inferences are to be made, and methodological rigor in both qualitative and quantitative data collection and analysis. These needs are more likely to be met through inter-disciplinary collaborations that include (among others) anthropologists, social demographers, and clinicians who have disciplinary expertise pertaining to female genital practices and/or practicing populations. With this collaborative structure in mind, six priorities for research merit discussion.

First, researchers need to examine the motivations of various actors who are involved either in the perpetuation of female genital practices or in the processes of social change. Such an examination would require parallel efforts to understand: (1) the social, cultural, religious, and economic contexts that give rise to certain understandings about gender, gender relations, and family relations more broadly; and (2) the social fabric in which these practices are perceived as important for the social identity and economic security of women. One goal of this broader, critical analysis would be to delineate the "local logic" for behaviors that to outsiders seem anomalous or even morally reprehensible.

Second, researchers need to make a concerted effort to understand the perceptions of men regarding to the causes of, justifications for, and consequences of various forms of the practice. To date, the bulk of research on female genital practices has ignored the views of men because women are seen as both the "perpetrators" and "victims" of the practice. However, if the origins of female genital cutting are founded in patriarchal family relations, or the intersection of these relations with class and/or religious ideologies, then attention to men as implicit or explicit actors in either the continuation of the practice or the process of social change is critical.

Third, future efforts to understand the health consequences of female genital practices require more rigorous study designs. All such studies should include detailed classifications of female genital cutting that capture major points of variation in the practice within particular cultural contexts, but permit cross-cultural comparisons. Such studies should also gather information about the timing and exact nature of the first and any subsequent genital procedures so that the frequency of the practice can be considered in analyses of its health effects. Finally, studies that are population-based and that include representative samples of women need to be conducted in parallel with clinic-based studies so that observed associations between various forms of the practice and specific health consequences can be generalized to identifiable population groups.

Fourth, structured instruments that have been used in cross-sectional surveys of female genital cutting may be enhanced in ways that will permit rigorous analysis of the effects of various forms of female genital cutting on marital stability through their effects on fertility, health, marital sexuality, and marital gender roles. Current instruments, for example, include only general questions about the circumcision status of women and may or may not ask about the specific form of the procedures performed. Because a woman may experience circumcision more than once in her life, future instruments should include a "circumcision history" that consists of questions about the timing and nature of all procedures performed. (One advantage of having this data would be to determine the extent to which women who experience less severe forms of genital cutting undergo subsequent procedures just prior to or after marriage.) In addition, standard national demographic and health surveys tend to include questions only about the current marital status of ever-married women of reproductive age. In order to link temporally a particular genital procedure with a particular marital event (e.g. first marriage, formal or informal separation, polygynous marriage of the husband, divorce, remarriage), future instruments should include detailed marital histories of all women. These same instruments should also continue to include standard pregnancy histories, and unless politically unfeasible, sampling frames should be expanded to include never-married women (at least for a subset of the survey questions). Together, these detailed data would allow researchers to examine the temporal associations between circumcision, fertility, and marriage in ways that until today have not been possible.

Fifth, greater attention needs to be given to the less visible but equally salient psychological consequences of female genital practices. While exposing the most extreme consequences of more severe forms of the practice may serve useful political purposes for those whose interests lie primarily in eradication of the practice, the less visible psychological and emotional consequences for women who experience any form of the practice deserve broader attention. An understanding of these less visible effects is likely to be achieved through in-depth interviews with women who have experienced various forms of genital cutting and who are at various stages of pre-marital and married life.

Finally, increasing attention needs to be given to the implications for marriage of change in the prevalence of female genital practices. With evidence in certain settings of declines in the overall prevalence of the practice or with the spread of less severe forms, studies are needed that allow researchers to specify if and how girls who are genitally cut and those who are not genitally cut secure marital partners. In this context, researchers will need to consider seriously models that allow them to determine whether underlying factors that have caused one of these changes (e.g. adoption of less severe cutting) also underlie other trends (e.g. changes in the age at marriage). Assuming this issue of simultaneous determination can be addressed, an understanding of the implications for marital formation of social change in the practice may best be achieved through a longitudinal follow-up of initially uncircumcised girls to determine if the age-specific probability of marriage differs between those who are and are not eventually circumcised. In parallel, qualitative interviews should be conducted with never-married and engaged young women and men to understand the extent to which these groups see female genital cutting as a pre-requisite for marriage.

At this stage, the literature provides insufficient evidence to permit us to describe the extent to which female genital cutting is demographically significant. As a consequence, questions of "whether" and "how much" remain ones for future, systematic, and sensitive investigation. At the same time, the literature clearly suggests that female genital cutting in its many forms is a culturally significant practice. Therefore, future social demographic inquiry into female genital practices needs to work at the nexus of understanding social constructs and social changes part in parcel with understanding rates of marriage, divorce, and children ever born.

NOTES

1. The 28 countries are: Benin, Burkina Faso, Cameroon, Central Africa Republic, Chad, Côte d'Ivoire, Djibouti, Egypt, Ethiopia, Eritrea, Gambia, Ghana, Guinea, Guinea Bissau, Kenya, Liberia, Mali, Mauritania, Niger, Nigeria, Senegal, Sierra Leone, Somalia, Sudan, Tanzania, Togo, Uganda, and Zaire.

2. See also Barstow (1999), Black and Debelle (1995), Brady (1999), Eke and Nkanginieme (1999), Elchalal et al. (1999), Ford (2001), Fourcroy (1998), Gibeau (1998), Johnson and Rodgers (1994), Jordan (1994), Kiragu (1995), Ladjali et al. (1993), McCaffrey, Jankowska, and Gordon (1995), Morris (1999), Omer-Hashi (1994), Omer-Hashi and Entwistle (1995), Ortiz (1996), Rendell (1999).

3. Gordon's (1991) and Lyons' (1981) analyses are constructed around this very point. Lyons (1981) notes that relativism was introduced into anthropology as a moral posture; in the case of genital practices, it was historically important for the purpose of removing the racist basis and content of the discussion. Ironically, Lyons notes, that what was useful for moral posturing is now "being decried for its lack of moral initiative" (p. 514). Gordon (1991) more generally remarks that "cultural relativism, although it is not generally considered to be so, is also a position of advocacy" (p. 13) and tries to situate the debate on female circumcision in the anthropological literature somewhere between humanist positivism and contextual non-positivism (or relativism). Also see the commentaries of Boddy (1991), Morsy (1991), and Schepper-Hughes (1991) on Gordon's essay, and Gruenbaum (1982, 1991) and van der Kwaak (1992), for additional related comments.

4. "Sunna" means conforming to traditions that existed during the lifetime of Prophet Mohammed (Gruenbaum, 2001).

5. Agugua and Egwuatu (1982) find in their Nigerian study that excision may result in labial fusion (in 30% of the 55 pediatric cases that presented themselves), thus making it similar to infibulation.

6. Explanatory figures or pictures may be found in Hicks (1993) and Toubia (1993) among others.

7. An even more radical form, called introcision, exists. This form involves cutting into the vagina or splitting the perineum, either digitally or with a sharp instrument. This type has been reported only among Aboriginal populations of Australia (Lyons, 1981; Verzin, 1975; Worsley, 1938). According to Hosken (1978), the Australian medical authorities state that these practices no longer exist (p. 150).

8. According to Toubia (1993), the law against these practices in Sudan was omitted from a 1991 legal revision, rendering the current legal status unclear (p. 45).

9. Hicks (1993, p. 11) points out that "postpartum re-stitching (closure of what, in fact, is an open wound) has inadvertently become interpreted as re-infibulated."

10. There is some question, however, as to whether the infibulations were outstanding prior to enslavement or undertaken by the captors (Widstrand, 1964).

11. For example, in contrast to male circumcision, which is celebrated with great fanfare, in the Sudanese village Boddy studied, female circumcision is celebrated by "the briefest and most subdued of ceremonial feasts: morning tea" (1982, p. 683). Sami (1986, p. 104) notes that "the size of the celebration depends on the family's means but, in general, male circumcision is a bigger ceremony." Also see Kennedy (1970) and Ammar (1954). Others report a range of ceremonies, including some elaborate ones (e.g. Cloudsley, 1983; El Dareer, 1982).

12. Lightfoot-Klein (1989b) suggests the use of a traditional smoke and oil ceremony allows women to manifest their sexuality and receptivity to sexual relations with their husbands, in a culture where women believe they cannot (and apparently do not) otherwise initiate sexual relations. She suggests that women can, on the margins, manipulate their (sexual) environment, thus maintaining some control over it.

13. Gruenbaum (1991, p. 642) tells the following story: "Several of the older women, however, still considered pharaonic circumcision the key to marital bliss, using infibulation as a means of sexually frustrating one's husband, and thereby exciting both partners. Another woman I spoke with even claimed that if my husband ever had the chance to experience sex with a Sudanese wife, he'd send me away."

14. For a general discussion of marital exchange, see Lewis (1994). With regards to female genital cutting in particular, the literature does a poorer job of clarifying these exchange relationships, although many authors note their existence and importance.

15. Case studies with this evidence are fairly common (e.g. Barclay, 1964; Cloudsley, 1983). Related evidence is given by Shandall (1967, pp. 195–196).

16. Use of urban residence or education as markers of class is problematic for two reasons. First, Hicks (1993) notes that persistence of female genital practices in urban settings may in fact be the result of persistent social ties with rural areas. Second, modernization theory proposes that increasing urbanization is associated with decreasing emphasis on landed wealth and the inheritance of property, which is presumed among modernization theorists to be the source of women's access to resources and the consequent need for markers of marriageability.

17. In a subsequent review, we were able to identify more studies of varying quality that assess the effects of female genital practices. The basic conclusions about study quality and effects do not vary markedly between this review and the subsequent review, however. Please contact the authors to receive a copy of the subsequent review, which

at the time of this publication, is in preparation for submission to a peer-reviewed journal.

18. Because RTI and PID are among the leading causes of infertility, the presence of these infections in circumcising populations is reviewed more closely in the next section.

19. There does not seem to be an obvious relationship between those countries (or regions) that practice female circumcision and those that do not (using Toubia's list of 27 countries) and the percentage of women at the end of their childbearing years who are childless (found in Frank, 1983). (Frank does not have data on 15 out of 27 countries on Toubia's list.) However, Frank's (1983) data are intended to represent national level fertility and childlessness, whereas, female circumcision varies quite a bit in severity and by locality, ethnicity, and family system within most societies.

20. As an exception, Mammo and Morgan (1986) include a single footnoted comment that isolates one group as practitioners of female genital cutting – the Christian Ahmaras. According to the evidence in Hicks (1993), however, Mammo and Morgan (1986) would be mistaken to isolate the Christian Amharas as the only group practicing female circumcision in Ethiopia. For example, most Galla (apparently also called Oromo) populations, who are Ethiopia's largest ethnic group, "circumcise" females (Hicks, 1993); however, the evidence on which type(s) of circumcision they practice is unclear. Hicks (1993) claims that while most groups in Ethiopia do not practice infibulation, many groups, including the Galla, practice excision.

21. It is important to note that infibulation creates a barrier to coitus. Because an inability to have coitus due to infibulation would generally occur in the first weeks or months of marriage, however, it is expected that this barrier would only increase the interval between marriage and first birth among infibulated women without substantially affecting overall fertility. Notably, these effects of coital difficulty would likely be greater if they lead to unsterile procedures (e.g. use of unhygienic instruments to cut open the infibulation or to widen the vaginal opening) that increase the risk of infection (El Dareer, 1982; Shandall, 1967). At the time this chapter was written, however, there are no studies that examine differences in coital frequency between infibulated and un-infibulated women and the subsequent use of interventions to facilitate sex.

22. De Silva's study design has some basic problems, however: The treatment population is an immigrant group and likely self-selected on several relevant criterion, such as marital and socioeconomic status (including a preponderance of urban-dwellers), and, therefore, circumcision characteristics. Of these, De Silva has data only on circumcision status, which clearly shows that his sample is not representative of Sudan (e.g. the rates of those who are not circumcised and those who have the *sunna* and intermediate types are much higher than is representative of Sudan). Divisions between type of circumcision are not maintained throughout the analysis (probably because the cell sizes would be too small); however, this may explain why the obstetric effects of circumcision are less than one might expect to find in a largely infibulating population.

23. This is perhaps because both groups of women received ante- and neonatal care.

24. A more recent study found no differences among 233 Sudanese and 92 Somali women delivering in King Abdulaziz University Hospital in Jeddah, Saudi Arabia in any of following characteristics of labor and delivery: duration of first-, second-, and third-stage labor; rates of episiotomy; rates of vaginal laceration; APGAR scores; blood loss; maternal stay (Rouzi, Sindi et al., 2001).

25. It is not entirely clear that the denominator (e.g. total number of pregnancies) is 48, although she reports that the mean number of pregnancies to eight women is six.

These stillbirths occurred to two women. Additionally, one child was reported to have died one day after birth. It is unfortunate that the authors do not associate the stillbirths (or other outcomes in their study) with the circumcision characteristics: one woman was not circumcised, four had *sunna* circumcisions, and seven were infibulated.

26. In an oft-cited paper, Mustafa (1966, p. 304) claims that "20–25% of the cases of infertility in the Sudan are due to infibulation, which may cause chronic pelvic infection or may prevent sexual intercourse." As he offers neither data nor citations to support his claim, we do not give weight to it here.

27. Belsey and Ware (1986) report that studies from the U.S. and Sweden indicate that gonorrhea is shown to be the cause of inflammation of the fallopian tubes in less than half of the patients with PID and that a previous delivery, abortion, or curettage has been associated with about 20% of such cases.

28. Meuwissen does not report having data on the circumcision status or history of his patients. Toubia (1993) suggests that the prevalence of circumcision in Ghana is about only 30% and Hosken (1981) suggests that in Ghana, it is practiced only in the north.

29. Tubal factor infertility refers to that resulting from post-inflammatory damage to the fallopian tubes such as by PID.

30. Larsen does not consider the decline in the prevalence of infibulation in the interval but sees this decline as part of a trend in Africa in the declining prevalence of sterility.

31. Women who experience vesicovaginal fistula as a result of the practice also are likely to be ostracized not only by their husbands but also by their communities (Warsame, 1989 in Toubia, 1994).

32. El Din (1977) makes the related point that when a Sudanese woman bears no children (or none that survive) a husband may ask for a refund of half of the marriage cattle (e.g. bride wealth paid from the groom's family to the bride's) to help him find another wife more likely to bear children.

33. Lightfoot-Klein (1989b) provides case evidence of divorce occurring without ramifications in Sudan when it occurs to women after they have proven their fertility or is for reasons unrelated to fertility and beyond the woman's control. Lewis (1994) suggests that divorce is generally accepted in Somali society, but does not comment on its acceptability when it is due to infertility.

ACKNOWLEDGMENTS

For comments on earlier versions of this manuscript, the authors thank Frank Zimmerman, Lindy Williams, and Zeinab Khadr. The authors also thank Nikki Denise Khanna and Anne Mackay Austin for their assistance in the final preparation of this manuscript.

REFERENCES

Abdalla, R. H. D. (1982). *Sisters in affliction: Circumcision and infibulation of women in Africa.* London: Zed Press.

Abd el Salam, S. (1999). Roundtable on cutting women's genitals. Language is both subjective and symbolic. *Reproductive Health Matters*, *7*(13), 121–123.

Abu Daia, J. M. (2000). Female circumcision. *Saudi Medical Journal*, *21*(10), 921–923.

Abu-Sahlieh, S. A. A. (1994). To mutilate in the name of Jehovah or Allah: Legitimization of male and female circumcision. *Medicine and Law*, *13*, 575–622.

Agugua, N. E. N., & Egwuatu, V. E. (1982). Female circumcision: Management of urinary complication. *Journal of Tropical Pediatrics*, *28*, 248–252.

Allam, M. F., de Irala-Estevez, J., Fernandez-Crehuet Navajas, R., Serrano del Castillo, A., Hoashi, J. S., Pankovich, M. B., & Rebollo Liceaga, J. (2001). Factors associated with the condoning of female genital mutilation among university students. *Public Health*, *115*(5), 350–355.

Allam, M. F., de Irala-Estevez, J., Navajas, R. F.-C., del Castillo, A. S., Hoashi, J. S., Pankovich, M. B., & Liceaga, J. R. (1999). Students' knowledge of and attitudes about female circumcision in Egypt [letter]. *New England Journal of Medicine*, *34*, 1552–1553.

Almroth, L., Almroth-Berggren, V., Hassanein, O. M., Al-Said, S. S. E., Hasan, S. S. A., Ulla-Britt, L., & Berstrom, S. (2001). Male complications of female genital mutilation. *Social Science and Medicine*, *53*, 1455–1460.

Althaus, F. A. (1997). Female circumcision: Rite of passage or violation of rights? *International Family Planning Perspectives*, *23*, 130–133.

Ammar, H. (1954). *Growing up in an Egyptian village: Silwa, province of Assam*. London: Routledge & Kegan Paul.

Arbesman, M., Kahler, L., & Buck, G. M. (1993). Assessment of the impact of female circumcision on the gynecological, genitourinary and obstetrical health problems of women from Somalia: Literature review and case series. *Women and Health*, *20*(3), 27–42.

Assaad, M. B. (1980). Female circumcision in Egypt: Social implications, current research, and prospects for change. *Studies in Family Planning*, *11*(1), 3–16.

Assaad, M. B. (1999). Roundtable on cutting women's genitals. Challenging the terminology and overcoming the culture of silence. *Reproductive Health Matters*, *7*(13), 126–127.

Aziz, F. A. (1980). Gynecologic and obstetric complications of female circumcision. *International Journal of Gynecology and Obstetrics*, *17*, 560–563.

Baasher, T. (1979). Psychological aspects of female circumcision. In: *Traditional Practices Affecting the Health of Women and Children*. Alexandria, Egypt: World Health Organization.

Baker, C., Gilson, G., Vill, M., & Curet, L. (1993). Female circumcision: Obstetric issues. *American Journal of Obstetrics & Gynecology*, *169*, 1616–1618.

Balk, D. (2000). To marry and bear children? The demographic consequences of infibulation in Sudan. In: B. Shell-Duncan & Y. Hernlund (Eds), *Female "Circumcision" in Africa: Culture, Controversy, and Change* (pp. 55–71). Boulder: Lynne Reinner.

Balk, D. (2001). *The role of class in circumcision and infibulation in Sudan*. Unpublished manuscript.

Barclay, H. B. (1964). *Buurri Al Lamaab: A suburban village in the Sudan*. Ithaca, NY: Cornell University Press.

Barstow, D. G. (1999). Female genital mutilation: The penultimate gender abuse. *Child Abuse and Neglect*, *23*(5), 501–510.

Belsey, M. A. (1979). Biological factors other than nutrition and lactation which may influence natural fertility: Additional notes with particular reference to sub-Saharan Africa. In: H. Leridon & J. Menken (Eds), *Natural Fertility*. Liege: Ordina Editions.

Belsey, M. A., & Ware, H. (1986). Epidemiological, social, and psychological aspects of infertility. In: V. Insler & B. Lunenfeld (Eds), *Infertility: Male and Female*. Edinburgh: Churchill Livingston.

Beradi, J., Teillet, J., Godard, J., Laloux, V., Allane, P., & Franjou, M. H. (1985). Consequences obstetricales de l'excision feminine. *Journal de Gynecologie, Obstetrique et Biologie de la Reproduction*, *14*(6), 743–746.

Berhane, Y. G., Emmelin, M., & Hogberg, U. (2001). Women's health in rural setting in societal transition in Ethiopia. *Social Science and Medicine*, *53*(11), 1525–1539.

Black, J. A., & Debelle, G. D. (1995). Female genital mutilation in Britain. *British Medical Journal*, *310*(6994), 1590–1592.

Boddy, J. (1982). Womb as oasis: The symbolic context of pharaonic circumcision in rural Northern Sudan. *American Ethnologist*, *9*(4), 682–698.

Boddy, J. (1991). Body politics: Continuing the anticircumcision crusade. *Medical Anthropology Quarterly, New Series*, *5*(1), 15–17.

Bongaarts, J., Frank, O., & Lesthaeghe, R. (1984). The proximate determinants of fertility in sub-Saharan Africa. *Population and Development Review*, *10*(3), 511–538.

Brady, M. (1998). Female genital mutilation. *Nursing*, *28*(9), 50–51.

Brady, M. (1999). Female genital mutilation: Complications and risk of HIV transmission. *AIDS Patient Care and Stds*, *13*(12), 709–716.

Brisson, P., Haroon, P., & Feins, N. (2001). Female circumcision. *Journal of Pediatric Surgery*, *36*(7), 1068–1069.

Bureau of Statistics and Macro International (1997). *Tanzania demographic and health survey 1996*. Dar es Saalam, Tanzania: Bureau of Statistics Planning Commission and Calverton, MD: Macro International.

Calder, B. L., Brown, Y. M., & Rae, D. I. (1993). Female circumcision/genital mutilation: Culturally sensitive care. *Health Care for Women International*, *14*(3), 227–238.

Caldwell, J. C., & Caldwell, P. (1983). The demographic evidence for the incidence and cause of abnormally low fertility in tropical Africa. *World Health Statistic Quarterly*, *36*, 2–34.

Caldwell, J. C., Orubuloye, I. O., & Caldwell, P. (1997). Male and female circumcision in Africa from a regional to a specific Nigerian examination. *Social Science and Medicine*, *44*, 1181–1193.

Caldwell, J. C., Orubuloye, I. O., & Caldwell, P. (2000). Female genital mutilation: Conditions of decline. *Population Research and Policy Review*, *19*(3), 233–254.

Candib, L. M. (1999). Incest and other harms to daughters across cultures: Maternal complicity and patriarchal power. *Women's Studies International Forum*, *22*, 185–201.

Carr, D. (1997). *Female genital cutting: Findings from the demographic and health surveys program*. Calverton, MD: Macro International.

CEDPA-Egypt (1999). *The positive deviance approach in female genital mutilation eradication*. Final end-of-project report for PROWID to the Center for Development and Population Activities.

Chalmers, B., & Omer-Hashi, K. (2000). 432 Somali women's birth experiences in Canada after earlier female genital mutilation. *Birth*, *2*(4), 227–234.

Cloudsley, A. (1983). *Women of Omdurman: Life, love and the cult of virginity*. London: Ethnographica.

Constantinides, P. (1985). Women heal women: Spirit possession and sexual segregation in a Muslim society. *Social Science and Medicine*, *21*(6), 685–692.

Cook, R. (1979). Damage to physical health from pharonic circumcision (infibulation) of females: A review of the medical literature. In: *Traditional Practices Affecting the Health of Women and Children*. Alexandria, Egypt: World Health Organization.

Davis, G., Ellis, J., Hibbert, M., Perez, R. P., & Zimbelman, E. (1999). Female circumcision: The prevalence and nature of the ritual in Eritrea. *Military Medicine*, *164*(1), 11–16.

Daw, E. (1970). Female circumcision and infibulation complicating delivery. *The Practioner*, *204*, 559–563.

Demographic and Health Surveys (1991). *Sudan demographic and health surveys 1989/1990.* Department of Statistics, Ministry of Economic and National Planning, Khartoum, Sudan, and Institute for Resource Development/Macro International, Columbia, MD.

De Silva, S. (1989). Obstetric sequelae of female circumcision. *European Journal of Obstetrics, Gynecology, and Reproductive Biology*, *32*, 233–240.

Dewhurst, C., & Michelson, A. (1964). Infibulation complicating pregnancy. *British Medical Journal*, *2*, 1442.

Dirie, M. A., & Lindmark, G. (1991). Female circumcision in Somalia and women's motives. *Acta Obstetricia et Gynecologica Scandinavica*, *70*, 581–585.

Dirie, M. A., & Lindmark, G. (1992). The risk of medical complications after female circumcision. *East African Medical Journal*, *69*(9), 779–782.

Eke, N., & Nkanginieme, K. E. (1999). Female genital mutilation: A global bug that should not cross the millennium bridge. *World Journal of Surgery*, *23*(10), 1082–1086.

Elchalal, U., Ben-Ami, B., & Brzezinski, A. (1999). Female circumcision: The peril remains. *BJU International*, *83*(Suppl. 1), 103–108.

El Dareer, A. (1982). *Women, why do you weep*? London: Zed Press.

El Dawla, A. S. (1999). The political and legal struggle over female genital mutilation in Egypt: Five years since the ICPD. *Reproductive Health Matters*, *7*, 128–136.

El-Defrawi, M. H., Lotfy, G., Dandash, K. F., Rafaat, A. H., & Eyada, M. (2001). Female genital mutilation and its psychosexual impact. *Journal of Sex and Marital Therapy*, *27*, 465–473.

El Din, M. A.-A. G. (1977). The economic value of children in rural Sudan. In: J. C. Caldwell (Ed.), *The Persistence of High Fertility* (Vol. 2, pp. 617–658). Canberra: The Australian National University.

El-Gibaly, O., Ibrahim, B., Mensch, B. S., & Clark, W. H. (1999). The decline of female circumcision in Egypt: Evidence and interpretation. Policy Research Division Working Paper No. 132, The Population Council, New York, N.Y.

El-Gibaly, O., Ibrahim, B., Mensch, B. S., & Clark, W. H. (2002). The decline of female circumcision in Egypt: Evidence and interpretation. *Social Science and Medicine*, *54*, 205–220.

El Saadawi, N. (1982). *The hidden face of Eve*. Boston: Beacon Press.

El-Zanaty, F., Hussein, E. M., Shawky, G. A., Way, A. A., & Kishor, A. (1996). *Egypt demographic and health survey 1995*. Calverton, MD: MacroInternational.

Epstein, D., Graham, P., & Rimsza, M. (2001). Medical complications of female genital mutilation. *Journal of American College Health*, *49*(6), 275–280.

Erian, M. M., & Goh (1995). Female circumcision. *Australian and New Zealand Journal of Obstetrics and Gynaecology*, *35*(1), 83–85.

Ericksen, K. P. (1989). Female genital mutilations in Africa. *Behavior Science Research*, *23*(1–4), 182–204.

Ericksen, K. P. (1995). Female circumcision among Egyptian women. *Women's Health: Research on Gender, Behavior, and Policy*, *1*(4), 309–328.

Ford, N. (2001). Tackling female genital cutting in Somalia. *The Lancet*, *358*, 1179.

Fourcroy, J. L. (1998). The three feminine sorrows. *Hospital Practice*, July 15.

Frank, O. (1983). Infertility in sub-Saharan Africa: Estimates and implications. *Population and Development Review*, *9*(1), 137–144.

Gadallah, A., Zazour, A. H., El-Gibaly, O. M., AbdelAty, M. A., & Monazea, I. M. (1996). Knowledge, attitude, and practice of women teachers on female circumcision in Assiut governorate, Final report. Paper Presented at Rainbo Workshop on Female Genital Mutilation, November, Cairo.

Gausset, Q. (2001). AIDS and cultural practices in Africa: The case of the Tonga (Zambia). *Social Science and Medicine*, *52*(4), 509–518.

Gibeau, A. M. (1998). Female genital mutilation: When a cultural practice generates clinical and ethical dilemmas. *JOGNN*, *27*(1), 85–91.

Gordon, D. (1991). Female circumcision and genital operations in Egypt and the Sudan: A dilemma for medical anthropology. *Medical Anthropology Quarterly, New Series*, *5*(1), 3–28.

Grassivaro-Gallo, P. (1986a). Views of future health workers in Somalia on female circumcision. *Medical Anthropology Quarterly*, *17*(3), 71–73.

Grassivaro-Gallo, P. (1986b). *La circoncisione femminila in Somalia. Una ricerca sul campo*. Milan: F. Angeli.

Grassivaro-Gallo, P., & Viviani, F. (1992). The origin of infibulation in Somalia: An ethological hypothesis. *Ethology and Sociobiology*, *13*, 253–265.

Gray, C. S. (1998). A case-history based assessment of female genital mutilation in Sudan. *Evaluation and Programming Planning*, *21*, 429–436.

Gruenbaum, E. (1982). The movement against cliterodectomy and infibulation in Sudan: Public health policy and the woman's movement. *Medical Anthropology Newsletter*, *13*(2), 4–12.

Gruenbaum, E. (1988). Reproductive ritual and social reproduction: Female circumcision and the subordination of women in Sudan. In: N. O'Neill & J. O'Brien (Eds), *Economy and Class in Sudan*. Aldershot, England: Avebury.

Gruenbaum, E. (1991). The Islamic movement, development, and health education: Recent changes in the health of rural women in central Sudan. *Social Science and Medicine*, *33*(6), 637–645.

Gruenbaum, E. (1996). The cultural debate over female circumcision: The Sudanese are arguing this one out for themselves. *Medical Anthropology Quarterly (New Series)*, *10*(4), Dec.

Gruenbaum, E. (2000). Is female circumcision a maladaptive cultural pattern? In: B. Shell-Duncan & Y. Hernlund (Eds), *Female "Circumcision" in Africa: Culture, Controversy, and Change* (pp. 41–54). Boulder, CO: Lynne Rienner.

Gruenbaum, E. (2001). *The female circumcision controversy: An anthropological perspective*. Philadelphia: University of Pennsylvania Press.

Gulick, J. (1976). *The Middle East: An anthropological perspective*. Pacific Palisades, CA: Goodyear Publishing Co.

Hanley, M. G., & Ojeda, V. J. (1995). Epidermal inclusion cysts of the clitoris as a complication of female circumcision and pharaonic infibulation. *Central African Journal of Medicine*, *41*(1), 22–24.

Hansen, H. H. (1972/3). Cliterodectomy: Female circumcision in Egypt. *Folk (Dansk Etnographfisk Tidsskrift)*, 14–15, 15–26.

Hardy, D. B. (1987). Cultural practices contributing to the transmission of human immunodeficiency virus in Africa. *Reviews of Infectious Diseases*, *9*(6), 1109–1119.

Hayes, R. O. (1975). Female genital mutilation, fertility control, women's roles, and the patrilineage in modern Sudan: A functional analysis. *American Ethnologist*, *2*(4), 617–633.

Henin, R. A. (1981). Fertility, infertility, and sub-fertility in eastern Africa. *International Union for the Scientific Study of Population Conference Proceedings, Manila* (pp. 667–697). Liege: Ordina Editions.

Hezekiah, J., & Wafula, F. (1989). Major health problems of women in a Kenyan village. *Health Care for Women International*, *10*, 15–25.

Hicks, E. K. (1993). *Infibulation: Female mutilation in Islamic Northeastern Africa*. New Brunswick: Transaction Publishers.

Hosken, F. P. (1978). The epidemiology of female genital mutilations. *Tropical Doctor*, *8*, 150–156.

Hosken, F. P. (1981). Female genital mutilation in the world today: A global review. *International Journal of Health Services*, *11*(3), 415–430.

Hosken, F. P. (1982). *The Hosken Report: Genital and sexual mutilation of females* (3rd rev. ed.). Lexington, MA: Women's International Network News.

Huddleston, C. (1949). Female circumcision in the Sudan. *The Lancet*, *1*, 626.

Ibrahim, B. (personal communication, January, 2002).

Ibrahim, H. (1979). *The Shaiqiya: The cultural and social change of a northern Sudanese riverain people*. Wiesbaden, Germany: Franz Steiner Verlag GMBH.

Inhorn, M. C., & Buss, K. A. (1993). Infertility, infection, and iatrogenesis in Egypt: The anthropological epidemiology of blocked tubes. *Medical Anthropology*, *15*, 217–244.

Isa, A. R., Shuib, R., & Othman, R. S. (1999). The practice of female circumcision among Muslims in Kelantan, Malaysia. *Reproductive Health Matters*, *7*(13), 137–143.

Johnson, M. C. (2000). Becoming a Muslim, becoming a person: Female 'circumcision,' religious identity, and personhood in Guinea-Bissau. In: *Female Circumcision in Africa: Culture, Controversy, and Change* (pp. 215–233). Boulder: Lynne-Rienner.

Johnson, K. E., & Rodgers, S. (1994). When cultural practices are health risks: The dilemma of female circumcision. *Holistic Nursing Practice*, *8*(2), 70–78.

Jones, H., Diop, N., Askew, I., & Kabore, I. (1999). Female genital cutting practices in Burkina Faso and Mali and their negative health outcomes. *Studies in Family Planning*, *30*(3), 219–229.

Jordan, J. A. (1994). Female genital mutilation (female circumcision). *British Journal of Obstetrics and Gynaecology*, *101*(2), 94–95.

Kassamali, N. J. (1998). When modernity confronts traditional practices: Female genital cutting in northeast Africa. In: H. L. Bodman & N. Tohidi (Eds), *Women in Muslim Societies: Diversity within Unity* (pp. 39–61). Boulder: Lynne Rienner.

Kennedy, J. G. (1970). Circumcision and excision in Egyptian Nubia. *Journal of the Royal Anthropological Institute*, *5*(2), 175–191.

Khattab, H. A. (1992). The silent endurance: Social conditions of women's reproductive health in rural Egypt. Amman, Jordan, UNICEF, Regional Office of the Middle East and North Africa, p. 59.

Kheir, E.-H. H. M., Kumar, S., & Cross, A. (1991). Female circumcision: Attitudes and practices in Sudan. *Demographic and Health Surveys World Conference Proceedings* (Vol. 3. pp. 1697–1717), Columbia, MD: Macro International.

Kiragu, K. (1995). Female genital mutilation: A reproductive health concern. *Population Reports*, *41*(Suppl. 3), 1–4.

Knight, R., Hotchin, A., Bayly, C., & Grover, S. (1999). Female genital mutilation – experience of The Royal Women's Hospital, Melbourne. *Australian & New Zealand Journal of Obstetrics & Gynaecology*, *39*(1), 50–54.

Koso-Thomas, O. (1987). *The circumcision of women: A strategy for eradication*. London: Zed Books.

Kroll, G. L., & Miller, L. (2000). Vulvar epithelial inclusion cyst as a late complication of childhood female traditional genital surgery. *American Journal of Obstetrics & Gynecology*, *183*(2), 509–510.

Ladjali, M., Rattray, T., & Walder, R. J. W. (1993). Female genital mutilation. *British Medical Journal*, *307*(6902), 460.

Lane, S. D., & Meleis, A. I. (1991). Roles, work, health perceptions and health resources of women: A study in an Egyptian delta hamlet. *Social Science and Medicine*, *33*, 1197–1208.

Larsen, U. (1989). A comparative study of the levels and the differentials of sterility in Cameroon, Kenya, and Sudan. In: R. Lesthaeghe (Ed.), *Reproduction and Social Organization in Sub-Saharan Africa*. Berkeley: University of California Press.

Larsen, U. (1994). Sterility in sub-Saharan Africa. *Population Studies, 48*(3), 459–475.

Larsen, U. (1995). Differentials in infertility in Cameroon and Nigeria. *Population Studies, 49*(2), 329–346.

Larsen, U., & Yan, S. (2000). Does female circumcision affect infertility and fertility? A study of the Central African Republic, Cote d'Ivoire, and Tanzania. *Demography, 37*(3), 313–321.

Lax, R. F. (2000, Winter). Socially sanctioned violence against women: Female genital mutilation is its most brutal form. *Clinical Social Work Journal, 28*(4).

Laycock, H. T. (1950). Surgical aspects of female circumcision in Somaliland. *The East African Medical Journal, 27*, 445–450.

Lenzi, E. (1970). Damage caused by infibulation and infertility. *Acta European Fertility, 2*, 47–58.

Leonard, L. (1996). Female circumcision in southern chad: Origins, meaning, and current practice. *Social Science and Medicine, 43*, 255–263.

Leonard, L. (2000). Interpreting female genital cutting: Moving beyond the impasse. *Annual Review of Sex Research, 11*, 158–191.

Lesthaeghe, R. J. (Ed.) (1989). *Reproduction and social organization in sub-Saharan Africa*. Berkeley: University of California Press.

Lewis, I. M. (1994). *Blood and bone: The call of kinship in Somali society*. Lawrenceville, NJ: Red Sea Press.

Lightfoot-Klein, H. (1989a). *Prisoners of ritual: An odyssey into female genital circumcision in Africa*. New York: Hawthorne Press.

Lightfoot-Klein, H. (1989b). The sexual experience and marital adjustment of genitally circumcised and infibulated females in the Sudan. *The Journal of Sex Research, 26*(3), 375–392.

Lowenstein, L. F. (1978). Attitudes and attitude differences to female genital mutilation in the Sudan: Is there a change on the horizon? *Social Science and Medicine, 12*, 417–421.

Lyons, H. (1981). Anthropologists, moralities, and relativities: The problem of genital mutilations. *Canadian Review of Sociology and Anthropology, 18*(4), 499–518.

Mackie, G. (1996). Ending footbinding and infibulation: A convention account. *American Sociological Review, 61*, 999–1017.

Mackie, G. (2000). Female genital cutting: The beginning of the end. In: B. Shell-Duncan & Y. Hernlund (Eds), *Female "Circumcision" in Africa: Culture, Controversy, and Change* (pp. 253–282). Boulder, CO: Lyne Reinner.

Maendeleo Ya Wanawake Organization (1991). *A report on harmful traditional practices that affect the health of the women and their children in Kenya*. Report Supported by the Population Crisis Committee, Washington, DC.

Mammo, A., & Morgan, S. P. (1986). Childlessness in rural Ethiopia. *Population and Development Review, 12*(3), 533–546.

Mawad, N. M., & Hassanein, O. M. (1994). Female circumcision: Three years' experience of common complications in patients treated in Khartoum teaching hospitals. *Journal of Obstetrics and Gynaecology, 14*(1), 40–44.

McCaffrey, M. (1995). Female genital mutilation: Consequences for reproductive and sexual health. *Sexual and Marital Therapy, 10*(2), 189–200.

McCaffrey, M., Jankowska, A., & Gordon, H. (1995). Management of female genital mutilation: The Northwick Park Hospital experience. *British Journal of Obstetrics and Gynaecology, 102*(10), 787–790.

McCleary, P. H. (1994). Female genital mutilation and childbirth: A case report. [See comments.] [Erratum appears in *Birth*, 1995, Mar; *22*(1), 49.]. *Birth, 21*, 221–223.

McFall, J. A., & McFall, M. H. (1984). *Disease and fertility*. NY: Academic Press.

McLean, S., & Graham, S. E. (1983). *Female circumcision, excision, and infibulation: The facts and proposals for change*. London: Minority Rights Group (Report No. 47).

Mensch, B. S., Bagah, D., Clark, W. H., & Binka, F. (1999). The changing nature of adolescence in the Kassena-Nakana District of Northern Ghana. *Studies in Family Planning*, *30*(2), 95–111.

Meuwissen, J. H. J. M. (1966). Human infertility in West Africa. *Tropical and Geographic Medicine*, *18*, 147–152.

Ministry of Planning, Democratic Republic of Sudan (1979). *Sudan fertility survey 1978*. Standard Recode, Version 5 MROF. London: International Statistical Institute. (World Fertility Survey, revised version 1982.)

Missailidis, K., & Gebre-Medhin, M. (2000). Female genital mutilation in eastern Ethiopia. *The Lancet*, *356*, 137.

Momoh, C., Ladhani, S., Lochrie, D. P., & Rymer, J. (2001). Female genital mutilation: Analysis of the first twelve months of a Southeast London specialist clinic. *BJOG*, *108*(2), 186–191.

Moore, M. (2000). Severity of genital cutting is linked to complications experienced later in life. *International Family Planning Perspectives*, *26*(1), 45–46.

Morison, L., Scherf, C., Ekpo, G., Paine, K., West, B., Coleman, R., & Walraven, G. (2001). The long-term reproductive health consequences of female genital cutting in rural Gambia: A community-based survey. *Tropical Medicine & International Health*, *6*(8), 643–653.

Morris, R. I. (1999). Female genital mutilation: Perspectives, risks, and complications. *Urological Nursing*, *19*(1), 13–19.

Morsy, S. A. (1991). Safeguarding women's bodies: The white man's burden medicalized. *Medical Anthropology Quarterly (New Series)*, *5*(1), 19–23.

Mustafa, A. Z. (1966). Female circumcision and infibulation in the Sudan. *Journal of Obstetrics and Gynaecology of the British Commonwealth*, *73*, 302–306.

National Statistics Office (1997). *Eritrea demographic and health survey*. Asmara Eritrea: National Statistics Office, Department of Macro Policy and International Economic Cooperation, and Calverton, MD: Macro International.

Ntiri, D. W. (1993). Circumcision and health among rural women of the southern Somalia as part of a family life survey. *Health Care for Women International*, *14*, 215–226.

Obermeyer, C. M. (2003). The health consequences of female circumcision: Science, advocacy, and standards of evidence. *Medical Anthropology Quarterly*, *17*(3), 394–412.

Obermeyer, C. M., & Reynolds, R. (1999a). Female genital surgeries: The known, the unknown, and the unknowable. *Medical Anthropology Quarterly (New Series)*, *13*(1), Mar.

Obermeyer, C. M., & Reynolds, R. (1999b). Roundtable on cutting women's genitals. Female genital surgeries, reproductive health, and sexuality: A review of the evidence. *Reproductive Health Matters*, *7*(13), 112–120.

Olenick, I. (1998). Female circumcision is nearly universal in Egypt, Eritrea, Mali and Sudan. *International Family Planning Perspectives*, *24*, 47–49.

Omer-Hashi, K. H. (1994). Commentary: Female genital mutilation: Perspectives from a Somalian midwife. *Birth*, *21*(4), 224–226.

Omer-Hashi, K. H., & Entwistle, M. (1995). Female genital mutilation. *The Canadian Journal of Human Sexuality*, *4*(2), 137–147.

Ortiz, E. T. (1996). Female genital mutilation and public health: Lessons from the British experience. *Health Care for Women International*, *19*, 119–129.

Orubuloye, I. O., Caldwell, P., & Caldwell, J. (2000). Female "circumcision" among the Yoruba of southwestern Nigeria: The beginning of change. In: B. Shell-Duncan & Y. Hernlund (Eds),

Female "Circumcision" in Africa: Culture, Controversy, and Change (pp. 73–94). Boulder, CO: Lynne Reinner.

Ozumba, B. C. (1992). Acquired gynetresia in eastern Africa. *International Journal of Gynecology and Obstetrics*, *37*(2), 105–109.

Passmore, S. L. (1981). *Against the mutilation of women: The struggle to end unnecessary suffering*. London: Ithaca Press.

Rendell, B. (1999). Assault on women. *Nursing Standard*, *14*(7), 20.

Robertson, C. (1996, Spring). Grassroots in Kenya: Women, genital mutilation, and collective action, 1920–1990. *Signs*, *21*(3).

Rouzi, A. A., Aljhadali, E. A., Amarin, Z. O., & Abduljabbar, H. S. (2001). The use of interpartum defibulation in women with female genital mutilation. *British Journal of Obstetrics and Gynaecology*, *108*, 949–951.

Rouzi, A. A., Sindi, O., Radhan, B., & Ba'aqeel, H. (2001). Epidermal clitoral inclusion cyst after type I female genital mutilation. *American Journal of Obstetrics & Gynecology*, *185*(3), 569–571.

Rushwan, H. (1980). Etiologic factors in pelvic inflammatory disease in Sudanese women. *American Journal of Obstetrics and Gynecology*, *138*, 877–879.

Rushwan, H. (2000). Female genital mutilation (FGM) management during pregnancy, childbirth and the postpartum period. *International Journal of Gynecology and Obstetrics*, *70*, 99–104.

Sami, I. R. (1986). Female circumcision with special reference to the Sudan. *Annals of Tropical Medicine*, *6*, 99–115.

Santow, G. (1995). Social roles and physical health: The case of female disadvantage in poor countries. *Social Science and Medicine*, *40*(2), 147–161.

Sayed, G. H., Abd El-Aty, M. A., & Fadel, K. A. (1996). The practice of female genital mutilation in Upper Egypt. *International Journal of Gynecology and Obstetrics*, *55*, 285–291.

Schepper-Hughes, N. (1991). Virgin territory: The male discovery of the clitoris. *Medical Anthropology Quarterly (New Series)*, *5*(1), 25–28.

Sequeira, J. (1931). Female circumcision and infibulation. *The Lancet*, *2*, 1054–1056.

Shamma, A. O. (1949). Female circumcision in the Sudan. *The Lancet*, *1*, 544–545.

Shandall, A. (1967). Circumcision and infibulation of females. *Sudan Medical Journal*, *5*, 178–212.

Shaw, E. (1985). Female circumcision: Perceptions of clients and caregivers. *Journal of American College Health*, *33*(5), 193–197.

Shell-Duncan, B. (2001). The medicalization of female circumcision: Harm reduction or promotion of a dangerous practice? *Social Science & Medicine*, *52*(7), 1013–1028.

Shell-Duncan, B., & Herlund, Y. (2000). Female "circumcision" in Africa: Dimensions of the practice and debates. In: B. Shell-Duncan & Y. Hernlund (Eds), *Female "Circumcision" in Africa: Culture, Controversy, and Change* (pp. 1–40). Boulder, CO: Lyne Reinner.

Silberstein, A. J. (1977). Circoncision feminine en Côte D'Ivoire. *Annales de Societé Belge de Médicine Tropicale*, *57*(3), 129–135.

Slack, A. T. (1988). Female circumcision: A critical appraisal. *Human Rights Quarterly*, *10*, 437–486.

Spadacini, B., & Nichols, P. (1998). Campaigning against female genital mutilation in Ethiopia using popular education. *Gender and Development*, *6*, 44–52.

Talle, A. (1993). Transforming women into 'pure' agnates: Aspects of female infibulation in Somalia. In: V. Broch-Due, I. Rudie & T. Bleie (Eds), *Carved Flesh, Cast Selves: Gender Symbols and Social Practices*. Oxford: Berg.

TOSTAN (1999). *Ending female genital cutting in the Kolda Region*. Final end-of-project report for PROWID to the Center for Development and Population Activities.

Toubia, N. (1985). The social and political implications of female circumcision: The case of Sudan. In: E. W. Fernea (Ed.), *Women and the Family in the Middle East: New Voices of Change*. Austin: University of Texas Press.

Toubia, N. (1993). *Female genital mutilation: A call for global action*. New York: Women, Ink.

Toubia, N. (1994). Female circumcision as a public health issue. *New England Journal of Medicine*, *331*(11), 712–717.

Toubia, N. (1998). Female circumcision/female genital mutilation. *African Journal of Reproductive Health*, *2*(2), 6–8.

Tubiana, M.-J. (1984). Beri. In: R. Weeks (Ed.), *Muslim Peoples: A World Ethnographic Survey* (2nd ed., pp. 154–158). Westport, CT: Greenwood Press.

van der Kwaak, A. (1992). Female circumcision and gender identity: A questionable alliance? *Social Science and Medicine*, *35*(6), 777–787.

van Roosmalen, J., Reynerse, M. M., & Wiebenga, J. E. (1992). AIDS and women's health care in developing countries. *Tropical and Geographical Medicine*, *44*(3), 284–285.

Verzin, J. A. (1975). Sequelae of female circumcision. *Tropical Doctor*, *5*, 163–169.

de Villeneuve, A. (1937). Étude sur une coutume Somalie: Les femmes cousues. *Journal de la Societé des Africanistes*, *6*, 15–32.

Walker, L. R., & Morgan, M. C. (1995). Female circumcision: A report of four adolescents. *Journal of Adolescent Health*, *17*, 128–132.

Walley, C. (1997). Searching for voices: Feminism, anthropology, and the global debate over female genital operations. *Cultural Anthropology*, *12*(3), 405–438.

Widstrand, C. (1964). Female infibulation. *Studia Ethnographica Upsaliensia*, *10*(Varia I), 95–124.

Williams, L., & Sobieszczyk, T. (1997). Attitudes surrounding the continuation of female circumcision in the Sudan: Passing the tradition to the next generation. *Journal of Marriage and the Family*, *59*(4), 966–981.

World Health Organization (1996). *Female genital mutilation: Information pack*. Geneva: World Health Organization.

World Health Organization (1997). *Female genital mutilation: A joint WHO/UNICEF/UNFPA statement*. Geneva: World Health Organization.

Worsley, A. (1938). Infibulation and female circumcision: A study of a little-known custom. *Journal of Obstetrics and Gynaecology of the British Empire*, *45*, 686–691.

Yount, K. M. (2002). Like mother, like daughter? Female genital cutting in Minia, Egypt. *Journal of Health and Social Behavior*, *43*(3), 336–358.

Yount, K. M. (2004). Symbolic gender politics, religious group identity, and the decline in female genital cutting in Minya, Egypt. *Social Forces*, *82*(3), 1063–1090.

Yount, K. M., & Balk, D. L. (2002). Methodological and ethical issues in research on the health consequences of female genital cutting in Africa. Paper presented at the Conference to Advance Research on Female Genital Cutting, Bellagio, Italy, April 29 to May 3.

CONTRACEPTIVE TECHNOLOGY AND REPRODUCTIVE RIGHTS: THE IUD AT HISTORICAL AND GEOGRAPHICAL JUNCTURES

Chikako Takeshita

Contraceptives are what Foucault termed "disciplinary technologies," part of the "socialization of reproductive behavior" that can discipline such behavior in multiple ways. But, simultaneously, contraceptives can be means of liberation, offering strategies of resistance against related disciplines of gender as well as race, class, and global position.

The International Conference on Population and Development (ICPD) in Cairo in 1994 served as a turning point for the guidelines of the international family planning community. The Cairo Program of Action declares reproductive health as a central goal of family planning and recognizes women's empowerment as an important component of protecting reproductive rights.[1] Major international aid organizations such as the United Nations Population Fund (UNFPA) have since revised their promotional material to align themselves with the agreement made at the conference.[2] International family planning policies and practices, however, have long been guided by the principle that global population growth must be slowed down by distributing more contraceptive technologies in the developing world. Since old habits die hard, I believe that the newly acknowledged importance of women's social empowerment and rights to reproductive self-determination should continue to be emphasized. This paper does just that.

Gender Perspectives on Reproduction and Sexuality
Advances in Gender Research, Volume 8, 251–284

ISSN: 1529-2126/doi:10.1016/S1529-2126(04)08008-7

I use the intrauterine device (IUD) as a vehicle for my analyses to navigate historical and geographical examples demonstrating that reproductive norms of a particular time and place affect the role a contraceptive technology plays in women's struggles to control their own fertility. The role of the IUD shifts between an emancipating and an oppressive device depending on the social arrangements within which the device operates. Some of the characteristics of the IUD that I will describe may apply only to this particular contraceptive method. Nevertheless, the analyses I present in this paper are intended to provide insights into a more general conceptualization of the relationship between contraceptive technologies and women's control over their reproductive lives.

The IUD is the most prevalent reversible contraceptive method in the developing world. It is a small device that is inserted into the uterus to prevent pregnancy for up to 10 years. Side effects include increased menstrual bleeding and cramps. More severe health risks were prevalent in earlier models of the IUD, which are known to have been responsible for perforations of the uterine wall and aggravated pelvic inflammatory diseases (PIDs) resulting in infertility and deaths.[3] In order to extract an IUD safely and regain fertility, women must seek the attention of trained personnel. Population control advocates, whose primary focus has been to slow down Third World population growth, have promoted the IUD as one of the most efficient methods to decrease pregnancies of women who have little incentive to use contraceptives. Women's reproductive rights activists have opposed the method, concerned that it imposes serious health risks on the users and undermines a woman's right to freely make decisions about her reproductive life (Hartmann, 1995). Mirroring the emergence of the new language from the Cairo conference that resolved the tension between women's rights activist and population control advocates, the representation of the IUD has become less contentious. The device is now often characterized as one of a number of contraceptive choices that are offered to women who desire to limit the number of offspring.

The first half of the paper traces the parallel development of the IUD and social movements surrounding the issue of fertility control. I mainly focus on three historical intersections: the birth control movement in the 1920s and the perception of the Grafenberg IUD; the mobilization of the IUD by the population control movement in the 1960s; and the repositioning of the IUD in line with the 1994 international agreement on the women-centered approach to population issues. For each period, I illustrate how social movements shaped expectations about reproduction and constructed the role of the IUD. Simultaneously, I look for evidence that the IUD, with its features and availability, influenced the structure of policies and practices concerning fertility control. I argue that reproductive norms and desires, ideas about proper approaches to controlling fertility, and the perception and deployment of a contraceptive device have evolved cooperatively throughout time. The historical transformation of the IUD shows that the device is neither inherently empowering nor disempowering for its users. The roles it is conceived to play in reproductive struggles are actively constructed in conjunction with the dominant social ideals present at the time. I suggest that even the current popular understanding that a variety of contraceptives are necessary to fulfill the need for reproductive health can be viewed in part as an artifact of the reconciliation of the two conflicting positions between population control and women's rights.

Divergent reproductive norms and practices play a significant part in shaping the roles IUDs play in reproductive struggles at different geographical locations. In the second half of the paper, I use narratives told by scholars who have observed local values and practices regarding fertility control to generate insight into the variety of ways women use the IUD to gain control over their reproductive lives. Ethnographic accounts from Nigeria, China, Tajikistan, Uzbekistan, and Bangladesh suggest that women negotiate reproductive self-determination not only by manipulating the IUD but also by managing social tensions between women's own reproductive desires and interventions by others. Examples also show that the roles IUDs play in reproductive struggles are products of social conditions rather than of any essential quality of the contraceptive device. These observations lead to the conclusion that family planning programs which focus on contraceptive delivery and not on the context in which fertility is controlled may not result in improving the social conditions that prohibit women to take control of their reproductive lives.

In total, I demonstrate that whether and how a contraceptive method contributes to or undermines women's control over their reproductive lives is often shaped by social conditions that are particular to a time and place. I also challenge the idea that contraceptives are essentially a technology that universally improves women's reproductive choice by demonstrating how such characterization has been constructed. The availability of contraceptive methods is only one of the elements in a diverse array of women's reproductive struggles. The analyses in this paper reinforce the notion that women's social, economic, and political empowerment – not the distribution of contraceptives – should be considered the primary agent for protecting women's reproductive rights.

EMPOWERING OR DISEMPOWERING? HISTORICAL DEVELOPMENT OF REPRODUCTIVE RIGHTS AND THE SHIFTING ROLE OF THE IUD

Characterizing the Grafenberg IUD as an Emancipating Device

I begin my historical analysis of the co-evolution of reproductive norms and desires, approaches to fertility control, and the meaning assigned to contraceptives with an examination of the Grafenberg Ring, the first modern IUD. The Grafenberg ring, developed in the late 1920s by a German doctor, Ernst Gräfenberg, was a small ring made of silkworm gut and coiled silver that can be compressed to be inserted into the uterus. The Grafenberg ring appeared at a time when changes in social attitude towards sexuality had formed a favorable climate for a new contraceptive method. The device was greeted with much interest from the European birth control movement, and Gräfenberg was invited to speak at the Third Congress of the World League for Sexual Reform held in London in 1929 and at the Seventh International Birth Control Conference in Zurich in 1930 (Davis, 1971).

The concept of intrauterine contraception itself was not novel at the time of Gräfenberg's invention. In fact, it dates back to the ancient practices of Arabs and Turks, who knew that inserting a small stone through a tube into the uteri of camels would prevent pregnancy (FDA, 1978). Pessaries pre-existed the IUD as devices that are inserted into the uterus. They came in various materials and shapes, but commonly had a part that was inserted into the uterus and a stem remaining in the vagina. They were used in attempts to treat a wide range of gynecological complaints as well as to prevent pregnancy. By 1909, Ralph Richter had demonstrated the efficacy of intrauterine contraception. The medical community, however, was for the most part not interested in getting involved with fertility control (Davis, 1971). What helped Gräfenberg's ring to be accepted by the middle-class Europeans was the association he made with science and the sex reform movement.

Dugdale (1999, 2000) argues that a number of rhetorical moves and material changes associated with the Grafenberg ring helped negotiate its position as a device that supports the emancipatory movement of sex reform. First, Gräfenberg dissociated his IUD from traditional stem pessaries by eliminating the stem that remains in the vagina. This physical rearrangement of parts served to break the link between his intrauterine contraception and the sexual underworld that stem pessaries were often associated with. Secondly, Gräfenberg differentiated his device from traditional contraceptives that were inserted by midwives and lay-abortionists by marketing it as a modern scientific form of contraception that is medically inserted with gynecological instruments. Gräfenberg positioned his IUD as a *new* device that was suitable for "respectable" middle-class women that were part of the sex reform movement. Another important move, according to Dugdale, was to situate the Grafenberg ring as one possible contraceptive choice among many other methods such as the diaphragms, foams, and spermicidal jellies. The concept of choice sat well with the discourse of equality and with sexually confident women. Dugdale contends:

> In order to link the IUD with the sex reform movement, a particular mode of organization of the IUD had to be put into place, a conglomeration of physical parts, meanings and practices

> had to be produced that would enable a set of emancipatory meanings to become associated with this contraceptive technology (Dugdale, 2000, p. 169).

In other words, the Grafenberg ring was constructed as an emancipatory device with the assistance of a social climate that readily approved a "scientific" device and welcomed a new contraceptive method as a tool for meeting a socially acceptable goal.

Clarke (2000) points out that while women are usually not involved in the design or the process of technological development, women as users are often "clearly targeted and thereby configured by technoscience" (p. 40). In other words, when contraceptives are developed or constructed, it is commonly accompanied by the configuration of contraceptive users. Van Kammen (2000) and Oudshoorn (2000) show in their researches in contraceptive immunology and male contraceptives that the users configured by developers can be divided into social users and representation of users. Social users are those implicated in the process of contraceptive development as identifiable persons at the receiving end of the technology. Representations are the profiles of users imagined by actors involved in the design of technologies. Gräfenberg targeted his contraceptive device to a set of social users, the upper and middle-class women that identified themselves with the sex reform movement. Simultaneously, Gräfenberg represented his users as emancipated women. Dugdale (2000) contends that the Grafenberg ring produced "the body of the new woman," namely "the desiring body, subject to various tastes, part of a scientific world that promised a rational and equitable society, under the control of an active and informed reason" (p. 169).

The profile of the Grafenberg ring IUD begins to show that reproductive norms and desires, appropriate ways of fertility control, and meanings associated with a contraceptive method mutually reinforce one another. A positive relationship between the first modern IUD and women's reproductive self-determination evolved within the context of early twentieth century Europe, where support for women's autonomous decisions and scientific means of fertility control were rising.

Reconfiguring the IUD in a Movement to Limit Women's Control Over Fertility

A birth control movement similar to the European sex reform movement started in the United States in 1914. The movement deployed contraceptives as part of a struggle to support powerless women, the working class in particular (Gordon, 1990). "Birth control," a term coined by Margaret Sanger in 1915, signified fundamental rights for women, who not only sought "incremental improvements in their sex lives or medical care," but also sought to "transform the nature of women's rights ... to include free sexual expression and reproductive self-determination" (Gordon, 1990, p. 204). Advocates believed that obtaining control over reproduction was a step towards disrupting existing unequal distributions of power. This movement welcomed contraceptive technologies as a tool that facilitated their goals. The IUD, however, did not become popular in the United States due to the medical community's disapproval of the device, largely on the grounds of risk of infections (Davis, 1971). Gräfenberg himself, who had immigrated to the United States, was advised against using the method in the country and spent the rest of his career fitting cervical caps and diaphragms.

A revival of interest in the IUD surged after 1959 when favorable trials were reported from Israel and Japan. This time, however, the interest in the device was not part of a movement that greeted the device as a means to enhance options for women's reproductive choice and sexual freedom, but emerged within the agenda of population control, which had the opposite effect of undermining individual fertility choice. During the post-World War II years, both government and private organizations in the United States started to focus on the rapid growth of population in the developing world, regarding it as a threat to worldwide political and economic stability and as a cause of environmental degradation. The Population Council was founded in 1952 by John D. Rockefeller III with his conviction that "the relationship of population to material and cultural resources of the world represents one of the most crucial and urgent problems of the day" (Hartmann, 1995, p. 102). Population studies at U.S. universities began to be funded by large grants provided by private organizations including the Population Council and the Rockefellers. With great interest in limiting population growth in the developing world, these organizations monitored aggregate birth rates and supported the distribution of contraceptives, regarding them as an efficient solution to limiting birth. The population control ideology treated fertility control as a collective necessity rather than an individual right. Individual woman's reproductive desires and well-being were compromised in aggressive population control campaigns in which developing country governments supported by international institutions applied pressure on their citizens to accept contraception (Hartmann, 1995).

The need to develop a new contraceptive method was one of the impetuses for the establishment of the Population Council. The Council's conception of an "ideal" contraceptive included "low user-responsibility requiring minimal repetitive motion from the patient, long term effectiveness, and low cost to produce and use" (Onorato, 1990, p. 241). Under such criteria, the Council was beginning its research agenda in the late 1950s on the study of contraceptive immunology, or a vaccine against pregnancy that would be effective for at least a year once administered to the client. The 1959 favorable reports from Israel and Japan on the IUD inspired the Council to pursue this method as one that fulfills their ideal contraceptive criteria.

The Council sponsored the First International Conference on Intra-Uterine Contraception in 1962, which was attended by 48 IUD investigators from all over the world. The conference was convened to evaluate the suitability of the IUD as the tool for population control. When a participant suggested that a detailed medical history of the patient be taken prior to the insertion of the IUD in order to avoid PIDs, Chairman Alan Guttmacher, former president of the Planned Parenthood Federation, objected to it as too time-consuming and restrictive for use in underdeveloped countries. "We dare not lose sight of our goal," announced Guttmacher, "– to apply this method to large populations" (Tietze & Lewit, 1962, p. 122).

Medical complications of the IUD were still a serious concern and conference attendees were well aware that the majority of the medical community condemned the method. At least one participant ventured to explicitly state that the potential harm to individual users were expendable in the general scheme of the population of the world:

> Suppose one does develop an intrauterine infection and suppose she does end up with a hysterectomy and bilateral salphingo-oophorectomy. How serious is that for a particular patient and for the population of the world in general? Not very. Perhaps, we have to stop thinking in terms of individual patients and change our direction a bit (Dr. Robert J. Willson, in Tietze & Lewit, 1962, p. 124).

Others, however, pointed out that opposition from the medical profession must be overcome first. "Our first objective must be" stated Christopher Tietze, "to convince our colleagues outside of this room that intra-uterine contraception is a respectable medical procedure and not devil's work" (Tietze & Lewit, 1962, p. 123).

It was apparent to the Council that "a large-scale, scientifically impeccable, and very public field trial" was necessary for the rehabilitation of the IUD (Meldrum, 1996, p. 283). During the 1960s, the Population Council funded about 95% of the development cost of modern IUDs, allowing physicians such as Jack Lippes, inventor of the Lippes Loop IUD, to design and experiment with various models (Clarke, 1998). The organization also sponsored investigators who agreed to contribute data to a long-term statistical evaluation of the IUD. The evaluation project, Cooperative Statistical Program (CSP), was led by Christopher Tietze between 1963 and 1968 on five different models of IUD involving more than 30,000 women and 33 researchers. CSP had a great impact on establishing the IUD as a scientifically revalidated contraceptive method, although it was not without difficulty.

The evaluation project suffered methodical complications common in clinical trials of contraceptives. For one thing, randomized assignment of products to experimental subjects – a key concept for obtaining statistically meaningful results in clinical trials – was impossible to attain because subjects who were given information about various contraceptive options and IUD models made choices of their own product. Moreover, many women dropped out of the trial or switched to another method early on in the trial jeopardizing the original research design. Only 55% of the original subjects were still using the device at the end of the study. Tietze was compelled to reconstruct his research question and devise a new statistical technique. Nonetheless, he ultimately managed to demonstrate that the cumulative pregnancy for long-term IUD users was 6.5 per 100 users at the end of year 6.[4] Despite the problems of drop-outs, this statistical result "established the medical legitimacy of the IUD and provided the justification for the Population Council's introduction of the device into fertility control programs around the world" (Meldrum, 1996, pp. 291–292).

The IUD matched the method population control advocates were seeking – one that "did not require 'the birth control habit,' that could be used in a population without high motivation to practice contraception" (Reed, 1983, p. 427). IUD proponents rejected the pill as "too commercial, too expensive, and also user-dependent" (Meldrum, 1996, p. 283). Unlike the pill that can be discontinued at the user's will, once inserted, the IUD requires medical intervention to discontinue its use. The Population Council considered this provider-controlled aspect of the IUD as very desirable (Onorato, 1990). Christopher Tietze candidly admits this to his interviewer in 1971:

> There was such a feeling of urgency among professional people, not among the masses, but something had to be done. And this was something that you could do to the people rather than something people could do for themselves. So it made it very attractive to the doers (Reed, 1983, p. 307).

As Alan Guttmacher announced, "no contraceptive could be cheaper, and also once the damn thing is in, the patient cannot change her mind" (Quoted by Watkins, 1998, p. 70).

Dugdale (2000) argues that at this point the IUD was reconfigured into what she calls a "population-control-IUD," or was "transformed into a mass fertility control device" (p. 170). The realignment of the IUD as an effective tool for Third World fertility control was accompanied by the reconstruction of its users. Diverging from the Grafenberg ring users who were construed as liberated women with the freedom to select from multiple contraceptive options, the users of the population-control-IUD were now represented as the "unmotivated women" that this device had to be given to (Dugdale, 2000). The claimed advantage of the IUD, namely that the method only required a one time acceptance of the device and no continuous involvement by the user, relied on the notion that certain populations of women had to be managed. A 1968 Food and Drug Administration report, though less explicitly, emphasizes the point:

> Rebirth of interest in the IUD as an effective, acceptable method of contraception stems from two factors. [. . .] Second is the suggestion that the underprivileged woman is more effectively served when the need for recurrent motivation, required in most other forms of contraception, is removed (FDA, 1968, p. 1).

The representation of IUD users as women who either cannot or do not want to use methods that involve continued application persisted for many years in more subtle expressions. For example, the 1988 Population Reports suggests IUDs to women who "have trouble using barrier methods or remembering to take a pill every day and want a method with no bother" (Population Reports, 1988, p. 24).

The case of the population-control-IUD demonstrates that reproductive norms, approaches to fertility control, and assigned meanings of the IUD co-evolved, reinforcing one another to form a social arrangement that pursued population control. The idea that Third World reproduction must be limited to avoid overpopulation was accompanied by a conviction that fertility rates must be controlled by efficient scientific means and international oversight. The IUD was constructed as an ideal tool for ensuring user compliance, and the availability of the technology fueled the idea that such a goal was attainable. Construction of the users as women who needed to be served by a long-lasting method gave legitimacy to both the population control ideology and the IUD as a controlling device.

Health risks of IUDs continued to be a serious concern even though distributors of the method often downplayed them. The Dalkon Shield disaster most strongly impressed upon the U.S. public the danger of the IUD as well as the irresponsible corporate greed that took precedence over the well-beings of the users (Grant, 1992; Hawkins, 1997; Hicks, 1994; Mintz, 1985; Perry & Dawson, 1985). The Dalkon Sheild IUD was promoted by its inventor, Hugh Davis, as a breakthrough device with low rates of pregnancy and spontaneous expulsion from the uterus. The polyethylene device that looked like a shield with crab-like-legs caused much pain during insertion, use, and removal for the users. It sometimes embedded itself in the uterine wall. More hazards were caused by the thread, which was attached to the device and dropped through the cervix into the vagina. The open-ended multifilamented string became a conduit for bacteria to travel into the uterus causing serious infections that led to infertility, septic abortions, and even deaths.[5] Despite signs of complications, Dalkon Shield producer A. H. Robins Co. continued to market the product during the 1970s. Two-point-three million devices were sold in the United States alone, and a total of 4.5 million were distributed in 80 countries (Mintz, 1985). The company was strongly condemned for its actions in a court decision in 1984, which was followed by 300,000 claims for damage. Other IUD makers withdrew their products from the U.S. market in fear of liability suits.[6] After the 1980s, the IUD for the most part fell out of favor as a contraceptive option for American women.[7]

Women's health activists have expressed concerns over IUD's safety for women in remote places where health services are not optimal (Bandarage, 1997; Hartmann, 1995). Adequate healthcare facilities with equipment for insertion, supplies to disinfect the instruments, and trained staff are necessary for safe IUD insertion and removal. Furthermore, testing of sexually transmitted diseases (STDs) and PIDs that might be aggravated by IUD insertion should be performed to eliminate users with higher health risks. Should IUD users contract STDs, develop PIDs or other complications such as perforation of the uterine wall and unexpected pregnancy with the IUD in place, they require adequate medical attention to avoid permanent injuries, infertility, and death. Increased menstrual bleeding, a common side effect of the IUD, may degrade the health of anemic women. "Despite these risks," laments Hartmann, "the IUD continues to be promoted heavily in many Third World family planning programs, not only because of its efficacy in preventing pregnancy, but because women lack control over the device" (p. 219).

The abuse of the IUD by state programs aimed at limiting fertility is a significant concern for the wellbeing of women. Coercion and incentives to accept the device undermine women's rights to make their own reproductive choice since once the device is inserted the user has little control over its removal. Even if trained personnel were accessible, they may refuse to remove the device. It is even possible for medical staff to insert the IUD in women who have just given birth or had an abortion without their knowledge or proper consent (Ortega et al., 1998). A number of countries are reported to have employed the IUD in state programs to enforce population control. The Chinese government has been severely criticized for its aggressive fertility control campaigns involving IUD insertion, sterilization, and forced abortion (Aird, 1990). India has heavily promoted the Lippes Loop IUD during the 1960s (Hartmann, 1995). In Mexico, the device seems to have been targeted at indigenous population in Chiaps (Thompson, 2000). As Bandarage (1997) contests, in certain countries, "the population control objective has prevailed over women's health and safety in the heavy promotion of the IUD" (p. 82).

In light of women's rights to reproductive health and self-determination, the population-control-IUD stands in stark contrast to the Grafenberg ring. The Grafenberg ring, as a part of the sex reform movement, was conceived to liberate women by improving their reproductive choice. The IUD in the context of population control evolved into an oppressive device for women who are exposed to its health risks and are directed by their governments and international aid to limit their fertility regardless of their own wishes. The conflicting roles between the emancipating IUD and the population-control-IUD mirror the tension between the birth control movement that aimed at increasing women's reproductive self-determination and the population control movement that sought the opposite. I maintain that both IUDs are neither essentially liberating nor oppressive. The meanings assigned to the device's design, usage, value, and users were social constructs that embodied political ideologies prevalent at a particular time and place. The next historical stage redefines the IUD as a neutral method offered to women with *needs*, aligning the device with the move to reframe population policy through women's rights.

RECONCILING THE TENSION: IUD AS A CHOICE THAT MEETS CONTRACEPTIVE NEEDS

The Transition of the Relationship Between Reproductive Rights and Population Control

By the 1960s, when the population-control-IUD was established, the terms "birth control," "family planning," and "population control" had come to be used interchangeablly in the U.S. (Gordon, 1990). The phrase "birth control" has been sometimes used to describe what is more properly called "population control," or the targeting of "poor, working-class, minority and Third World people, in the United states and abroad, in the form of prescriptive, even coercive, programs urging birth-rate reduction" (ibid, p. xviii). Gordon contends that "birth control" and "population control" should be clearly distinguished as separate political agendas with a separate history, claiming that the term "birth control" should be used to signify the political struggle for self-determination of women. I, too, have used the terms in compliance with Gordon's definition, and positioned the two movements at opposite ends of political ideologies in the two previous sections of this paper. The history of the two movements, however, is not so clearly distinguishable: they have from time to time shown a tendency to merge with each other.

The idea that decreasing fertility is a solution to poverty, which is at the base of the argument that population control benefits developing countries, existed since the early days of the birth control movement. Margaret Sanger herself pursued both aims: she advocated women's reproductive self-determination and the use of contraceptive technologies at the same time she believed that the number of children had to be curtailed in order for poor women and men to overcome poverty. Therefore, in the early days of the birth control movement, decreasing the fertility of the poor and helping women avoid unwanted pregnancy were pursued as compatible goals. Sanger, however, later shifted away from protecting women's reproductive control and catered towards embracing "eugenicist and elitist view of the poor, and adopted a top-down approach to the delivery of services" and "paved the way for the coming of population control" (Hartmann, 1995, p. 101). The mid-century population control movement silenced the call for reproductive self-determination, at least for women that were targeted as responsible for population explosion, and pressed for their compliance with fertility control.

During the 1980s and 1990s, women's rights activists challenged population policies that concentrated on reducing aggregate birth rates and employed strict measures to accept contraception at the expense of women's health and wellbeing. They started to develop concepts that redefined family planning in light of women's rights rather than birthrates and contraceptive prevalence. Dixon-Mueller (1993), for instance, suggests the concept "reproductive health," which she characterizes as follows:

> Reproductive health incorporates a clear feminist and human rights focus for its full realization. It moves birth control out from under the umbrella of "family planning" and "planned-parenthood," with their patriarchal connotations, into the realm of individual rights to sexual and reproductive health (204).

Just before the 1994 International Conference on Population and Development (ICPD) in Cairo, the International Women's Health Coalition (IWHC) published *Population Policies Reconsidered: Health, Empowerment, and Rights* (Sen et al., 1994). The collection of contributions attempted to articulate new directions for population policies based upon the goals of health, empowerment, and human rights. Issues brought up in the IWHC publication such as "human rights and reproductive rights," "women's empowerment," "reproductive and sexual health," and "women-centered approach to fertility control" became central concepts in the Program of Action documented in the Cairo meeting. Efforts by women's health activists bore fruit when the Cairo Program of Action was endorsed as the "consensus" on a new framework for a women-centered approach to population policy by a diverse group of participants, including population control constituencies, women's rights activists, and the Catholic Church.

During the years preceding the ICPD, advocates of population control were also busy trying to build support for their objectives as well. In the 1970s and 1980s, the population control establishment tried to impress upon developing country governments that population control and development were inseparable problems, claiming that rapid population growth is both the cause and effect of poverty (Hartmann, 1995). In preparation for the ICPD, population control advocates allied with environmentalists and appealed that overpopulation caused environmental degradation (ibid). The population constituency was helped at the conference by the Vatican's opposition to any reference of abortion. The Vatican, who opposed any reference to abortion and weakened passages on reproductive and sexual rights, made the population constituency appear progressive. The battle over abortion resulted in drawing the conference's attention away from critiques from women's groups, who maintain that fundamental inequity and economic and political realities were the major source of infringement on reproductive rights.

Hartmann (1995) maintains that the consensus was in effect carefully orchestrated by the coalition of population control advocates and environmentalists even though "the Program of Action contains many strong articulations of women's rights perspectives" (p. 151). The agreement falls short of pushing for fundamental changes to overthrow social inequities that hinder women's rights. Instead the Cairo consensus settled at the middle-ground where it can incorporate varying objectives of different actors and agendas. The Program of Action indeed reflects the pressure applied by women's health activists and has reframed population policies under women's rights to health and self-determination. At the same time, however, key concepts left room for interpretation that allowed population policy makers and family planning programs officers to apply the consensus to existing programs without extensive conceptual changes.

"Women's empowerment," for instance, is a concept that, at least rhetorically, became an accepted norm at the conference. "No set of actors," however, "has been able to capture and stabilize its meaning" (Halfon, 2000, p. 103). The concept originated from a radical critique of development practice that perpetuated existing power structures. In the original context, women's empowerment signified a collective movement of women's struggles to demand the "transformation of structures of subordination through radical changes in law, property rights, and other institutions that reinforce and perpetuate male domination" (Sen & Grown, 1987, p. 129, quoted by Halfon, 2000, p. 107). In this sense, empowerment was a political goal in itself, and a precondition for guaranteeing women's reproductive rights.

When women's empowerment was read in the context of population and development, the term was interpreted for policy-making purposes and it began to focus somewhat narrowly on reproductive issues. Nafist Sadik, former UNFPA director, for instance, defines empowering women as extending "choices" about marriage, education, employment, social and physical environment, pregnancy, and family size (Halfon, 2000). Often, a gesture is made to suggest that a specific focus on reproductive rights and health contributes to the broader goal of empowerment (ibid). Halfon quotes a program officer, who states: "with reproductive freedom and choice come opportunities for women to participate in the affairs of family and society that are otherwise closed off to them" (p. 111). The speaker implies that reproductive choice leads to empowerment, rather than vice versa as the Cairo document argues. The term lost its original intention to be a political movement to challenge existing power differentials when it is applied to projects related to family planning and population policy. Now, empowerment programs "primarily focus on contraceptives development and delivery and reproductive health-care, with some emphasis on education and job opportunities and challenging legal or family structures" (Halfon, 2000, p. 127). The flexibility of the term has allowed parties with various agendas to appear to have a consensus, while employing the concept in divergent ways.

"Unmet need" is another concept that has held together various constituencies. Only this time, the term was not so open to flexible appropriation because of its deep connection with established practices. Halfon (2000) observes that because it already had a long history, the concept of "unmet need" was able to mediate between the population establishment and women's rights activists and to serve as an "important bridge between the old regime and the women's empowerment regime" (Halfon, 2000, p. 182).

The concept "unmet need" originated in a demographic technique of the 1970s employed to quantify the need for contraceptives. The idea was to quantify women with unmet need, or women who expressed a desire to limit childbirth but were not using contraceptives, in order to justify the distribution of contraceptives. Demographic surveys were strongly driven by the motivation to count women whose pregnancy may be prevented. Hence, at least initially, demographers tended to count all women who expressed any wish to have fewer pregnancies as "women with unmet need" even when they had expressed no desire to use contraceptives or intended to leave fertility to God's will.[8] Over the years, the notion has been revisited and suggestions have been made in order for the concept to more accurately reflect "need." Suggestions include incorporating a broader set of needs such as reproductive health delivery and explaining factors that prevent women's access to contraceptive methods (Halfon, 2000). "Unmet need," in the post-Cairo population discourse, became a concept that held together multiple actors and agendas. Rather than resisting the concept as driven by demographic objectives, women's health activists attempted to bridge the gap between population control and women's health by expanding the notion of "need." Dixon-Mueller and Germain (1992), for instance, suggest that the notion be expanded to include the needs of unmarried women and the needs for a broader range of services including infertility services, abortion services, prevention of STDs, and related reproductive health problems. By applying "unmet need" to satisfying a variety of women's individual needs, the concept reconciled individual rights with achieving social objectives. However, as Halfon (2000) points out, even though attempts have been made to use "unmet need" expansively as the surrogate concept for broader need, because it has been strongly associated with the narrow practice of contraceptive delivery in the past, such a practice may continue to take precedence.

Increasing the variety of contraceptive offerings has been expressed as one of the needs that must be fulfilled to assure women's reproductive choice.[9] This concept of "choice" also holds together the people focusing on the management of population growth and women's rights activists. From the perspective of population control, increasing the variety of contraceptives increases the chance of contraceptive acceptance (Oudshoorn, 1996). While not all women's health activists endorse all types of contraceptive methods,[10] from the perspective of women's health and rights, a variety in the choice of contraceptives is to be welcomed provided that the methods are safe, health care services are adequate, and users are informed of the different methods. The idea that there is a "need" for a variety of contraceptives situates contraceptive methods neatly into the discourse of unmet need and the related idea that women are empowered by having their needs met. Within this context, all contraceptives, provided that they are safe, become neutrally enabling tools for women with a desire to limit fertility.

Reconstructing the IUD as a Contraceptive "Choice"

The IUD has joined other contraceptives as a neutral enabler after a series of material and rhetorical rearrangements were made, including physical changes, dissociation from negative images of the past, and the construction of a new representation of IUD users. During the 1960s a *T*-shaped polyethylene IUD wrapped with copper wire and/or embedded with copper plates was developed. The design was conceived after a study of rabbits demonstrated the effectiveness of copper in preventing pregnancy and another study showed that the *T*-shaped polyethylene IUDs decreased pain, bleeding, and spontaneous expulsions (Schmidt et al., 1994). Copper-releasing IUDs were called medicated IUDs, and were differentiated from plastic and steel ring IUDs, which were considered inert. Copper-releasing IUDs with different loads of copper were designed and tested during the 1970s and 1980s (Rowe, 1994). The Population Council's Copper-T 380A has been the most prevalent model with 25 million devices distributed to 70 countries by 1991 (Schmidt et al., 1994).

Having attained a high rate of success in preventing pregnancy with the Copper-T, IUD developers emphasized that they have shifted their attention to identifying appropriate users and providing high-quality medical counseling to maximize safety and acceptability (Population Reports, 1988). Various studies on not only the effectiveness, but also on side effects (bleeding and pain), infections, expulsion, perforation of the uterine wall, and unintended and ectopic pregnancy were conducted to improve efficacy and acceptance of the Copper-T. Population Reports (1995) promotes that the Copper-T IUDs are more effective, long-lasting and have fewer side effects than previous IUD models, and that women who use them have found them to be very effective, safe, and convenient.

The Population Council fought off the dangerous image created by the Dalkon Shield and subsequent withdrawals of other IUDs from the U.S. market. By 1988, scientists affiliated with the organization singled out the Dalkon Shield as "a no-longer marketed device" that had five times more likelihood of pelvic inflammatory disease and two times more likelihood of tubal infertility than other IUDs (Population Reports, 1988, p. 14).[11] The same report also stressed that the withdrawal of IUDs from the U.S. market was a business decision, not because safety was a concern. Furthermore, the 1995 Population Reports explicitly responds to the concern over pelvic infections, stating that "it is now clear that an increased risk of pelvic inflammatory disease is concentrated in the first month after IUD insertion and among women exposed to STDs" (Population Reports, 1995, p. 2). It also assures that there is no increased risk of infertility for a woman using a copper IUD who has a mutually monogamous relationship and thus is not exposed to STDs, and that IUDs help protect against ectopic pregnancy while in use. Through physical changes in the device and scientific claims made about its safety, the IUD has been reconstructed as a safe and effective method. Simultaneously, IUD developers repositioned the IUD as one of the valid choices for contraceptive users, refraining from the characterization of the method as one that best carries out the agenda of the provider who hopes to manage population growth. Population Reports (1995) advises that "Family planning programs should offer IUDs along with other methods of contraception and help clients choose the methods that best suit them" (p. 25). The aspect of the device that hands over control to the provider is rephrased as a provider-dependent method that requires trained staff to insert and remove the device. The importance of ensuring the option to remove the device whenever and for whatever reason the woman desires is also emphasized. The IUD is now one of the methods offered to meet the need for a variety of contraceptive choices – sitting well with the new discourse of women-centered fertility control.

Along with the material and the rhetorical rearrangement of the device, the users of the IUD were also reconfigured to be suitable for the new device. The new ideal IUD users are women with a certain medical and behavioral profile whose needs are met by the IUD. The Copper-T 380A IUD that was introduced in the United States under the brand name ParaGard in 1988 has been carefully targeted towards women that have already had children, have no history of PID, and are in a monogamous relationship.[12] The Population Council does not limit Copper-T 380A users in developing countries to women that have already given birth. It does note, however, that non-married young women may be less likely to have a mutually faithful sexual relationship, in which case she may face a risk of STDs and subsequent infertility that can be increased by IUD use. IUD is not recommended to women with high risk of contracting STDs and with a recent history of pelvic infections (Population Reports, 1995). The population-control-IUD used to be coupled with the "unmotivated" users who had to be serviced by a contraceptive method that does not require users' continuous involvement. The term "IUD acceptors" has been employed in reports discussing IUD users, implying that family planning programs were trying to motivate women to accept the insertion of the device.[13] This expression suggested that women passively received contraceptives rather than actively seeking them out. Now, the Cairo consensus presents women as people with rights to choice and adequate reproductive services. Potential IUD users have come to be represented as women who recognize their need for contraceptives and appreciate being able to choose from a variety of methods. The interest in the contraceptive device is now presented as the woman's rather than as a solution to the problem of overpopulation. The Cairo language transformed the representation of IUD users from someone that something had to be "done to" and passive acceptors of the IUD to someone who wants to choose a contraceptive method for themselves. Through these rhetorical reconfigurations, the IUD has resolved the tension between its conflicting roles – an emancipating tool on the one hand and an oppressive device on the other – and settled in a new position that allows the device to be regarded as a neutral fertility control method. It has now become a device that is a good "choice" for many women who "need" contraceptives, the availability of which leads to the "empowerment" of women who are enabled to limit their fertility. While the physical improvements of the IUD are not to be neglected, significant social rearrangements took place in repositioning the device as a more acceptable method. The IUD was reconstructed to correspond with the consensus that was negotiated between the population establishment and women's rights activist in Cairo. In other words, this neutral representation of the IUD is in part an artifact of the resolution that was reached between groups with divergent positions on fertility control.

Representations of the IUD and its users have co-evolved with changing norms concerning reproduction and fertility control. Social movements have defined the context in which the IUD was developed, interpreted, and deployed. As the representations of women's roles in fertility control shifted from active to passive then back to active, the significance of the IUD transformed accordingly, its role constructed through social alignments that were particular to time and place.

Currently, the IUD is represented by the Population Council and other family planning programs as a valid method that should be offered as a contraceptive choice, provided that the method is safely managed and is provided to women at their will. Emphasizing the distribution of a contraceptive in the developing world as a neutral and universal method, however, hides the social and cultural conditions that inhibit women from taking control of their reproductive lives. The following section addresses what the generalized representation of the IUD makes invisible: the various ways in which women anchor power through the use or rejection of the IUD.

IUDs AND REPRODUCTIVE STRUGGLES IN THE DEVELOPING WORLD: WOMEN'S DESIRE, REPRODUCTIVE NORMS, AND POPULATION POLICY

Women in developing countries comprise the majority of IUD users.[14] Have these women been subjected to population control and oppressed by the provider-controlled feature and health risks of the IUD? Or have IUDs offered women opportunities to control their own fertility as autonomous individuals? Are these women now rational users that welcome more choice and accessibility to contraceptives? Or are they experiencing the tension felt between the two contradictory goals of granting individual reproductive rights vs. limiting population growth? How do women themselves manipulate the IUD to pursue their own desires? What kind of negotiations are women involved in when engaging with contraceptives? A number of anthropological works attest that women in different parts of the world engage in various kinds of struggles over reproductive choice within a complex network of nested interests over fertility (Ginsburg & Rapp, 1995; Greenhalgh, 1995; Petchesky & Judd, 1998; Russell, Sobo & Thompson, 2000). Ethnographic accounts of IUD users provide vivid images of women and their reproductive struggles that are unavailable otherwise. The rest of the paper turns to narratives told by researchers who have observed local values and practices of fertility control as a part of their demographic research, development project, and/or anthropological work. I retell their stories to illustrate the variety of ways in which women struggle for reproductive self-determination using or rejecting the IUD. These stories show that women who use the IUD are not best characterized as users who simply choose the IUD to meet their need for contraceptives. Women's liberty to decide on their reproductive lives and the choices they make are significantly influenced by cultural values, social norms, state policies on fertility control, and interests of others who have a stake in women's fertility. The position the IUD occupies in each woman's reproductive struggle is a complex function of reproductive norms constructed through policy and culture, other contraceptives that are available, and conflicting desires of women, their family, and health care workers. Because their reproductive struggles are embedded in the society in which they live, helping women negotiate reproductive self-determination will take far more than distributing reliable contraceptives.

Displacing and Reinterpreting the IUD: Etiki Women in Nigeria

I start this section with Renne's (1997) account of the contrasting perception of the IUD between Nigerian health care workers and Etiki Yoruba village women in southwestern Nigeria. The Nigerian family planning officials have adopted the view that family planning is desirable and that fertility should be scientifically and safely managed by modern contraceptive technologies. They associate the IUD with positive implications related to Western technology and perceptions of progress. The Etiki village women, however, have a completely different set of expectations about fertility control and the role of IUD. They are more interested in protecting their fertility and relate to the IUD with concerns of infertility. This example rather clearly shows that offering the IUD as a neutrally enabling method for women who want to limit birth is not always interpreted as such in the local context.

Etiki women's reproductive desires are constructed through their cultural values, which deems it important for a woman to "demonstrate her fertility through the regularly spaced birth of children rather than attempting to limit fertility, for such life and death matters are ultimately up to God" (Renne, 1997, p. 1142). Some Etiki women consider controlling fertility morally wrong as an affront to god and as a sign of neglecting motherhood. Most importantly, they fear infertility since women who cannot bear children have a greater social disadvantage.

In Etiki women's cultural framework, the IUD is associated with infertility caused by external intervention rather than viewed as an effective contraceptive that meets a woman's need to limit fertility. In the Etiki language, the IUD is called "turning the uterus," which is an indigenous concept that refers to infertility brought on through agency of someone with supernatural power at the behest of an ill-intentioned individual. Only individuals with extraordinary knowledge, such as traditional divine healers and witches, are believed to be capable of causing the uterus to turn and make a woman infertile. Only these powerful individuals can "turn back" the uterus to restore fertility. Women relate to the IUD with this traditional belief because IUDs require an insertion into the uterus by another powerful stranger, the medical doctor, and fear that the IUD may lead to an indefinite infertility. Renne points out that there are other factors that contribute to the Nigerian women's aversion to the IUD, such as distrust in the government to continue providing health care that women may need for treating side-effects and removing the IUD. She asserts, however, that the cultural association of the IUD to "turning the uterus" plays a significant role in Ekiti women's resistance to the IUD.

In this particular cultural and geographical context, the IUD is not seen as a contraceptive that fulfills the need of women who want to prevent unplanned pregnancy. Ekiti women have displaced the IUD from the scientific framework that deems it an effective contraceptive method and have reassigned it a culturally meaningful significance. From their perspective, resisting the IUD and thereby resisting the intervention by powerful individuals – whether they are witches, medical doctors, or the government – is a significant part of maintaining control over their own fertility.

Resisting the IUD and State Control: The Case of Rural Chinese Women

IUD use in China is an example in which the government deliberately mobilized the device to control fertility in its country. Chinese women comprise 60–70% of the more than 100 million IUD users around the world (Mauldin & Segal, 1994). China's population control policy has been known to be very stringent and is often described as oppressive to individuals.[15] Since the state set its goal in 1979 to reduce the average fertility rate to one child per couple and achieve a negative population growth, the government has taken elaborate direct and indirect measures to meet its goal. Techniques include economic incentives for limiting births and economic disincentives for having more than one child as well as reproductive policing activities carried out by local birth control cadres who are assigned birth quotas and targets. As a result, contraception usage leapt from near zero to 50 or 60% in two decades. Although the government officially disapproves of coercive practices such as involuntary sterilization and forced abortion, reports of such practices have been made by the media, human rights activists, and anti-abortionists. As a result, China's population policy has received much international criticism.[16]

State policies have had a great impact on the reproductive norms and desires of Chinese citizens. Greenhalgh (1994) points out that Chinese village women's fertility desires are shaped by what the community considers as the norm or ideal, which is strongly influenced by the state mandate. Villagers in Shaanxi province during the late 1980s considered one boy and one girl an ideal family size, believing that it was crucial for their wellbeing to raise two children, at least one of whom was a son.[17] While the number of children that the villagers generally desire exceeded the state's one-child-per-couple mandate, the villagers' view on the ideal family composition was in fact strongly colored by the long-term state propaganda for small families and reflected the villager's acceptance that reproductive possibilities are limited under strong state control. Furthermore, as Greenhalgh contends, "by embodying state demands in their conscious reproductive aspirations, the peasants were not only accepting, they were also unwittingly reproducing state control over their childbearing" (p. 12).

The Chinese government has positioned the IUD as one of the major tools of fertility control, much the same way as it was conceived by the U.S. and international population control advocates of the 1960s. During the past few decades, the IUD, along with sterilization and abortion, became an indispensable tool for local birth cadres, who were directly responsible for controlling fertile bodies under strong pressure from the government to achieve low birth rates (Greenhalgh, 1994). The two low-cost, highly effective, provider-controlled procedures, namely IUD insertion and sterilization, which involve only one-time application and little or no attention afterwards, are for the most part the only methods available to the rural population.[18] User-controlled contraceptives such as the pill that allow users to terminate the method whenever the users wish never accounted for more than 2 or 3% of contraceptive use in the villages that Greenhalgh studied. Pills were only available to women physically unable to use an IUD – a choice made by local health officials, not by the women themselves.

The Chinese government's intention to remove control over reproduction from its citizens is apparent in the design of the IUDs developed in China. According to Mauldin and Segal (1994), Chinese delegates visited the Population Council in the 1960s and took samples of the Lippes Loop and Ota Ring IUDs. Since then, China has developed their own IUDs including the stainless steel ring, *V*-shaped, and uterine cavity-shaped models. Stainless steel rings are the most widely used contraceptive method in China (Gu et al., 1994). These IUDs were deliberately designed without strings, making them tamperproof: they are difficult for users to check the device's location and pull it out on their own (Greenhalgh, 1995).[19] Non-clinical removal of any IUD is unsafe, but the self-removal of a stringless IUD can be even more physically dangerous.

Chinese women have not simply passively accepted contraception imposed by the state. Greenhalgh (1994) reports from villages in Shaanxi province that Chinese village women resist policy provisions by illegally removing the IUD. She believes that the heavy penalties stipulated for unauthorized IUD removals suggests that such practice is common and is a problem for the population policy enforcers. Among the 18 women who lost their IUDs in 1988 in villages in the northwestern province of Shaanxi, two thirds of them told Greenhalgh that the

IUDs were spontaneously expelled or simply fell out. Women are unlikely to voluntarily disclose that they have unlawfully and intentionally removed their IUDs, and therefore it is difficult to assess how many IUDs were actually spontaneously expelled. Greenhalgh argues that the loss of the IUDs could well have been motivated by a desire to conceive, judging from the fact that the majority of women who lost their IUDs became pregnant within three months. Greenhalgh surmises that the response "it fell out" may be a convenient gloss for "it was illegally removed," and suggests that unauthorized IUD removal is a strategy women use, despite the health risk that it entails, to resist the state policy's provisions to allow them to only have one child.

These resistances, however, should not be interpreted as an "autonomous decision" or a purely individual choice. Greenhalgh points out that a woman's decisions to "resist" or "accept" the IUD may be influenced by whether or not her family composition meets the community norm of two children with at least one son. The number of children they had at the time the IUD was inserted suggests that the women who told Greenhalgh that the device fell out desired another child, especially a son. In other words, these women's reproductive aspirations were shaped by the community norm, and when they resisted state control over their fertile bodies, they were acting as an agent of their families while also asserting individual reproductive choice.

Local birth-planning cadres play an important roll in reproductive struggles in rural china. Cadres are more often than not cornered into a tight spot that requires them to mediate between the state mandate and desires of village women and families. Croll (2000) reports that Chinese villagers assisted other villagers who were trying to have a son by helping them carry their second or third pregnancy to term without being detected by birth officials. In one of the villages, resistance from the villagers pressured the birth cadres to keep "one eye open and one eye closed" (p. 84) to unauthorized pregnancies. The local birth planning cadres in the villages Greenhalgh studied also faced strong resistance from villagers who desired more than one child and at least one son. The birth cadres were compelled to negotiate new terms of policy enforcement whereby they would exercise stricter control over those who attempted to exceed the village norm but offer leniency towards villagers who had not yet met the ideal family composition even though this violates the formal policy (Greenhalgh, 1994). In other words, unauthorized IUD removals and subsequent pregnancies were tolerated when they were conducted by women whose families were too small by community standards. Birth cadres were less likely to allow a woman who already has two children with one son to have another child after she illegally removed her IUD.

At first glance, the IUD in Chinese villages appears as an oppressive tool that removes control over reproduction from women. In a number of cases, however, women resist state intervention and strive to meet their reproductive goal by escaping the fertility control of local birth control cadres or by pressuring them to redefine the terms of reproduction. Greenhalgh's account demonstrates that negotiation over reproduction in rural China takes place among a network of interests woven by state mandates, community standards, local health officials, family expectations, and individual desires. IUDs are manipulated in these negotiations to impose government control over fertility, to resist state intervention, and to punish or tolerate women who contravene community norms. The IUD plays a fluid role in the negotiations over reproductive choices rather than solely as an agent of power for the authorities.

On a slightly different note, China has been experimenting with incorporating the Cairo consensus into their population policy.[20] The United Nations Population Fund (UNFPA) is working on a four-year, $20 million project with China on an experimental program in 32 model counties, where birth quotas are eliminated, health officials are trained to cater to individual choices, and a variety of methods are offered to clients (Takeshita, 2001; UNFPA, 1997). As a part of this project, rural women were provided with literacy training and micro-credits to earn their own income, which in turn raised the status of the women in their families and led them to become aware of their ability to take an active role in making reproductive choices.[21] We have yet to see whether the UNFPA project will render results that satisfactorily meet the Chinese government's expectation to curtail population. Whether or not the concept of voluntarism will pan out in this country also remains to be seen. A group of observers that recently visited some of the counties where the UNFPA/China project is being implemented reported to the U.S. government that they found no evidence of coercive fertility control practices.[22] Yet, the Chinese government has put a law in effect in September 2002 that continues to mandate "social compensation fees" or "fee for society to bring up children" for families that exceed their birth quota. The law also requires that the woman receive sterilization after the second child. Couples that commit to having only one-child are rewarded.[23] Hence, while new variety of contraceptive methods may be added to Chinese women's reproductive choices and physically coercive fertility control may diminish, coercion based on economic control may continue to impinge on women's reproductive self-determination.

Negotiating IUD Insertion: Tajikistan, Uzbekistan, and Bangladesh

The story of Zulfia, a Tajik woman, epitomizes reproductive struggles of women in the developing world who face pressure from family members to produce more children. Harris (2000) gives a brilliant account of how Zulfia used a clever tactic to convince her husband that she needed to be on birth control. Her husband wanted her to keep trying to have a son after she had given birth to three daughters. When she was in labor with her fourth child, instead of sending for a midwife, she made her husband stay and attend the birth by himself. Harris recounts Zulfia's story that filled the room full of Tajik women with laughter:

> Throughout my whole labor, I did not let go of my husband, no matter how bad things got. When finally it was all over and my fourth daughter had been born, he turned to me and said: "That was absolutely horrible. I can't let you go through it again. As soon as the 40 days are up you are to go to the doctor to be fitted with an IUD. It doesn't matter that we don't have a son. I can't face such a childbirth again." Since then I have never become pregnant again and my husband never mentions having a son (p. 1).

This story is a reminder that reproductive self-determination is often hard won by the women in Tajikistan as in many parts of the world and that while women have much to endure, they also "deal with their lives with ingenuity, imagination, strength, and above all laughter" (Harris, 2000, p. 1).

Harris provides other accounts of Tajik women's reproductive struggles that involved the IUD. Even within the same cultural setting, each reproductive negotiation differs slightly depending on the woman's relationships and circumstances. While Zulfia's husband responded promptly with an understanding of his wife's hardship, another husband could have continued to insist on having a son. While another Tajik woman, Tahmina, took the initiative to have an IUD inserted regardless of her husband's consent, another woman Tillo was pressured by her husband to extract her IUD so as to conceive another child. Tozagul obtained an IUD without her husband's knowledge after she had given birth to six children in seven years. When her husband tried to divorce her on account of infertility after several years, she informed him that she had been using the IUD. Her husband divorced her immediately, outraged that years of efforts to express his masculinity through his wife's fertility was lost in "years of empty sex" (Harris, 2000, p. 221).[24]

Reproductive norms in Tajikistan had long been characterized by the large family tradition and pro-natalist policy under the former Soviet Union. As a product of strict gender roles, women's reproductive desires have traditionally conformed to the social expectation that they will marry an arranged partner and bear many children, including sons, to support the couple (Harris, 2000). After independence, the government of Tajikistan, influenced by UN organizations and other international agencies, accepted policies that support women who regulate their fertility (Harris, 1998). The UNFPA provided a variety of free contraceptives and funds for the government to set up nation-wide family planning centers.

Procurement of contraceptives, however, has not necessarily become easy for women due to ineffective information distribution, indifference in the medical community, and expense for the users. Since the IUD was the only available reversible contraceptive method available during the Soviet era, the device remains the preferred method for a majority of women due to its familiarity (Harris, 1998). Obtaining an IUD to prevent unwanted pregnancies, which sometimes requires negotiation with their husbands, is an important part of Tajik women's control over their own fertility.

The IUD plays a similar role in Uzbekistan. Krengel and Greifeld (2000) provide the social context in which the IUD is characterized and utilized in Uzbekistan. Uzbekistan, like Tajikistan, is a predominantly Islamic nation that became independent in 1991. Reversing the pronatalist ideology of the Soviet era, the Uzbekistan government launched a large family planning program, regarding improvement of maternal and child health as one of the strategies towards strengthening the new nation. The high rate of anaemia in women caused by environmental problems and high birth rates are now officially seen as major causes of the unsatisfactory state of reproductive health. Changes in government family planning policy as well as the comeback of the Islamic culture serve as an important backdrop to the ways in which reproductive preferences are negotiated through the manipulation of the IUD.

Values and practices surrounding reproduction in Uzbekistan were transformed with the socio-economic transitions accompanying the nation's independence from the Soviet Union. Abortion, which used to be practiced widely as a form of birth control, is now disapproved of by the Islamic religion and increasingly carried out secretly outside the public health service. Women's roles in the family and as mothers are now more emphasized compared to their role as workers. Many respondents (male and female of various ages) of Krengel and Greifeld's (2000) study expressed their belief that reproductive choice is subordinate to the wishes of husbands and elder males of the family, or alternatively to God. Two boys and two girls, or three boys and two girls are considered the ideal family composition. Krengel and Greifeld's respondents indicated that they would continue to reproduce if the couple has no children of one of the sexes even if the total number of children already had reached four or five.

Midwives are assigned to community health facilities to monitor the reproductive health of local women. Some midwives are responsible for up to 1,000 women while others care for 100 to 150 women. Midwives keep notes on all women of fertile age and manage them according to the classification of the national program, which consists of women who can freely conceive, women who should temporarily avoid pregnancy because they have just given birth to a child, and women who should not become pregnant due to illness or age. This last category implicitly includes women who have already had many (five or more) children, who are assumed to be in bad health due to their fecundity.

Apart from abortion, IUD was practically the only reversible contraceptive that was known or available under the Soviet Union. Since it has become difficult for women to seek safe abortions at hospitals, the role of IUD in birth control has become even greater. A 1996 survey showed that over 50% of married women were using modern contraceptive methods, and close to 90% of them used the IUD. A small number of women were using sterilization, condom, injection, or pills. IUDs are overall very well accepted mainly due to familiarity and practicality: "they were well known, simply procured, easy to care for, have high efficacy rates, and are invisible" (Krengel & Greifeld, 2000, p. 213).

Women's reproductive desires vary: some desire a larger family than the state policy stipulates, and others wish to limit the number of offspring. Midwives and the IUD, the former being the official manager of fertility and the latter being the most prevalent contraceptive method, play a large part in mediating women's reproductive desires. Uzbek midwives have reported that they take advantage of the surreptitiousness of the IUD to intervene and relieve women of pressure from their family to continue having more children. Quoting a midwife, Krengel and Greifeld (2000) write: "in some such cases, it is a big relief for the woman when we say, 'sit down, I shall insert an IUD for you.' The husband will not know about it. For a good purpose one can also deceive" (p. 212). The goal of the state to limit births and a woman's desire to control her fertility converged using the same means, the IUD. The midwife, whose role is to ensure that the number of births is limited per woman, became an ally for the woman who wished to avoid pregnancy in this case.

Midwives may occasionally allow women who already have enough children or who were past their reproductive age to carry through their pregnancy. Krengel and Greifeld refer to a case of a woman of about forty years, who still wanted a baby and somehow managed to get rid of her IUD to get pregnant. Her midwife explained that she did not report this woman to the authorities because she believed that the woman was still healthy despite having had many children and thus there was insufficient reason to discontinue her pregnancy. Much like the Chinese village health officials, midwives in Uzbekistan are often forced into a position to negotiate the tension between a woman's individual reproductive desire to continue to have children and the government's policy to limit childbirth. While giving different reasoning for closing their eyes to unauthorized IUD self-extraction, Chinese birth cadres and Uzbek midwives, who are both in charge of monitoring women's fertility for the government, mediated the negotiation between the individual woman's reproductive choice and state provisions.

In many social and cultural circumstances, women are expected to follow their husbands' and elders' will, and openly defying them may be socially disadvantageous. In these places, women often use their wits to negotiate spacing births or limiting the number of children with the help of modern contraceptives (as with Zulfia's case introduced at the beginning of this section). Stark (2000) recounts a story of Komola, a Bangladesh woman, who convinced her husband to take her to the clinic to treat her sick child and obtained an IUD during the visit without her husband's knowledge. Later, when she feared that she might develop problems with the device and need his help, she informed her husband of her contraception. Although her husband initially expressed disapproval, he acquiesced to the use of contraception when she pointed out that the couple could not afford to have more children. In Stark's study, Bangladesh women who knew that their husbands would not permit contraceptive use obtained one first without their consent and confessed afterwards. Stark explains that confessing to the husband after having secretly obtained an IUD is a strategy women use to control their fertility without upsetting their social relationships. The act of confession acknowledges the control of the husband and neutralizes his anger. Furthermore, this is a way to save face for the husband, who would then be able to claim that he never approved or knew of his wife's contraception.

As Stark (2000) points out, women and men have a great deal of ambivalence towards using contraceptives. A woman often considers limiting births as a necessity to maintain her physical health and to reduce the economic burden imposed by a large size family. While pursuing contraceptives, women take risks of physical abuse and divorce, endure the guilt of defying household and religious authority, and potentially experience uncomfortable side effects from the contraceptive method. Men's concerns around maintaining family status in the community and their own position of power in the household often conflict with contraceptive use. An IUD may contribute to the empowerment of a woman who successfully pursues her contraceptive goals, but can also be a threat to her social and physical wellbeing. Contraceptive usage involves a great deal of negotiation between the woman, who must weigh her desire to control her fertility against potential social and physical risks, and family members and health care providers, whose interests may conflict with the woman's contraceptive use or non-use.

The secrecy that the IUD offers is a major benefit for a woman in societies where social status and security are exchanged for adherence to social hierarchy and the avoidance of openly contradicting authority figures. Not only secret insertion, but secret removal to get pregnant against a husband's desire, is another possible manipulation of the IUD that meets a woman's reproductive goal.[25] Contraceptive injections, which can easily be administered every three months by a health care worker who calls on village users or by a clinic where users can pay a visit, also offer surreptitiousness and thus are often favored. Preference for the injection method has been reported from many regions including Bangladesh. There, Depo-Provera was indicated as the most popular method, one that was "easy and left no evidence" (Stark, 2000, p. 185). Surreptitiousness was not an intentional character of the original design of the IUD, but turned out to be a rather serendipitous advantage that contributes to a woman's attempt to control her own fertility.

Subversive strategies such as secret insertion of the IUD do not challenge the social subordination of women. Tactics such as informing the husband later about IUD use to restore his authority only contributes to perpetuating the existing power structure that subordinates women's reproductive wishes to those of men's. Still yet, whether sought openly or secretly, an IUD can become a device that is manipulated to meet the goal of women who wish to limit their fertility. Indeed, as Stark contends, attempts by women to "control their fertility, and thus their social world, by using contraception" is "indicative of active, goal-oriented behavior in the face of many obstacles within the society that restrict their personal autonomy" (p. 186). These women's behavior to seek the IUD to limit their fertility may be interpreted as examples of women being empowered by having their unmet need for contraceptives fulfilled by the IUD. Granted that making contraceptive methods available to women is a necessary condition for women to be able to use them, women's struggles over fertility control and empowerment in societies such as Tajikistan and Bangladesh are not resolved simply through delivering contraceptives to remote areas, or "meeting unmet contraceptive needs." Women in many societies must struggle over the limited control over their fertility that is granted to them. Hence, women's social and political empowerment must be considered the primary need before women are able to freely and safely make reproductive choices.

CONCLUSION

The construction of the relationship between contraceptives and reproductive self-determination has transformed over the years as ideas and interests guiding approaches to fertility control changed. The birth control movement in the 1920s viewed contraceptive technologies as a means for women to take control of their own fertility, whereas the population control movement of the 1960s positioned contraceptives as efficient tools for controlling fertility in the developing world. Contraceptives were once again reconceptualized over the recent decades, this time as a response to the needs of women. The tension between the interests of population control advocates and women's reproductive rights activists was reconciled through reframing international population policy through the language of a women-centered approach to family planning. I argue that the currently prevalent representation of contraceptive offerings as a response to women's unmet needs is in part a byproduct of the resolution made in Cairo.

A contraceptive method is neither a politically neutral device nor a device that empowers only one set of actors in a monolithic manner. Rather, a contraceptive mediates women's reproductive desires in multiple ways by facilitating alliances between social actors in the networks woven around interests over fertility. When an Uzbek midwife helped a woman secretly use an IUD, the IUD facilitated an alliance between the state, midwife, and the woman against the husband. When another Uzbek midwife tolerated a woman's IUD self-removal, an alliance between the midwife and woman was made against the state provision. In Bangladesh, the woman who secretly inserted an IUD and her husband who acquiesced to it formed an alliance against societal expectations that encourage fecundity. In China, the alliance was formed between the woman, her family, and the villagers against the state and the local cadre, who ultimately accepted the community norm and tolerated illegal IUD removals. Far from the image that the IUD is a neutral "choice" for women who wish to avoid pregnancies, the device is the point of contention in these negotiations over fertility control. The IUD can be an empowering or disempowering device for women who obtain or reject it depending on how and by whom the method is being mobilized. The extent of contribution that the IUD makes to women's empowerment ultimately relies on the situated negotiations that women engage in an attempt to pursue their reproductive choices while abiding by local norms and ensuring that the outcome secures her social economic status.

The cases from different geographic locations I cited above all point out in one way or another that "reproductive rights are given meaning by the specific culture, social space, and political context in which a right is exercised" (Dawla et al., 1998, p. 99). Cultural ideas about ideal family composition and decision-making authority as well as government policy and practice shape the meaning and means of controlling reproduction. For a woman in parts of the world where the community is placed above the individual, the western idea that an individual woman should make rational decisions about her reproductive preferences using a scientific contraceptive does not correspond with a culturally ideal way for women to take control of their fertility. Each woman's social relations and circumstances determine what counts as an empowering way for a woman to take control over fertility. In order to strive for a world in which women can freely and safely decide on their reproductive lives, providing them with contraceptive choices is essential but insufficient, especially in areas where the liberty for women to make decisions is constrained in many ways. Empowering women and working towards eliminating barriers that hinder women's reproductive self-determination must be considered a fundamental part of winning women's reproductive rights.

NOTES

1. For a complete documentation, see Program of Action, International Conference on Population and Development (1994).

2. See for example: http://www.unfpa.org.

3. The Dalkon Shield IUD (discussed later in this paper) was particularly hazardous, being responsible for at least 20 deaths (Hicks, 1994) and numerous complications including septic abortions, birth defects and infertility (Mintz, 1985). The Majzlin Spring IUD, first marketed in 1968, was seized by federal agency in 1973 for being unsafe with a high rate of uterine perforation (Perry & Dawson, 1985). Other IUDs such as the Lippes Loop IUD are also reported to have perforated the uterine wall and migrated to abdominal areas (Simcock, 1985).

4. For the pregnancy rate cited, see Christopher Teitze, "Intrauterine Contraception: A Research Report," *Studies in Family Planning*, 1968, 36: 11–12.

5. The cervical thread on the IUD, sometimes called the tail, should be made of monofilamented fiber to avoid bacteria travelling from the vagina to the uterus between the filaments inside the string. The Dalkon Shield, however, had a tail made of an open-ended multifilament string – a design decision made because a single-filament string was supposedly too weak – which became the deadly conduit of bacteria travelling into the victim's uterus. See Mintz (1985, pp. 131–148) for more details.

6. Ortho Pharmaceuticals withdrew the Lippes Loop in 1985 because of fears of liability. G. D. Searle withdrew their Copper-7 and Tatum-T in 1986 when their liability insurance lapsed (source: http://www.ralbm.tripod.com/ALL_Encyclopedia/encyc032.txt).

7. IUDs never exceeded 10% usage rate in the U.S. even during the 1970s when they were most popular. Two IUD models remained on the market after the 1980s. Usage during the 1990s was around 1%. There have been indications of revived interest in the IUD in the U.S. after the introduction of Mierna, a new hormone-releasing IUD. See Anonymous (2001a, b).

8. See Halfon (2000) for details on how unmet need was defined in the 1975–1976 Bangladesh Fertility Survey carried under the World Fertility Survey program. Using interview transcripts from the survey, he presents examples of women who fit the category of unmet need in terms of her reproductive desires, but explicitly states that they will not use contraceptives and/or invoke the will of God.

9. For example, the Population Council states that the organization is "testing new approaches to safe, effective, and reversible contraception and thus expanding the choices that may be available to future generations" (http://www.popcouncil.org). UNFPA raises "failure to offer a wide selection of methods" as one of the reasons that contraceptive services are not being utilized by women in developing countries (http://www.unfpa.org).

10. Feminist perspectives on contraceptives vary. Due to concerns over safety and abuse, some women's health activists reject certain methods such as implants, injections, contraceptive immunology, and the IUD.

11. During an interview, Sheldon Segal of the Population Council told Halfon that the Population Council always opposed the Dalkon Shield. (Personal communication with Saul Halfon, 2002).

12. http://www.paragardiud.com.

13. For example, the title of Fisher and de Silva (1986) reads: "Satisfied IUD acceptors as family planning motivators in Sri Lanka."

14. Based on the 1990 statistics in Mauldin and Segal (1994), at least 83% of the users reside in the developing world.

15. For more discussion on fertility control in China by feminist scholars, see Anagnost (1988), Greenhalgh (1994), and Greenhalgh and Li (1995).

16. For an exemplary critique of China's population policy, see Aird (1990). The United States government has withheld funding to the UNFPA, perceiving the organization as colluding with the coercive Chinese population policy. (While UNFPA works in China, it denounces all forms of coercion in family planning.) Also U.S. policy makers often use their opposition to China's population policy as a political tool to negotiate family planning aid policies (Takeshita, 2001).

17. Son preference in rural China has been extremely strong to the extent that giving birth to baby girls have led to violence against or the abandonment of the mother and daughter (Croll, 2000).

18. China's country-wide statistics according to the Center for Reproductive Law and Policy indicate: 41.1% IUD, 36.6% tubal ligation, 11% male sterilization, 3.8% pills. http://www.crlp.org.

19. While the Grafenberg ring did not have a thread that drops through the cervix into the vagina, most of the later IUD models (with exceptions such as the Ota ring and the Chinese IUDs) have a cervical thread. The thread (about 1–2 cm long) stays in the vagina near the cervix, and helps to check that the device is in place. The thread is also used when the device is removed.

20. According to the UNFPA website (2001): http://www.unfpa.org/regions/apd/countries/china.htm "China attended the International Conference on Population and Development (ICPD) in 1994 and is a party to its Programme of Action. Prior to the ICPD, the Government announced its intention to move from an administrative family planning approach to a reproductive health/family planning service-oriented approach, focused on the needs of clients. This new orientation was reflected in the Guidelines on Family Planning Work in China, 1995–2000."

21. Personal communication with UNFPA representative, March 2001.

22. Report to the United States Department of State, June 22, 2002 (http://www.house.gov/maloney/issues/UNFPA/unfpausreport.pdf).

23. From the website of the United Nations Economic and Social Commission for Asia and the Pacific: http://www.unescap.org/pop/database/law_china/ch_record052.htm.

24. The stories of these individual women are elaborated in Harris's extensive ethnographic work in Tajikistan, in which she documented women's experience with reproductive struggles and their subjection to gender roles.

25. For instance, Dawla, Hadi and Wahab (1998) refers to Egyptian women who suggested that the IUD can be secretly removed to conceive against her husband's desire to have no more children.

ACKNOWLEDGMENT

I am greatly indebted to Saul Halfon for his critical comments on this paper.

REFERENCES

Aird, J. S. (1990). *Slaughter of the innocents: Coercive birth control in China*. Washington, DC: AEI Press.

Anagnost, A. S. (1988). Family violence and magical violence: The woman as victim in China's one-child family policy. *Women and Language*, *11*(2), 16–22.

Anonymous (2001a). Rediscovering the benefits of the IUD. *Contraceptive Technology Update*, *22*(1), 5–6.

Anonymous (2001b). The IUD: Is it on the comeback trail? *Contraceptive Technology Update*, *22*(9), 109–111.

Bandarage, A. (1997). *Women, population and global crisis: A political-economic analysis*. London: Zed Books.

Clarke, A. E. (1998). *Disciplining reproduction: Modernity, American life sciences, and "the problem of sex"*. Berkeley: University of California Press.

Clarke, A. E. (2000). Maverick reproductive scientists and the production of contraceptives, 1915–2000+. In: A. R. Saetnan, N. Oudshoorn & M. Kirejczyk (Eds), *Bodies of Technology: Women's Involvement with Reproductive Medicine* (pp. 37–89). Columbus: Ohio State University Press.

Croll, E. (2000). *Endangered daughters: Discrimination and development in Asia*. London: Routledge.

Davis, H. J. (1971). *Intrauterine devices for contraception: The IUD*. Baltimore: Williams & Wilkins.

Dawla, A. S. E., Hadi, A. A., & Wahab, N. A. (1998). Women's wit over men's: Trade-offs and strategic accommodations in Egyptian women's reproductive lives. In: R. P. Petchesky & K. Judd (Eds), *Negotiating Reproductive Rights: Women's Perspectives Across Countries and Cultures* (pp. 69–107). London: Zed Books.

Dixon-Mueller, R. (1993). *Population policy and women's rights: Transforming reproductive choice*. Westport, CT: Praeger Publishers.

Dugdale, A. (1999). Inserting Grafenberg's IUD into the sex reform movement. In: D. MacKenzie & J. Wajcman (Eds), *The Social Shaping of Technology* (2nd ed.). Buckingham: Open University Press.

Dugdale, A. (2000). Intrauterine contraceptive devices, situated knowledges, and making of women's bodies. *Australian Feminist Studies*, *15*(32), 165–176.

Fisher, A. A., & de Silva, V. (1986). Satisfied IUD acceptors as family planning motivators in Sri Lanka. *Studies in Family Planning*, *17*(5), 235–242.

FDA (1968). *Report on intrauterine contraceptive devices*. Washington, DC: Food & Drug Administration.

FDA (1978). *Second report on intrauterine contraceptive devices*. Washington, DC: Food & Drug Administration.

Ginsburg, F., & Rapp, R. (Eds) (1995). *Conceiving the new world order: The global politics of reproduction*. Berkeley: University of California Press.

Gordon, L. (1990). *Woman's body, woman's right: Birth control in America* (2nd ed.). New York, NY: Penguin Books.

Grant, N. J. (1992). *The selling of contraception: The Dalkon Shield case, sexuality, and women's autonomy*. Columbus: Ohio University Press.

Greenhalgh, S. (1994). Controlling births and bodies in village China. *American Ethnologist*, *21*(1), 3–30.

Greenhalgh, S. (Ed.) (1995). *Situating fertility: Anthropology and demographic inquiry*. Cambridge: Cambridge University Press.

Greenhalgh, S., & Li, J. (1995). Engendering reproductive policy and practice in peasant China: For a feminist demography of reproduction. *Signs*, *20*(3), 601–641.

Gu, S., Zhuang, L. et al. (1994). Chinese IUDs. *Proceedings from the Fourth International Conference on IUDs*. W. C. Bardin and D. R. Mishell. Boston, Butterworth-Heinemann: 1–10.

Halfon, S. (2000). *Reconstructing population policy after Cairo: Demography, women's empowerment, and the population network*. Unpublished Dissertation, Cornell University, Ithica, NY.

Harris, C. (1998). Theory and practice in reproductive health: An example from the Bokhtar women's health project, Tajikistan. In: A. Hardon (Ed.), *Beyond Rhetoric: Participatory Research on Reproductive Health* (pp. 50–58). Amsterdam: Het Spinhuis.

Harris, C. (2000). *Control and subversion: Gender, Islam, and socialism in Tajikistan*. Unpublished Dissertation, University of Amsterdam.

Hartmann, B. (1995). *Reproductive rights and wrongs: The global politics of population control*. Boston: South End Press.

Hawkins, M. F. (1997). *Unshielded: The human cost of the Dalkon Shield*. Toronto: University of Toronto Press.

Hicks, K. M. (1994). *Surviving the Dalkon Shield IUD: Women vs. the pharmaceutical industry*. New York: Teachers College Press.

Krengel, M., & Greifeld, K. (2000). Uzbekistan in transition – Changing concepts in family planning and reproductive health. In: A. Russell, E. J. Sobo & M. Thompson (Eds), *Contraception Across Cultures: Technologies, Choices, Constraints* (pp. 199–220). Oxford: Berg.

Mauldin, W. P., & Segal, S. J. (1994). IUD use throughout the world: Past, present, and future. In: W. C. Bardin & D. R. Mishell (Eds), *Proceedings from the Fourth International Conference on IUDs* (pp. 1–10). Boston: Butterworth-Heinemann.

Meldrum, M. L. (1996). "Simple methods" and "determined contraceptors": The statistical evaluation of fertility control, 1957–1968. *Bulletin of the History of Medicine*, *70*(2), 266–295.

Mintz, M. (1985). *At any cost: Corporate greed, women, and the Dalkon Shield*. New York: Pantheon Books.

Onorato, S. A. (1990). *Organizational legitimacy and the social construction of contraceptives: The politics of technological choice*. Dissertation in Sociology, Duke University.

Ortega, A. O., Amuch·stegui, A., & Rivas, M. (1998). "Because they were born from me": Negotiating women's rights in Mexico. In: R. P. Petchesky & K. Judd (Eds), *Negotiating Reproductive Rights: Women's Perspectives Across Countries and Cultures*. London: Zed Books.

Oudshoorn, N. (1996). The decline of the one-size fits-all paradigm, or, how reproductive scientists try to cope with postmodernity. In: N. R. B. Lykke (Ed.), *Between Monsters, Goddesses and Cyborgs: Feminist Confrontations with Science, Medicine and Cyberspace*. London: Zed Books.

Oudshoorn, N. (2000). Imagined men: Representations of masculinities in discourses on male contraceptive technology. In: A. R. Saetnan, N. Oudshoorn & M. Kirejczyk (Eds), *Bodies of Technology: Women's Involvement with Reproductive Medicine* (pp. 123–145). Columbus: Ohio State University Press.

Perry, S., & Dawson, J. (1985) *Nightmare: Women and the Dalkon Shield*. New York: Macmillan.

Petchesky, R. P., & Judd, K. (Eds) (1998). *Negotiating reproductive rights: Women's perspectives across countries and cultures*. London: Zed Books.

Population Reports (1988). IUDs – A new look. *Population Reports*, *B*(5). New York: Population Council.

Population Reports (1995). IUDs – An Update. *Population Reports*, *B*(6). New York: Population Council.

Reed, J. (1983). *The birth control movement and American society: From private vice to public virtue*. Princeton, NJ: Princeton University Press.

Renne, E. P. (1997). Local and institutional interpretations of IUDs in southwestern Nigeria. *Social Science and Medicine*, *44*(8), 1141–1148.

Russell, A., Sobo, E. J., & Thompson, M. (Eds) (2000). *Contraception across cultures: Technologies, choices, constraints*. Oxford: Berg.

Schmidt, F., Sivin, I., & Waldman, S. (1994). The copper T 380 IUD. In: W. C. Bardin & D. R. Mishell (Eds), *Proceedings from the Fourth International Conference on IUDs*. Boston: Butterworth-Heinemann.

Sen, G., Germain, A., & Chen, L. C. (Eds) (1994). *Population policies reconsidered: Health, empowerment, and rights*. New York: International Women's Health Coalition.

Sen, G., & Grown, C. (1987). *Development, crisis, and alternative visions: Third world women's perspectives*. New York: Monthly Review Press.

Simcock, B. W. (1985). IUD Complications. In: H. Hasson, W. A. A. van Os & E. S. E. Hafez (Eds), *Biomedical Aspects of IUDs*. Lancaster: MTP Press.

Stark, N. (2000). My body, my problem: Contraceptive decision-making among rural Bangladeshi women. In: A. Russell, E. J. Sobo & M. Thompson (Eds), *Contraception Across Cultures: Technologies, Choices, Constraints* (pp. 179–198). Oxford: Berg.

Takeshita, C. (2001). Localizing global concepts in family planning: The case of China and UNFPA. Paper presented at the Globalizing Interdisciplinary Pedagogy and Research, October 2001, Roanoke, VA.

Tietze, C., & Lewit, S. (1962) *Intra-uterine contraceptive devices*. Proceedings of the Conference April 30–May 1, 1962. New York City, NY: Excerpta Medica Foundation.

Thompson, M. S. (2000). Family planning or reproductive health? Interpreting policy and providing family planning services in highland Chiapas, Mexico. In: A. Russell, E. J. Sobo & M. S. Thompson (Eds), *Contraceptives Across Culture: Technologies, Choices, Constraints*. Oxford: Berg.

UNFPA (1997). Recommendation by the Executive Director Assistance to the Government of China, United Nations Population Fund Proposed Projects and Programmes. Executive Board of the United Nations Development Programme and the United Nations Population Fund. DP/FPA/CP/196, 8 July 1997.

Van Kammen, J. (2000). Do users matter? In: A. R. Saetnan, N. Oudshoorn & M. Kirejczyk (Eds), *Bodies of Technology: Women's Involvement with Reproductive Medicine* (pp. 90–122). Columbus: Ohio State University Press.

Watkins, E. (1998). *On the pill: A social history of oral contraceptives, 1950–1970*. Baltimore: Johns Hopkins University Press.

ABOUT THE AUTHORS

Deborah L. Balk is a social demographer at Columbia University's Center for International Earth Science Information Network (CIESIN). Her prior work has focused on fertility, marriage, health and gender in Asia and north Africa. Her current work integrates demography with geography, applying both geospatial and demographic data and techniques to one another. Her current research includes a study of climate, health and migration interactions in sub-Saharan Africa, and analysis of the global spatial distribution of population with particular attention to estimates of urban extents.

Alejandro Cervantes-Carson is assistant professor of sociology at Mary Washington College. Born in Mexico City, he studied both in Mexico and the United States, obtaining a Ph.D. in sociology from the University of Texas, at Austin. His primary areas of interest and research are political sociology, social inequality, and Latin America. He has written articles on gender, human rights, population policies and reproductive rights in Mexico. He is currently part of a research team studying a transnational community that connects northern Virginia, U.S., and southern Puebla, Mexico, and developing a project on deliberative democracy in the Zapatista movement.

Denise A. Copelton is visiting assistant professor of sociology at Franklin and Marshall College in Lancaster, Pennsylvania where she teaches courses on women's health, medical sociology, and sociology of families. She received her Ph.D. in sociology from Binghamton University (SUNY) in 2003. Her dissertation examined the social experience of pregnancy in the U.S., focusing both on the social construction of prenatal norms in popular pregnancy advice books and on the ways in which pregnant women accommodate and resist these norms in their daily lives.

Vasilikie Demos is professor emeritus of sociology at the University of Minnesota-Morris. She has studied ethnicity and gender in the United States and is currently completing a monograph on her study of Kytherian Greek women based on interviews in Greece and among immigrants in the United States and

Australia. With Marcia Texler Segal, she is co-editor of the Advances in Gender Research series and *Ethnic Women: A Multiple Status Reality* (General Hall, 1994). She is a past president of Sociologists for Women in Society and of the North Central Sociological Association, and has been an Honorary Visiting Professor at the University of New South Wales.

Lara Foley is assistant professor of sociology and governing board member of the women's studies program at the University of Tulsa. Among the courses she teaches are Sociology of Medicine and Sociology of Reproduction and Birth. Her work in this volume is based on her dissertation research examining the work narratives of midwives. Another article from this project, co-authored with Christopher Faircloth, entitled "Medicine as a Discursive Resource: Legitimation in the Work Narratives of Midwives" appears in *Sociology of Health and Illness*, 2003, *25*, 165–184. She is currently working on a book project examining the experiences and roles of male partners in pregnancy and childbirth.

Jennie Jacobs Kronenfeld is professor in the Department of Sociology, Arizona State University. She conducts research in the areas of health policy, health across the life course, health behavior including preventive health behavior, and research into AIDS in geographically mobile populations. She has recently authored Health Care Policy: Issues and Trends (Praeger, 2002). She has conducted research in a variety of topics related to child health, including recruitment into CHIP (child health insurance program) and has published a book on the impact of school-based health clinics, Schools and the Health of Children (Sage, 2000). She is a past president of Sociologists for Women in Society and past chair of the Medical Sociology Section of the American Sociological Association.

Marcia Texler Segal is Associate Vice Chancellor for Academic Affairs, Dean for Research and professor of sociology at Indiana University Southeast. Her research and consulting focus on education and on women in Sub-Saharan Africa and on ethnic women in the United States. With Vasilikie Demos, she is co-editor of the Advances in Gender Research series and *Ethnic Women: A Multiple Status Reality* (General Hall, 1994). She is a past president of the North Central Sociological Association and past chair of the American Sociological Association Sections on Sex and Gender and Race, Gender and Class.

Chikako Takeshita is a Ph.D. candidate in the Graduate Program in Science and Technology Studies at Virginia Tech University. Her research interests include socio-cultural and political aspects of biodiversity prospecting and indigenous rights. She is the author of the article "Bioprospecting and its Discontents: Indigenous Resistances as Legitimate Politics" (*Alternatives*, 2001, *26*, 259–282). More recently, she has been researching the social and scientific development of intrauterine devices, politics of medical representations of female bodies, and reproductive rights and population policies from a gender perspective. She has a M.S. degree from the Science and Technology Studies at Virginia Tech, an M.B.A. from INSEAD in Fontainebleau, France, and a B.A. from Keio University in Tokyo.

Carol A. B. Warren is Professor Emerita and former chair of sociology at the University of Kansas. Her former appointment was as associate to full professor of sociology at the University of Southern California. Among her recent publications are *Gender Issues in Ethnography* with Jennifer K. Hackney (Sage, 2000), "Qualitative Interviewing" in the *Handbook of Interview Research* (J. Gubrium & J. Holstein (Eds), Sage, 2002), *Pushbutton Psychiatry: A History of Electroshock in America* with Timothy Kneeland (Praeger, 2002) and "Sex and Gender in the 1970s," in *Qualitative Sociology* (Winter 2003). She is working on a book, *Discovering Qualitative Methods: Field Research, Interviews, and Images*, with Tracy X. Karneer, to be published by Roxbury, and on articles (with Timothy Kneeland) on "Mineral Magnetism in Psychiatric Treatment" and "Natural Electricity in Psychiatric Treatment: Amber, Fish and Eels."

Terri A. Winnick earned a B.S. in psychology at Indiana University-Purdue University, Indianapolis (IUPUI), and an M.A. and Ph.D. in sociology at Indiana University, Bloomington. She is an Assistant Professor at The Ohio State University, Mansfield. Her area of interest is medical sociology, with a focus on professions; she is currently doing research on the reaction of the established medical profession to alternative medicine.

Kathryn M. Yount is a social demographer specializing in the measurement of morbidity and mortality in less developed settings and in the integration of qualitative and quantitative data in sociodemographic analysis. She is currently an Assistant Professor in the Departments of International Health and Sociology and Affiliated Faculty of the Department of Women's Studies at Emory University. Her research focuses primarily on multi-method case studies and comparative analyses of the determinants of disparities by gender in survival, health, and access to care over the life course. Yount has received grants from the National Science Foundation, the University Research Committee at Emory, and the National Institute on Aging to study these issues in the Middle East.

SUBJECT INDEX